Liposomes

The Practical Approach Series

Related **Practical Approach** Series Titles

Essential Cell Biology Vol 2
Essential Cell Biology Vol 1
Cell-Cell Interactions 2/e
Essential Molecular Biology V2 2/e
Basic Cell Culture 2/e
Receptors
Protein Purification Applications 2
Protein Purification Techniques 1
Essential Molecular Biology V1 2/e
Animal Cell Culture 3/e
Membrane Transport
Gene Targeting 2/e
Protein Phosphorylation 2/e
Gel Electrophoresis of Proteins 3/e
Light Microscopy
Cell Separation

Please see the **Practical Approach** series website at
http://www.oup.com/pas
for full contents lists of all Practical Approach titles.

No. 264

Liposomes
Second Edition
A Practical Approach

Edited by

Vladimir Torchilin and
Volkmar Weissig

Department of Pharmaceutical Sciences,
School of Pharmacy,
Bouve College of Health Sciences,
Northeastern University, Boston, MA, USA

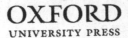

OXFORD
UNIVERSITY PRESS

*This book has been printed digitally and produced in a standard specification
in order to ensure its continuing availability*

OXFORD
UNIVERSITY PRESS

Great Clarendon Street, Oxford OX2 6DP

Oxford University Press is a department of the University of Oxford.
It furthers the University's objective of excellence in research, scholarship,
and education by publishing worldwide in

Oxford New York

Auckland Cape Town Dar es Salaam Hong Kong Karachi
Kuala Lumpur Madrid Melbourne Mexico City Nairobi
New Delhi Shanghai Taipei Toronto
With offices in
Argentina Austria Brazil Chile Czech Republic France Greece
Guatemala Hungary Italy Japan South Korea Poland Portugal
Singapore Switzerland Thailand Turkey Ukraine Vietnam

Oxford is a registered trade mark of Oxford University Press
in the UK and in certain other countries

Published in the United States
by Oxford University Press Inc., New York

ISBN 978-0-19-963654-9

Preface

More than ten years have passed since the first set of liposome technology-related protocols was published as a book *Liposomes: a practical approach*. Dr Roger New assembled and edited a very useful set of experimental protocols to meet the demand of that still young but fast growing scientific community involved in liposome investigation and application. Since no similar book was available at that time, Dr New's book was sentenced to success, and has for years remained the source of practical knowledge for liposomologists. However, since the first edition was published, many new protocols have appeared in established areas of liposome research, many new areas of liposome research have appeared with whole new sets of their own experimental protocols, and many new researchers have entered the challenging area of liposomology. The natural idea to prepare a new, updated edition of a 'practical' book on liposomes was in the air. Dr New himself clearly realized the need for the updated edition and several years ago started to work on one with Oxford University Press and even collected some chapters for the future book.

Unfortunately, because of personal reasons, he was unable to finish this edition, and the publisher suggested to us that we continue and finish what Dr New had started. With full understanding of the high demand for such a book, we accepted this offer. We decided to update the chapters from Dr New's portfolio and to expand the book by including a whole set of new chapters related to emerging areas of liposome research. We contacted many leading scientists in the field of liposomes asking for their contributions and their response was most favourable and encouraging. As a result, we have succeeded in collecting an outstanding set of contributions reflecting all the key areas of liposomology. The final structure of the book is as follows.

The first section of the book includes ten contributions covering numerous important experimental protocols in such heavily studied and important areas as preparation of liposomes; characterization of liposomes; application of various physical methods for liposome research; sterilization, stability, and storage of liposomes; encapsulation of drugs into liposomes; modification of the liposome surface for different purposes including the preparation of targeted liposomes; long-circulating liposomes; the behaviour of liposomes in biological systems; and the use of liposomes as transfection vectors.

The second section of the book includes five contributions addressing certain specific areas of liposome research and application. This section includes contributions considering specific issues of pH-sensitive liposomes; liposomes for diagnostic imaging; liposomal DNA vaccines; isothermic titration calorimetry of liposomes; and vesicular phospholipid gels.

We have also added a List of suppliers to the book and provided the book with a Subject index.

Current liposomology is a huge and still progressing area. In one single volume, even with the participation of the leading scientists from the field, one can hardly assemble a set of papers covering all possible aspects of liposome preparation, properties, and application. The editors realize that some potential readers may be disappointed by not finding in this book certain protocols they might be looking for. However, we strongly believe that everyone working in this exciting field of research, and especially those who are just beginning their scientific career, will still be able to use this volume as a helpful source for all the key protocols in a variety of liposome-related areas. If this is the case, and the book is a really useful practical handbook, the contributors to this book shall receive all possible credit while the editors are ready to take the blame for any omissions and drawbacks. Any comments from readers will be highly appreciated.

Boston, Massachusetts
June 2002

V. T.
V. W.

Contents

CONTENTS

Protocol list

Preparation methods

Preparation of hand-shaken multilamellar lipid vesicles

Preparation of sonicated liposomes

Entrapment of labelled transferrin during the preparation of freeze-dried rehydration liposomes (FRVs)

Preparation of liposomes by reverse-phase evaporation

Preparation of detergent-depleted liposomes by cross-flow filtration

Preparation of extruded liposomes

Purification of liposomes

Isolation of proteoliposomes by gel filtration

Separation of REV proteoliposomes from non-bound protein

Separation of low molecular weight solutes from liposomes by centrifugation through a minicolumn

Chemical analysis of liposomal components

The Bartlett assay for determination of inorganic phosphate

The Stewart assay for determination of phospholipids

TLC of lipids

HPCL analysis of (phospho)lipids

HPLC analysis of cholesterol and α-tocopherol

GC analysis of fatty acids

UV absorbance method for determination of conjugated dienes and trienes

TBA method for determination of endoperoxides

Iodometric method for the determination of hydroperoxides

Physical characterization of liposomes

Minicolumn centrifugation method

Protamine aggregation

Arsenazo III method for measurement of percentage release

Preparation and utilization of carboxyfluorescein liposomes

Preparation and utilization of glucose-containing liposomes

Miscellaneous methods

Bligh and Dyer-extraction

Sep-Pak minicolumn extraction

Preparation of carboxyfluorescein solution

Preparation of calcein solution

Abbreviations

A_{MFH}	amplitude of maximum heat flow
A_{MHR}	amplitude of maximum heating rate
A	area of membrane occupied by one lipid
ADA	acidic double-chain amphiphiles
al-NIPA	acidic and lipid-anchored copolymer of *N*-isopropylacrylamide
α-T	α-tocopherol
α-TS	α-tocopherol hemisuccinate
AUC	area under the curve
B	constant in the PCS correlation function
BDP	beclomethasone dipropionate
BHF	bis(6-hemisuccinyloxyhexyl) fumarate
BHT	butylated hydroxytoluene
BrPC	dibromooleoylphosphatidylcholine
CAIPEI	cetylacetylimidazoleylmethyl-poyethyleneimine
CF	carboxyfluorescein
CHE	cholesteryl hexadecyl ether
CHEM(S)	cholesterol hemisuccinate
Chol	cholesterol
CL	cardiolipin
CMC	critical micellar concentration
CMM	cylindrical mixed micelles
C_p	heat capacity
CPRG	chlorophenol red β-D-galactopyranoside
cryo-EM	cryo-electron microscopy
Γ	PCS decay constant
D	diffusion constant
DAPC	diarachidylphosphatidylcholine
DASG	diacylsuccinylglycerol
DBPC	dibehenylphosphatidylcholine
DC-Chol	*N*-[(*N'*,*N'*-dimethylamino)ethane]carbamoyl cholesterol
DCCI	dicyclohexylcarbodiimide
DF	deferoxamine

ABBREVIATIONS

dFdC	gemcitabine (2,2′-difluorodesoxycytidine)
dFdU	2,2′-difluorodesoxyuridine
DIP	dodecylimidazolylpropionate
DLPC	dilaurylphosphatidylcholine
DMAP	dimethyl aminopyridine
DMPC	dimyristoylphosphatidylcholine
DODAC	N,N-dioleoyl-N,N-dimethyl-ammonium chloride
DODAP	1,2-dioleoyl-3-dimethylammonium propane
DOPA	dioleoylphosphatidic acid
DOPC	dioleoylphosphatidylcholine
DOPE	dioleoylphosphatidylethanolamine
DOSG	dioleoylsuccinylglycerol
DOTAP	1,2-dioleoyloxypropyl-3-N,N,N-trimethylammonium chloride
DPPC	dipalmitoylphosphatidylcholine
DPPG	dipalmitoylphosphatidylglycerol
DPSG	dipalmitylsuccinylglycerol
DPX	p-xylene-bis-pyridinium bromide
dQ/dt	heating rate
DSC	differential scanning calorimetry
DSPC	distearoylphosphatidylcholine
DTA	differential thermal analysis
DTPA	diethylenetriamine pentaacetic acid
DTT	dithiothreitol
EDC	1-ethyl-3(3-dimethylaminopropyl)carbodiimide
EDTA	ethylenediaminetetraacetic acid
EMM	ellipsoidal mixed micelles
ePC	phosphatidylcholine from egg yolk
EPC	egg phosphatidylcholine
ePE	phosphatidylethanolamine from egg yolk
EPR-effect	enhanced permeability and retention effect
EYL	egg yolk lecithin
FA	fatty acids
FFA	free fatty acids
[18F]-FDG	[18F]fluorodeoxyglucose
FFTEM	freeze-fracture transmission electron microscopy
FITC	fluorescein isothiocyanate
FOX	ferrous ion oxidation in xylenol orange
FRET	fluorescence resonance transfer
FRV	freeze-drying rehydration vesicles
FTIR	Fourier-transform infrared spectroscopy
GALA	peptide with 30 amino acids, major repeat sequence Glu-Ala-Leu-Ala
GemConv	conventional Gemcitabine solution
GemLip	redispersed Gemcitabine containing VPG
GFP	green fluorescence protein
GLC	gas-liquid chromatography

GPC	glycero phospho compounds
G-6-PDH	glucose-6-phosphate dehydrogenase
GSH	reduced glutathione
G(t)	PCS correlation function at a given time
ΔH	enthalpy
HBS	HEPES-buffered saline
HEPES	N-2-hydroxyethylpiperazine-N'-2-ethane sulfonic acid
HHW	half height width of a transition peak
HMPAO	hexamethylpropyleneamine oxime
HPLC	high performance liquid chromatography
HPTS	8-hydroxy-1,3,6-pyrenetrisulfonate
H_R	heating rate
HSDSC	high sensitivity DSC
HYNIC	hydrazino nicotinamide
Hz	hydrazide
%ID	percentage of injected dose
I	current
ITC	isothermal titration calorimetry
i.v.	intravenous
k	Boltzmann's constant
K	scattering vector in PCS
keV	kilo electron volt
LPC	lysophosphatidylcholine
LPE	lysophosphatidylethanolamine
LPG	lysophosphatidylglycerol
Luc	firefly luciferase gene
LUV	large unilamellar vesicle
m	melting
MBPE	m-maleimidobenzoyl-N-hydroxysuccinimide
MDSC	modulated differential scanning calorimetry
MLV	multilamellar large/lipid vesicles
MOPS	3-(N-morpholino)propanesulfonic acid
MPa	megaPascal
MTD	maximum tolerated dose
MTDCS	modulated temperature DSC
MVV	multivesicular vesicle
n	reaction stoichiometry
N	Avogadro constant
N	intensity of the PCS signal
η	solvent viscosity
NGPE	N-glutaryl-phosphatidylethanolamine
NHS	N-hydroxysuccinimide
N-Rh-PE	N-rhodamine-phosphatidylethanolamine
N-SCA	N-stearoylcysteamine
NTA	nitrilotriacetic acid

ABBREVIATIONS

OA	oleic acid
ODN	oligodeoxynucleotide
O-glutaryl-CL	*O*-succinyl cardiolipin
OGP	octyl-glucopyranoside
OLV	oligolamellar large vesicles
ONPG	*o*-nitrophenyl-β-galactopyranoside
p	period
P	power
PA	phosphatidic acid
PBS	phosphate-buffered saline
PC	phosphatidylcholine
$P_{chamber}$	applied chamber pressure of the freeze-dryer
PCS	photon correlation spectroscopy
PE	phosphatidylethanolamine
PEG	poly(ethylene glycol)
PEGCer	PEG-ceramide
$PEGCerC_{14}$	PEGCer containing a 14-carbon fatty acyl chain
$PEGCerC_{20}$	PEGCer containing a 20-carbon fatty acyl chain
PEG-COOH	carboxylated PEG-derivative
PEG-PE	poly(ethylene glycol)-phosphatidylethanolamine
PEG-Osu	poly(ethyelene glycol) hydroxysuccinimide ester
PET	positron emission tomography
P_{front}	vapour pressure at the sublimation front in a freeze-dryer
PG	phosphatidylglycerol
ΔpH	transmembrane pH gradient
PHC	palmitoylhomocysteine
PI	phosphatidylinositol
POE	polyoxyethylene
POP	polyoxypropylene
POPC	palmitoyloleoylphosphatidylcholine
POPE	palmitoyloleoyl-phosphatidylethanolamine
PS	phosphatidylserine
PSL	pH-sensitive liposomes
ΔQ	heat differential
QQELS	quasi-elastic light scattering
R	resistance
RES	reticulo endothelial system
RET	resonance energy transfer
REV	rehydration–evaporation vesicles
R_h	mean hydrodynamic radius
rhodamine-PE	*N*-(lissamine rhodamine B sulfonyl)phosphatidylethanolamine
ROI	region-of-interest
R_{sat}	(saturating) surfactant/lipid ratio
R_{sol}	membrane dissolving surfactant/lipid ratio
R_T	thermal resistance

RT	room temperature
ΔS	entropy
SALP	stabilized antisense–lipid particle
SAXS	small angle X-ray scattering
s.c.	subcutaneously
SEAP	secreted alkaline phosphatase
SM	sphingomyelin
SMM	spherical mixed micelles
SMPB	N-succinimidyl-(4-[p-maleimidophenyl]) butyrate
SPC	soya lecithin
SPDP	N-succinimidyl pyridyl dithio propionate
SPECT	single photon emission computed tomography
SPLP	stabilized plasmid–lipid particle
SPM	sphingomyelin
sulfo-NHS	N-hydroxy-sulfosuccinimide
SUV	small unilamellar vesicle
$\Delta T_{1/2}$	half height width of a transition peak
t	half-life
TBA	thiobarbituric acid
TBS	Tris-buffered saline
T_c	temperature of the gel to liquid-crystalline phase transition
TCA	trichloroacetic acid
T_{dev}	temperature of devitrification
TEP	tetraethoxypropane
T_{front}	temperature at which ice is sublimated in a freeze-dryer
$T_{g'}$	glass transition temperature
TGA	thermogravimetric analysis
THS	tocopherol hemisuccinate
TLC	thin-layer chromatography
T_m	temperature at the peak of a transition
TNBS	trinitrobenzene sulfonic acid
TNP-PE	trinitrophenylated phosphatidylethanolamine
T_o	onset temperature of a transition
TPE	PE prepared from ePC by transesterification
T_{plate}	temperature of the freeze-dryer plate
TPP	triphenylphosphine
T_R	reference temperature
T_s	softening or collapse temperature of a freeze-dried cake
T_S	sample temperature
VPG	vesicular phospholipid gel

I General methods

Chapter 1
Preparation of liposomes

J. Lasch
Martin-Luther-University Halle-Wittenberg, Institute for Physiological Chemistry,
Halle(Saale), Germany.

V. Weissig
Northeastern University, Bouve College of Health Sciences, School of Pharmacy,
Boston, MA, USA.

M. Brandl
University in Tromso, Institute for Pharmacy, Department of Pharmaceutics,
9037 Tromso, Norway.

1 Handling and storage of lipids (adapted from ref. 1)

(a) Store organic solutions of phospholipids in a glass container layered with argon or nitrogen below −20 °C, preferably at −78 °C. The closure for the vial should be lined with Teflon. Alternatively, the vial can be sealed with Parafilm®. Never store organic solutions in polymer or plastic containers as this will leach impurities out of the container material (2). When transferring a portion of the material, remove the container from the freezer and allow it to reach room temperature before opening the bottle.

(b) For transferring organic solutions of lipids, always use glass, stainless steel, or Teflon. Never use plastic pipette tips.

(c) Saturated phospholipids, i.e. lipids composed of fatty acids that are completely saturated, are stable as powders. However, storage of these lipids in a glass container under identical conditions as described above for organic solutions is highly recommended.

(d) Unsaturated phospholipids are extremely hygroscopic as powders and will quickly absorb moisture and become gummy upon opening the storage container. Always dissolve such lipids in a suitable solvent (preferably chloroform) and store it in a glass container at −78 °C.

(e) Do not store phospholipids for long periods of time as aqueous suspensions.

2 Preparation methods

Various types of liposomes (MLV, SUV, LUV, FRV) can be prepared by very different methods implying that thare are several mechanisms operating in the liposome formation (Scheme 1).

2.1 Hand-shaken vesicles

In order to produce liposomes (of whatever kind) lipid molecules must be introduced into an aqueous environment.

It is an accepted view that dry lipid films form spontaneously large multilamellar vesicles upon addition of an aqueous phase. This is, however, erroneous. When dry lipid films are hydrated the lamellae swell and grow into myelin figures (thin lipid tubules) but in general do not detach from the support. Only mechanical agitation provided by shaking, swirling, pipetting, or vortexing causes the thin lipid tubules to break and reseal the exposed hydrophobic edges resulting in the formation of liposomes. In order to produce smaller and less lamellar liposomes, additional energy has to be dissipated into the system (see Sections 2.2 and 2.6).

In the original procedure a thin lipid film is deposited on the walls of a round-bottomed flask and shaken in excess of aqueous phase (Figure 1).

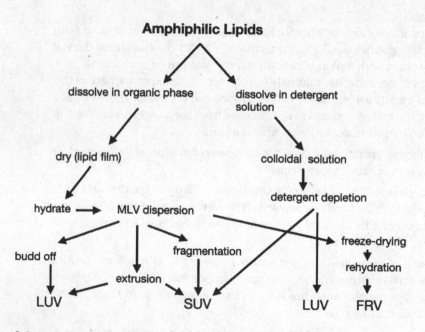

Scheme 1 General classification of various liposome preparation methods. SUV, small unilamellar vesicles; MLV, multilamellar large vesicles; LUV, large unilamellar vesicles; FRV, freeze-drying rehydration vesicles.

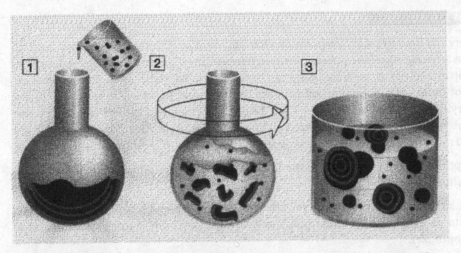

Figure 1 Schematic representation of the three stages of formation of MLVs. 1: Addition of an aqueous phase to a dry thin lipid film. 2: Swelling and peeling of the lipid film under vigorous agitation. 3: Milky suspension of equilibrated MLVs.

Protocol 1

Preparation of hand-shaken multilamellar lipid vesicles (MLVs)

Equipment and reagents

- Round-bottomed flask with a ground-glass neck of appropriate size (25–2000 ml)
- A container of pressurized inert gas (nitrogen or argon)
- Small glass or Teflon beads (1–3 mm)
- Dry chloroform and methanol (analytical grade)
- D,L-α-tocopherol (vitamin E, MW 430.7 g/mol) (Calbiochem-Novabiochem GmbH)

Method

1 Weigh out 5–60 mg of dry lipid(s), possibly add cholesterol (at the very most 30 mol% of the lipid used, say, maximally 9 mg to 60 mg PC), and a lipophilic antioxidant (e.g. 0.1 mg, α-tocopherol, vitamin E) into the round-bottomed flask (if the lipids are delivered in chloroform solution it can be done volumetrically).

2 Lipids are dissolved in an appropriate amount of chloroform. If charged lipids are present, add methanol (about 20–30 vol%) to facilitate or enable dissolution. Alternatively, a chloroform/methanol solvent mixture (2:1, v/v) can be used. Hydrohilic lipids such as glycolipids might require warming and/or addition of some drops of water, toluene, or n-butanol to trigger dissolution.

Protocol 1 continued

3   Dry the lipid by rotary evaporation (400–700 mmHg) with temperature set at 30 °C (in any case above the phase transition temperature T_m of the lipid). A good suction tap or a low grade vacuum pump can be used. Care has to be taken that solvents do not build up in the pump oil (run the pump on gas ballast). Alternatively, flush-drying with an inert gas can be used. To this end employ a capillary placed into the tubing connected to a pressurized gas container. Continue the drying in any case for 10 min after the dry residue first appears.

4   Optionally, add glass beads to the lipid solution in order to increase the surface-to-volume ratio of the dry film.

5   As a matter of routine remove the traces of solvent by high vaccum, e.g. put the flask into an exsiccator for some hours or overnight or attach it to the manifold of a lyophilizer.

6   Hydrate by 5–200 ml of the appropiate aqueous solution. Pre-warm the aqueous phase in case of lipids with a high phase transition temperature.

7   Agitate the suspension for minutes up to hours, depending on the lipid concen-tration, by shaking, swirling, or vortexing.

8   The liposomes formed are predominantely very heterogeneous large MLVs (milky suspension). The size distribution in these vesicle populations is around several microns (cf. Figure 2).

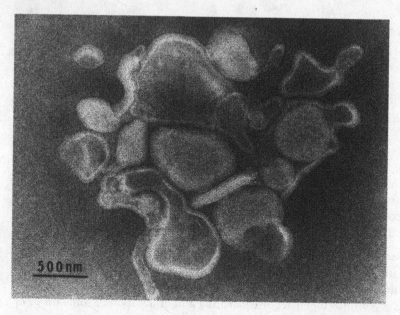

Figure 2 Electron micrograph of hand-shaken vesicles after negative staining with 2% ammonium molybdate.

Notes:

(a) Neutral lipids often yield in saline as compared to distilled water aggregates of MLVs. In general, charged lipids yield smaller and less lamellar liposomes. Besides lipid composition, the organic solvent, the rapidity of evaporation, the size of the flask, the composition of the aqueous phase, as well as the power of agitation influence the size distribution and the lipid homogeneity of the prepared MLVs.

(b) The addition of methanol should be avoided if not necessary, because methanol forms hydrogen bonds with polar head groups and is definitely more difficult to remove.

(c) Keep in mind that chloroform contains 1% ethanol as a preservative, and that pure chloroform may cause lipid peroxidation.

2.2 Sonicated vesicles

Sonication of various aqueous phospholipid dispersions was, historically, among the first mechanical treatments of amphiphilic lipids (3). The sample has not to be warmed above the phase transition temperature because of local heating and high enery input.

There are two techniques: either the tip of a sonicator is immersed into a liposome dispersion or a sample in a tube or beaker is placed into a bath sonicator.

Tip sonication is still probably the most widely used method for the preparation of SUVs on a small scale. This method is the one with the highest enery input into lipid dispersions and can be applied directly to MLVs (3). The dissipation of energy at the tip results in local overheating. Consequently, the vessel must be immersed into an ice/water-bath. Caveat, during sonication up to 1 h more than 5% of the lipid can de-esterify.

Protocol 2

Preparation of sonicated liposomes

Equipment and reagents

- A simple desktop centrifuge
- Special home-made conical tubes made from Pyrex glass (normal flasks, e.g. 25 ml or 50 ml round-bottomend flaks can be used as well)

- Branson sonifier®, model W-250 (Branson Ultrasonics Corp.)
- 1-Palmitoyl-2-oleoyl-sn-glycero-3-phosphocholine (Sigma, Taufkirchen, Germany)

Method

1 Place a sample of 1–10 ml of a MLVs dispersion (see Protocol 1) into the conical tube which in turn is placed into a 0 °C water-bath.

2 Immerse the transducer tip of the Branson sonifier into the sample adjusting it accurately to at least 1 cm (0.4 inch) above the botton of the vessel.

Protocol 2 continued

3 Flush with nitrogen (especially important, if unsaturated lipids are used).

4 Switch on the sonifier, adjust the sonication power gauge to about 100 W power output.

5 Set the timer to 10–60 min with 50–100% effective sonication time. The dispersion must turn from milky to opalescent—turning to daylight, you should be able to recognize the window-frame behind the sample!

6 Remove metallic particles shedded from the transducer tip (titanium) and larger particles (<3%) by centrifugation with a simple desktop centrifuge, 12 000 r.p.m. for 10–15 min.

Figure 3 shows a negative staining of sonicated liposomes without further purification.

Notes:

(a) Sonicated small vesicles (d < 40 nm) are usually metastable. The high curvature energy of the lipid bilayer is relaxed by fusion to vesicles of a diameter of 60–80 nm (4). Therefore it is recommended to keep the vesicles overnight at room temperature in the dark. To remove the small percentage of MLVs after probe sonication spin them down for an hour at 100 000 g. Many of the possible molecules to be encapsulated do not survive the vigorous sonication unharmed.

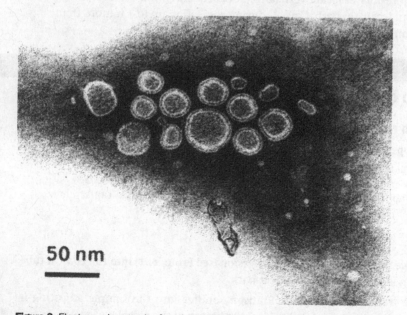

50 nm

Figure 3 Electron micrograph of sonicated liposomes after negative staining with 2% ammonium molybdate.

2.3 Freeze-dried rehydration vesicles

Freeze-dried rehydration vesicles (FRVs) are formed from preformed vesicles. Very high entrapment efficiencies, even for macromolecules, can be achieved. Drying brings the lipid bilayers and material to be encapsulated into close contact. Upon reswelling the chances for entrapment of adhered molecules are larger. Dehydration is best performed by freeze-drying. Rehydration must be done extremely carfully (see Protocol 3).

Excellent preparations of liposomal antigens are obtained by the combination of three techniques: generation of sonicated liposomes (see Protocol 2); their use for preparation of DRVs (dehydration–rehydration vesicles) according to the procedure given by Kirby and Gregoriadis (5); and finally homogenization and reduction of liposome size by extrusion through polycarbonate filters (Extruder LiposoFast®).

Protocol 3

Entrapment of labelled transferrin during the preparation of freeze-dried rehydration liposomes (FRVs)

Equipment and reagents

- Lyophilizer (Lyovac GT2, AMSCO Finn-Aqua)
- Extruder LiposoFast™ or LiposoFast™ – Pneumatic from Avestin
- Transferrin (Calbiochem-Novabiochem) labelled with ^{14}C by acetylation with [^{14}C]-acetanhydride yielding a specific radioactivity of 8.5×10^6 dpm/mg protein

- Phospholipon 90®: 96% soyaPC and 4% neutral lipid plus 0.2% α-tocopherol (Nattermann)
- Liposomes sonicated in PBS pH 7.4

Method

1 Freeze 1 ml of concentrated sonicated liposomes (12 mg Phospholipon 90/ml) plus 1 ml of radioactively labelled transferrin (2.1 mg protein = 17.85 dpm) after mixing as a thin film by slowly rotating the liposome dispersion in a 25 ml round-bottomed flask with a ground-glass neck immersed in a cryobath (dry ice in methanol).

2 Connect the flask to the lyophilizer, apply the vacuum, and sublimate the water completely.

3 Rehydrate the lipid immediately after disconnecting the flask from the lyophilizer with buffer or physiological saline solution or any other suitable buffer.

4 Add the aqueous phase in very small portions with a micropipette. Start with 2×100 µl portions and increase successively to 200 and 500 µl. Then fill up the difference to the final volume. After each addition swirl and vortex thoroughly. Wait between the additions several minutes. After adding the aqueous phase let the dispersion equilibrate for 30 min. In general, the total volume used for rehydration (1 ml in this protocol) must be smaller than the starting volume of liposome dispersion.

Protocol 3 continued

5   Extrude through polycarbonate membranes (large pore diameter) with the Lipo-soFast®; use 200 μm nominal pore diameter and/or larger. Extrusion is facilitated by applying very mild sonication to the sample in a bath sonicator.

6   Separate entrapped from non-entrapped transferrin by column filtration (see Section 3.1). Count radioactivity of the sample applied to the column and the pooled eluting liposome fraction. Result: 21% of the transferrin is entrapped in the FRVs.

Notes:

(a) This procedure is well suited to prepare liposomal peptide antigens because of its high entrapment efficiency. In general, mix 10 mg PC (sonicated in 5 ml aqueous phase) with 1 mg peptide antigen before lyophilization.

2.4 Reverse-phase evaporation

The procedure for preparation of 'REV liposomes', i.e. liposomes with a large internal aqueous space and high capture by reverse-phase evaporation, was introduced by Szoka and Papahadjopoulos in 1978 (6). Historically, this method provided a breakthrough in liposome technology, since it allowed for the first time the preparation of liposomes distinguished by a high aqueous space-to-lipid ratio and able to entrap a large percentage of the aqueous material presented. REV liposomes can be made from a whole variety of lipids or lipid mixtures including cholesterol and have aqueous volume-to-lipid ratios that are approximately 30 times higher than SUVs (see Section 2.2) and four times higher than multi-lamellar or hand-shaken vesicles (see Section 2.1). At low salt concentrations (1μM PBS) and under optimal conditions, up to 65% of the aqueous phase is entrapped within the vesicles, encapsulating even large macromolecular assemblies with high efficiency. Although the encapsulation efficiency depends to some degree on the chemical nature of the lipid, on the lipid concentration, as well as on the lipid / organic solvent (see below) / buffer ratio, routinely, an encapsulation efficiency between 30–45% can be achieved for such macromolecules as albumin, alkaline phosphatase, and ferritin (at 10 mg/ml initial concentration each) (6). The main drawback of this method is the exposure of the material to be encapsulated to an organic solvent, which, for example, may lead to denaturation of proteins.

The procedure is based on the formation of 'inverted micelles', i.e. small water droplets which are stabilized by a phospholipid monolayer and which are dispersed in an excess of organic solvent. Such inverted micelles are formed upon sonication of a mixture of a buffered aqueous phase, which contains the water soluble molecules to be liposomal encapsulated, and an organic phase in which the amphiphilic phospholipid molecules have been solubilized. Slow removal of the organic solvent leads to transformation of these inverted micelles into a viscous gel-like state. At a critical point in this procedure, the gel state collapses and some of the inverted micelles disintegrate. The resulting excess of phospholipid, in turn, contributes to the formation of a complete bilayer around the remaining micelles, which results in the formation of vesicles, i.e. REV liposomes.

REVs are mainly unilamellar, though some vesicles in each preparation may consist of several concentric bilayers, thus constituting oligolamellar vesicles. The size of REVs depends on the type of lipid and its solubility in the organic solvent, the interfacial tension between aqueous buffer and organic solvent, and on the relative amounts of water phase, organic solvent, and lipid. For REV liposomes composed of phosphatidylglycerol/phosphatidylcholine/cholesterol (1:4:5) in 0.1 PBS, a size range between 200–1000 nm with a mean size of 460 nm has been described (6). Filtration of this preparation through a 200 nm Unipore filter gave a more uniform vesicle population of between 120–300 nm with no loss of lipid (6). Because of the unpredictable and heterogeneous size distribution anywhere between 100–1000 nm of REV liposomes, the mean vesicle size of such preparations should be determined for each individual batch. A detailed physicochemical characterization of REV liposomes can be found in ref. 7.

Protocol 4

Preparation of liposomes by reverse-phase evaporation

Equipment and reagents

- Round-bottom flask of appropriate size, which is 25 ml for the protocol given below, i.e. for the use of 1 ml aqueous phase and 3 ml organic phase. Use any larger size if scaling up is required. Note that the surface-to-volume ratio appears to be important during the process of slow solvent evaporation, i.e. during the transformation of the inverted micelles into the viscous gel-like state.

- Rotary evaporator connected to a water aspirator. For better reproducibility of the preparation conditions, i.e. for the slow solvent evaporation, a KNF Laboport vacuum system with solid state vacuum controller (Fisher Scientific), or any other device allowing relatively precise vacuum control, is recommended.

- Bath sonicator
- Pressurized inert gas (nitrogen or argon)
- Peroxide-free diethyl ether (alternatively, isopropyl ether, halothane, or trifluorotrichloroethane may be used to form the organic phase with the solubilized phospholipid)

Method

1 Transfer an appropriate amount of phospholipids (as powder or as chloroform solution) into the round-bottom flask. The final lipid concentration in the aqueous liposome suspension may vary widely, anywhere between 10–100 mmol/ml. A typical REV liposome preparation as originally described by Szoka and Papahadjopoulos (6) contains 33 mmol of phospholipid and 33 mmol of cholesterol in 1.0 ml of aqueous phase.

Protocol 4 continued

2   Remove any solvent, either by rotary evaporation or by flush-drying with an inert gas.

3   Redissolve the lipid mixture in 3 ml diethyl ether. When some of the lipids have low solubility in ether, small amounts (up to about 0.25 ml) of chloroform or methanol may be added to increase their solubility.

4   Add 1 ml of the aqueous phase, containing any water soluble molecules to be liposomal encapsulated and keep the system continuously under inert gas. Note that the ratio 1 ml aqueous phase to 3 ml ether phase must be maintained for maximal encaspulation efficiency. However, it can be scaled down or up without any change in the characteristics of the resulting liposomes.

5   To form the inverted micelles, sonicate the two-phase system in a bath sonicator until the mixture becomes either a clear one-phase dispersion or a homogeneous opalescent dispersion. Usually, 2–5 min sonication time is sufficient. However, it is crucial that the homogeneous dispersion of inverted micelles in the organic phase remains stable, i.e. does not separate, for at least 30 min after sonication. Try to keep the sonication temperature below 10 °C.

6   Place the mixture on the rotary evaporator and remove the organic solvent (diethyl ether) under reduced pressure at room temperature, rotating at approx. 200 r.p.m.

    Very important: The formation of foam or bubbles during the solvent evaporation must be avoided entirely! Increase the pressure immediately as soon as signs of bubbles or foam appear; better still, start the procedure again. The total removal of the organic phase may take up to 30 min.

7   As the majority of the solvent has been evaporated, the material forms a highly viscous gel, sticking almost completely to the glass surface of the round-bottom flask. At a critical point, however, the gel collapses and within 5–10 min it becomes an aqueous suspension. At this point, excess water or buffer may be added, but it is not necessary. Note, that when the lipid mixture lacks cholesterol and/or the lipid concentration is very low, the gel phase and especially its collapse into a lipid-in-water suspension may not become apparent.

8   Rotate the mixture under further decreased pressure for an additional 15 min to remove traces of solvent.

9   For separation from non-encapsulated material, the REV liposomes can be dialysed, passed through a Sepharose 4B column, or centrifuged at 20 000 g.

2.5 Detergent depletion

Dialysis is used for the removal of small molecular weight material from liposome dispersions which escaped entrapment (Section 3, purification of lipsomes) as well as for the slow complete removal of detergents from mixed detergent-lipid micelles which leads to the formation of very homogeneous lipsomes. While pratically all lipids below their phase transition temperature can be used with this preparation technique only a few detergents are well suited. The detergent depletion tecchnique is very flexible, i.e. it allows the preparation of a great variety of liposomes and proteoliposomes. It is a very mild treatment which even sensitive proteins survive, i.e. proteins which lose their function (enzymic activity, binding of physiological ligands, etc.) by physical (sonication, extrusion) and chemical treatment (organic solvents) can be incorporated into lipid bilayers by this technique.

Most popular are sodium cholate, alkyl(thio)glucosides, and alkyloxypoly-ethylenes.

The starting solution in these methods is a colloidal solution of mixed micelles with a molar ratio detergent/phospholipid of 2:10. Mixed micelles are prepared by the addition of concentrated detergent solution to MLVs (the final detergent concentration must be well above its CMC), or hydrating lipid with detergent solution, or drying of both lipid and detergent from organic solution. Equilibration of mixed micelles in the aqueous phase might take quite a time and is not as short as many researchers assume.

Detergent depletion is achieved by one of four classical approaches:

(a) Dilution (8).

(b) Dialysis (9).

(c) Gel filtration (10).

(d) Adsorption.

For gel filtration see Section 3.1. Quantitative selective adsorption of detergent, first described by Holloway (11), is achieved by shaking or twirling of the mixed micelle solution with beaded organic polystyrene detergent adsorbers (Bio-Beads SM2 or XAD-2 beads). The advantage of detergent adsorbers is that they can also remove detergents with low CMC values which are not completely depleted by dialysis or gel filtration which remove only monomers. Surprisingly, they do not substantially adsorb lipids. Besides organic beaded adsorbers there are also suitable inorganic materials, such as zeolithes.

The use of different detergents results in different size distributions of the vesicles formed as well as in different ratios of LUVs/OLVs (oligolamellar vesicles)/MLVs. Cholate and deoxycholate produce the most homogeneous liposome populations. The mean size also depends on the type of detergent used. But above all, it is the kinetics which influence the size: faster depletion rates produce smaller vesicles, which is borne out by the data shown in Table 1. One reason is that slow fusion due to residual detergent in the lipid membranes causes increase and heterogeneity of vesicle size (12).

Dialysis is either performed as equilibrium dialysis in bags immersed in large detergent-free volumes of saline solution or buffer, or by using continuous flow cells, hollow fibre cartridges (13), diafiltration or, more recently, by cross-filtration (14), which enables an accelerated and efficient detergent removal, can be carried out continuously under sterile conditions, and scaled up to commercial dimensions. A schematic drawing of the tangential filtration device is shown in Figure 4.

13

Table 1 Characteristics of vesicles produced by different detergent depletion techniques and types of detergents.

Detergent	Phospholipid	Diamater (Å)	Detergent removal	Reference
CHAPS [a]	EYL [b]	2900	Very slow (dialysis)	[15]
OG [c]	EYL	2400	Very slow	[16]
CHAPS	EYL	2080	Slow (gel chromatography)	[16]
Triton X-100	EYL-EPA [d] (9:1)	1500	Slow (adsorbent beads)	[17]
GCh [e]	DMPC [f]	1300/380	Fast (dilution): gel state/liquid crystalline state	[7]
C12 E8 [g]	EYL	600	Medium (adsorbent beads)	[12]
OG	EYL	610	Fast (dilution)	[18]
C12 E8	EYL	560	Fast (adsorption)	[21]
OG	EYL	300	Extermely fast (dilution)	[19]
SCh [h]	EYL	300	Medium (gel Chromatography)	[20]

[a] 3-(3-Cholamidopropyl)-dimethylammonio-1propanesultfonate.

[b] Egg Yolk Lecithin.

[c] Octylglucoside.

[d] Egg Yolk Phospatidic Acid.

[e] Glycocholate.

[f] Dimyristoyl Phosphatidyl Choline.

[g] n-Dodecyl nonaethylene glycol monoether.

[h] Sodium cholate.

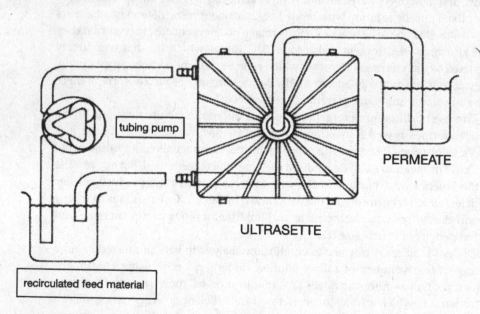

Figure 4 Self-contained tangential filtration device with parallel fluid path design (feed and retentate path are identical). Collection of fluid through the tube fitting at the centre of the device (ULTRASETTE™ is a product of FILTRON).

Protocol 5

Preparation of detergent-depleted liposomes by cross-flow filtration (adapted from ref. 14)

Equipment and reagents

- Tangential Flow Casette System (FILTRON) consisting of the MINISETTE Stainless Steel Casette Hardware w/sanitary ports (code no. FS003K01) and the MINISETTE Casette Omega Screen channel 10 kDa (code no. OS01001, filtration area 0.75 ft², 700 cm²), or the MINISETTE simple Omega Membrane 10 kDa (filtration area 0.15 ft², 140 cm²)

- MASTERflex™ pump model (7524–05) (Cole-Parmer Instrument Com.), Tygon® tubings
- Soya lecithin (SPC) or egg yolk lecithin (EYL) (Lipoid GmbH)
- Detergents: sodium cholate, N-octyl-β-D-glucopyranoside, CHAPS (Merck)

Method

1 Dissolve 760 mg POPC and detergent in an organic solvent, preferably chloroform/methanol (50:50, v/v) in a 150 ml round-bottomed flask. Lipid/detergent ratios (mol/mol): 1:1.6 for sodium cholate, 1:5 for octylglucoside, and 1:3 for CHAPS.

2 Remove the organic solvent by rotary evaporation, then dry the lipid/detergent film under vaccuum for another 60 min (e.g. by attaching the flask to a manifold of a lyophilizer).

3 Add 100 g MOPS buffer (10 mM with 150 mM NaCl pH 7.3) and resuspend the film which results in a clear solution of mixed micelles.

4 Put this solution into the starting reservoir of the tangential filtration device (see Figure 4) and start to recirculate the feed material (identical to the retentate).

5 Adjust the flow rate to 75 or 250 ml/min and carry out the filtration at a retentate pressure P_R of 0.4 bar.

6 Substitute the volume filtered out by an equal volume of MOPS buffer (volumetric control).

Notes:

(a) Never use membranes with a cut-off > 50 kDa because the pores are too large to hold back all lipid/detergent associates.

(b) If desired, the residual detergent concentration of the liposomes formed can be assayed in the retentate by HPLC (15).

(c) The kinetics of detergent removal depend on a number of instrumental settings (see Table 2).

Table 2 The influence of cut-off of membrane pore diameter, filtration area, and flow rate on detergent removal kinetics and vesicle size [a].

Membrane cut-off (kDa)	Filtration area (ft ^{2})	Flow rate (ml/min)	Filtration time until molar ratio cholate/lipid <0.3 (min)	End of filtration (min)	Cholate/lipid (mol/mol)	Filtrate (ml)	Vesicle Size After production	After 10 months
10	0.15	250	240	360	0.09	530	47.4 ± 7.7	49.5 ± 13.3
50	0.15	250	270	360	0.19	450	55.0 ± 11.6	55.2 ± 11.3
10	0.75	250	12	60	0.01	300	45.7 ± 8.2	44.7 ± 10.9
10	0.75	75	27	60	0.08	400	47.6 ± 9.4	42.0 ± 10.5

[a] Modified from ref 14 with permisson from El sevier Science.

2.6 High pressure homogenization

2.6.1 Homogenizers used for liposome preparation

Among the homogenizers used for liposome preparation three categories may be discerned according to geometry of their of interaction device:

(a) High pressure machines with a ring-shaped gap valve as the French Pressure Cell, or the APV homogenizers.

(b) High pressure machines with an interaction chamber where two fluid streams collide as in the microfluidizers.

(c) High shear mixers as the Ultra-Turrax.

For technical details of some common machines and liposome-related references see Table 3. Schematic drawings are given in Figure 5. Both, the gap- and interaction-chamber machines achieve high levels of energy dissipation and thus small particles. The gap geometry tends to clog less with coarse raw material. Both APV and microfluidizer machines are being used for the manufacture of parenteral products for human use. The lower level of energy and resulting somewhat bigger particle sizes renders high shear mixers suitable for manufacture of liposomes for topical application and intermediates for further processing by a high pressure homogenizer.

2.6.2 Liposome manufacture by homogenizers

In principle homogenizers can be used for liposome manufacture in three different ways:

(a) To homogenize preformed liposomes, e.g. MLVs (34) or DRVs (38).

(b) To transfer blends of solid lipid and buffer into SUVs (one-step method) (27).

(c) To homogenize preparations during injection of organic lipid solutions into the aqueous phase (44).

Table 3 High pressure homogenizers used for liposome manufacture.

Apparatus	Manufacturer	Operation mode	Batch size	Throughput	Pressure range	References
High pressure homogenizers with gap valves						
French Press	SLM Aminco Inc., Urbana, USA	Discontinous	3.7 or 35 ml respectively[a]	Up to max. 11.4 ml/min [b]	Up to 275 or 138 MPa respectively[a]	21–25
Stansted Cell Disruptor	Stansted Fluid Power Ltd., Stansted, UK	Continuous		150 ml/min	Up to 14 or 210 MPa respectively[a]	26
Micron Lab 40	APV Homogeniser, D-Lübeck [c]	Discontinous	40 or 70ml respectively[a]		15–160 or 10–90 MPa respectively[a]	27–30
Mini Lab 8.30H	APV Homogeniser, DK-Albertslund	Continuous		6.5 litre/hour	Up to 150 MPa	30, 31
Gaulin Lab 60	APV Homogeniser, D-Lübeck [c]	Continuous		60 litre/hour	Up to 70 Mpa	29, 30
Gaulin 15M	APV Homogeniser, Wilmington, USA	Continuous		60 litre/hour	Up to 70 MPa	32
High pressure homogenizers with interaction chamber						
Microfluidizer 110	Microfluidics Corp., Newton, USA	Continuous	min 60 ml	250–600 ml/min	20–160 MPa	33–43
Microfluidizer 210	Microfluidics Corp., Newton, USA	Continuous	min 3.8 litre	Up to 5.6 or 1.6 litre/min respectively[a]	17–82 or 40–207 Mpa respectively[a]	40
Nanojet	Nanojet Engineering, D-Dortmund	Continuous			Up to 120 Mpa	23

[a] Different Set-ups.

[b] The flow rate is adjusted manually, slower flow rates yield better results; flow rates exceeding 11.4 ml/min let the pressure collapse (23).

[c] The Lübeck factory has been closed down, the Micron Lab 40 is not produced any more. Used machines may be available.

18

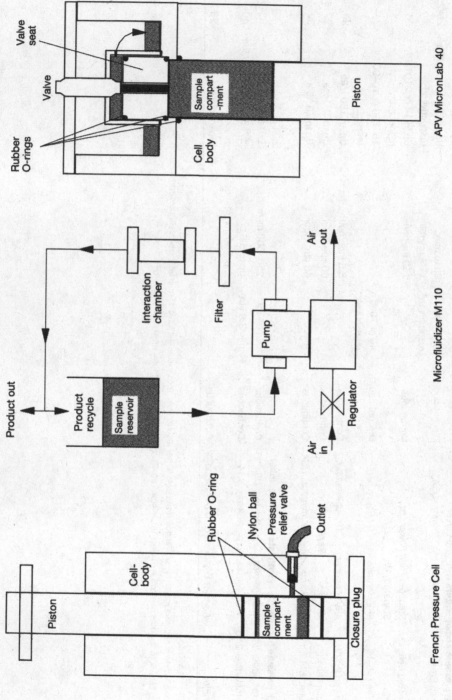

Figure 5 Schematic drawing of three common homogenizers. The figure is modified from refs 22, 30, and 34.

A protocol for liposome preparation by the French Pressure Cell is found in the 1st edition of this book (45). For liposome manufacture by the one-step technique Protocol 1 in Chapter 14 in this book may be used with slight modifications: Instead of 16 g of phospholipid in 24 g of buffer, as it is described for vesicular phospholipid gels, 4 g of phospholipid in 36 g of buffer are used to make SUV dispersions.

2.6.3 Reduction of liposome size and lamellarity

The main reason for homogenization is to make liposome sizes smaller and size distributions narrower and thus:

(a) To improve the macroscopic appearance of a preparation.

(b) To improve its physical stability in terms of sedimentation or floating.

(c) To achieve a preparation, which can be filtered through microbe-retentive filters (46).

The main biological advantage of smaller liposomes is that upon i.v. injection they are removed less rapidly from the bloodstream. Huang and co-workers demonstrated that even if the vesicles are sterically stabilized, smaller size (70–200 nm) and good size homogeneity is of advantage for prolonged circulation (47, 48).

When comparing liposome sizes of homogenized liposomes, as reported in the literature, one should be aware that the size analysis technique itself does influence the result to a great extent. Results gained by PCS differ from those gained by electron microscopy. Different PCS instruments may also yield quite different results on the very same sample (49). Although PCS is widely used, in our experience it is not an ideal technique to measure the size of homogenized liposomes. It often yields falsely too big vesicle diameters because very small vesicles (20–30 nm), that are typical for homogenized preparations, are near the detection limit of most commercial PCS analysers. Such small vesicles are underestimated or even neglected. They can only be detected properly if the number of particles per volume is quite high (concentrated dispersions) and if bigger particles are practically absent (50). Among the electron microscopic techniques cryo-electron microscopy has proven useful to determine not only the size but also the lamellarity of homogenized liposomes.

When determined by cryo-electron microscopy, the vast majority of vesicle sizes of homogenized dispersions range from 20–50 nm, whereas, when measured by PCS, average particle sizes of 50 nm up to hundreds of nanometres are found in the literature. All studies have the finding in common that high pressure homogenization causes a reduction of the average particle size. This may be due to two different mechanisms:

(a) A decrease in primary vesicle size.

(b) A reduction of the proportion of aggregates compared to single vesicles (27, 28, 34, 50).

Which of the two actually take place may be resolved by electron microscopy only. Homogenized vesicles are uni- to oligolamellar. After the first cycle average lamellarities, i.e. numbers of concentric lamellae per vesicle close to one, are already observed. A further decrease is seen with continued homogenization until unilamellar vesicles are formed throughout.

2.6.4 Influence of preparation variables on liposome size

The following process parameters have a major influence on vesicle size:

(a) Homogeneity of the starting material.

(b) Homogenizer type and valve.

(c) Homogenization pressure and number of cycles.

(d) Temperature.

(e) Lipid composition and content.

(f) Ionic strength of medium.

Usually there are preformed vesicles (MLVs or DRVs) homogenized. Alternatively the formation of liposomes and size reduction step can be carried out in one step if a blend of dry crystalline lipid and aqueous medium is processed by a high pressure homogenizer where the crystals are broken down and instantaneous swelling and formation of SUVs occur (one-step method) (27, 28). Such differences in the homogeneity of the starting materials influences the resulting vesicle sizes. Meyer found mean vesicle sizes of 343 and 253 nm for one-step vesicles and homogenized hand-shaken vesicles respectively (39). Sorgi attributed the fact that they were unable to achieve vesicle sizes below 200 nm even at highest possible pressures and after extended recycling to insufficient swelling of the lipids (33). In the same study filtration of homogenized vesicles through microbe retentive filters caused unacceptable loss of lipid when the swelling times before homogenization were too short.

As carried out above it is difficult to compare the performance of homogenizers in terms of vesicle sizes between different literature reports. A direct comparison between two microfluidizers (model 110 and 210) has been reported (40), between two APV homogenizers (Micron Lab 40 and Lab 60) (30), between French Press and Nanojet (23), and between microfluidizer 110 and APV Micron Lab 40 (43). Effects of different interaction device geometry have been studied for the Stansted (26), the microfluidizer (40), and APV Lab 60 (30).

Increased pressure yields smaller particles. Diameters also diminish by increasing the number of cycles, but not in the same way as with pressure. Along with the decrease in mean vesicle size the heterogeneity of vesicle sizes is reduced. After one or two homogenization cycles often bimodal size distributions are obtained by PCS, which upon continuation are converted to monomodal, whereas by electron microscopy exclusively monomodal size distributions are found for homogenized vesicles. Such electron microscopically determined size distributions show a broad, symmetric size distribution curve shape (Gaussian type) first, with a tendency to asymmetric, skewed shapes (steep to the left) after extended homogenization (27). Most reports indicate that vesicle sizes continuously decrease with continued recycling eventually approaching a constant value (37, 51). With certain lipid blends, however, liposome sizes reach a minimum (27, 28, 52) and re-increase with further homogenization cycles. This was attributed to secondary particle growth (28) (see below).

When long chain saturated phospholipids are used, process temperatures above the phase transition temperature of the phospholipids are recommended. A lower process temperature requires higher pressures to form small vesicles (32). The heat dissipation into the product by using a Gaulin Micron Lab 40 was determined to be in the magnitude of 0.25 degree per MPa and cycle (30). The liposome dispersion is thus subject to considerable warming up if the machine is not equipped with a heat exchanger.

After homogenization somewhat bigger vesicles are found with long chain saturated PCs than with fluid PCs (27). Inclusion of increasing amounts of cholesterol also leads to bigger vesicles (35). Increasing lipid concentrations leads to increasing mean vesicle sizes (31, 35). Vesicles of binary lipid mixtures prepared according to the one-step procedure show inhomogeneous lipid distribution (28) (see below).

2.6.5 Secondary particle growth

As already carried out a minimum in mean vesicle sizes may be observed during repeated homogenization especially with lipid blends of hydrogenated PC and cholesterol (27, 28). A re-increase of mean vesicle size, i.e. a secondary particle growth occurs. Either fusion of or so-called Ostwald ripening may be the reason for this. Ostwald ripening is gradual growth of the larger particles at the expense of smaller ones by means of molecular diffusion (53). Diederichs explained the secondary particle growth as an Ostwald ripening process (52). We assumed that the secondary particle growth represents a fusion phenomenon (27, 28) because the fraction of very small vesicles around 20 nm in diameter, which are found immediately after homogenization, disappears within minutes to hours. Such very small vesicles below 20 nm are unstable due to their extremely high membrane curvature especially if they contain stiff lipids such as long chain saturated PC or cholesterol.

2.6.6. Loading of liposomes by homogenization

The loading of liposomes is either carried out during swelling, homogenization, or in a separate step (remote loading). In order to avoid confusion, the terms encapsulation or entrapment are used here exclusively for hydrophilic compounds, which are located in the aqueous core of the liposome. The loading with amphiphilic or lipophilic compounds, which have a strong tendency to associate with the bilayer, is called incorporation.

A wide range of hydrophilic active compounds has been encapsulated within liposomes via high pressure homogenization. For a review on drugs see ref. 54. For a review on food technology see ref. 42. For a review on other biologically active macromolecules see Lelkes (22). Some typical encapsulation efficiencies and entrapped volumes of markers and active substances within homogenized liposomes can be found in ref. 54. They demonstrate how encapsulation of hydrophilic molecules into liposomes is influenced by the preparation variables. Encapsulation of hydrophilic substances follows a common rule: the higher the lipid concentration is and the bigger the liposomes are, the higher is the encapsulation efficiency. With increasing lipid concentration, more liposomes per volume are formed, a greater proportion of the total aqueous volume and thus active molecule ends up inside the liposomes, and the encapsulation efficiency is improved. With decreasing liposome size more but smaller liposomes form. As the volume of the liposomes is decreasing faster than their membrane area, a decrease in the entrapped volume per mole of lipid is observed. From vesicles sizes of 200 nm downward the decrease of encapsulation efficiency with decreasing vesicle sizes is very steep (40). This may be explained by the fact that with the very small vesicles a considerable portion of the total vesicle volume is taken by the membrane volume, i.e. the aqueous core represents only a minor part of the total vesicle volume. A comparison of calculated aqueous core volume of total vesicle volume to vesicle size can be found in ref. 30. The above mentioned rule that the encapsulation efficiency only depends on lipid concentration and vesicle size holds true only if the following conditions are fulfilled: there is no adsorption of the active molecule to the liposome surface, the number of lamellar layers around the aqueous core is one, the shape of the vesicles is spherical, all lipid is transformed into liposomes, i.e. no lipid crystals or lumps are present, and the steric hindrance between active molecule and liposome membrane is negligible.

Incorporation of amphiphilic or lipophilic materials within liposomes can also be achieved by homogenization, for examples see ref. 54. Such compounds are usually treated like lipids, i.e. dissolved in an organic solvent together with the lipid(s) and hydrated upon removal of the solvent before homogenization (28). For control of homogeneous incorporation see below.

2.6.7 Unwanted effects due to homogenization

There may occur degradation of both lipid and active compound, uneven distribution, as well as loss of lipid and erosion of the homogenizer.

Degradation of materials: Due to high intensities of energy dissipation and cavitation forces during high pressure homogenization the lipids may undergo hydrolysis and oxidation. Lysolecithin formation during homogenization up to 0.3% and 5% has been reported, whereas no oxidation could be detected (23, 51). Except nucleotides (30) and interferon α (55) most molecules, which are regarded as labile like haemoglobin, insulin, and enzymes, apparently can undergo high pressure homogenization without structural or functional damage (56, 57). For heat labile substances heating up should be avoided by cooling of the product during homogenization.

Loss of lipid: Literature data on this aspect are contradicting. Talsma found lipid recovery upon homogenization using a microfluidizer of 25–73% only. With higher lipid concentrations higher lipid loss occurred (37). Purmann reported that they were unable to process concentrations exceeding 157 mg/ml on a French Press due to the high viscosity (23). Lipid loss during repeated homogenization using a Nanojet machine was in the magnitude of 10–15%. The loss was explained by liposomal adsorption at the internal walls of the machine because it only occurred after extensive cleaning of the machine with ethanol (33). Even selective loss of one of the lipids (DC-Chol) of a binary mixture (DOPE/DC-Chol, 2:3) has been observed during homogenization using a microfluidizer despite the fact that a homogeneous film had been formed before hydration and microfluidization (33). We, in contrast, never saw any significant lipid loss (43).

Inhomogeneous incorporation of lipophilic substances within the bilayer: For lipid bilayers consisting of two or more lipids it is recommended to analyse whether all compounds are homogeneously distributed over the bilayer (27) especially in case of the one-step method. Bachmann (30) described an approach to analyse the homogeneity of membranes composed of binary lipid mixtures by DSC. Cholesterol for example results in a progressive broadening and flatting of the transition curve of PCs with concomitant decrease in phase transition enthalpy. From observed phase transition behaviour the degree of bilayer homogeneity can thus be judged.

Erosion of the homogenizer: There are several reports on contamination of liposome dispersions by rubber and metal particles probably originating from the homogenizers (23, 27). Quantitative data on contamination of liposome dispersions by metal traces upon homogenization are found in refs 30 and 43. The contamination found is in the ppm range, far below the toxic limits.

2.6.8 Shelf stability of homogenized liposomes

It is controversially discussed whether liposome dispersions can be stabilized for long-term storage in liquid form or whether freeze-drying is required. Some studies on long-term storage of homogenized liquid liposome preparations are promising: When the lipid composition contained small amounts of charged components constant average vesicle size and transmittance values over 60 days were found (29). Sorgi reported 18 months stability data of cationic liposomes made by a microfluidizer (33).

3 Purification of liposomes

Purification of liposomes has two things as its goal:

(a) Removal of low molecular weight material that was not entrapped into the aqueous liposomal interior (hydrophilic compounds) by encapsulation or escaped incorporation into the lipid bilayer (hydrophobic compounds).

(b) Removal of detergent from mixed micelles and mixed vesicles entailing liposome formation. In the latter case, only detergent monomers are removed.

3.1 Column filtration

Column filtration is in essence a diafiltration under the force of unit gravity or the hydrostatic difference between solvent reservoir and outlet orifice. Sephadex G-50 or G-100 are normally used but Sepharose 2B-6B or Sephacryl S200-S1000 can be employed as well. Liposomes do not penetrate into the pores of the beads packed in a column. They percolate through the interbead spaces. At slow flow rates and appropriate sample volumes the separation of liposomes from low molecular substances, including detergent monomers, is excellent. Liposomes elute in the void volume. Pre-treatment is necessary if one uses a column packed with more or less crosslinked polysaccharide beads swollen in the appropriate buffer for the first time. Surprisingly, freshly swollen polysaccharide beads adsorb substantial amounts of amphiphilic lipids. If liposome suspensions made from lecithins, labelled with ^{14}C in the head group are passed through a Sephadex G-50 or Sepharose 2B column, only 20–30% of the counts per minute (cpm) applied on the top of the column are rediscovered in the effluent. This high adsorptive lipid loss (unpublished results) illustrates in a quantitative manner the necessity of pre-treatment with empty liposomes. If *pre-saturation of the column by lipid* is done with empty liposome suspensions, column filtration can be used to separate liposomes from entrapped low molecular weight compounds (e.g. drugs, cytokines, enzyme inhibitors, substrates etc.), or proteoliposomes from residual free protein, or monomolecular detergent from mixed micelles (see Protocols 5 and 6).

Protocol 6

Isolation of proteoliposomes by gel filtration

Equipment and reagents

- Sepharose CL-4B column, 7×2 cm
- EDC (1-ethyl-3-(3-dimethylaminopropyl) carbodiimde)
- Proteoliposomes prepared by coupling of protein to liposomes containing activated carboxacylderivatives (e.g. O-succ- or O-glutaryl-cardiolipin) with EDC (58, 59)
- Reagents for protein determination: CBQCA protein quantitation kit (C-6667, Molecular Probes), which allows an ultrasensitive quantitation of proteins in lipid-containing mixtures

- Reagents for phospholipid determination: 10% ascorbic acid, 0.42% ammonium molybdate ($\times 4H_2O$) in 1 N H_2SO_4 (stable at room temperature), determination of phosphate after washing the sample with sulfuric acid/perchloric acid by measuring the absorbance of the reduced phosphomolybdate at 820 nm according to Ames (60)
- Commercial mouse IgG

Method

1. Pre-saturate the column with empty liposomes in 0.9% NaCl.

2. Apply a sample of proteoliposomes, volume: 300 μl.

3 Collect volume fractions of 400 μl and estimate their contents of lipid and protein according to Ames (23) (detection limit 0.01 μmole of phosphate) and with the CBQCA protein quantitation kit of Molecular Probes (detection limit 100 ng/ml), respectively.

4 In contrast to non-incorporated protein and low molecular weight material proteoliposomes are collected at the exclusion volume of the column.

Notes:

(a) Proteoliposomes with a high protein cargo of the liposomal membranes (e.g. IgG > 1 × 10^{-3} mol IgG/mol lipid) are prone to vesicle aggregation. Vesicle aggregates may clot the column. Density gradient centrifugation in a 40/30/0% (w/v) metrizamide [2-(3-acetamido-5-N-methyl-acetamido-2,4,6-triiodinebenz-amido)-2-deoxy-D-glucose] gradient can be used in such a case; proteoliposomes will enrich at the 30/0% phase boundary (see Protocol 7).

3.2 Purification of liposomes by centrifugation

Three different types of centrifugations can be applied for the purification of liposomes: Differential centrifugation, density gradient centrifugation, and centrifugation through molecular sieves. Differential high speed ultracentrifugation has been shown to eliminate larger liposomes from liposome mixtures and to yield high concentrations of SUVs in large amounts (61). The optimal centrifugation conditions for the isolation of small liposomes in the supernatant depend upon the lipid, the type of liposome preparation used, the buffer composition, and the temperature, and should be determined for each individual case. Usually, centrifugation times between 15–30 min at 100 000 to 160 000 g are sufficient to precipitate larger liposomes and to obtain a relatively homogeneous dispersion of small liposomes, e.g. SUVs, in the supernatant.

Likewise, differential centrifugation proved to be a fast and easy technique for separating large liposomes from non-encapsulated, especially from non-surface bound material, i.e. for 'washing' liposomes. For example, sugar-coated DRVs were separated from non-bound sugar by centrifugation at 100 000 g for 1 h and by washing the liposomal pellet repeatedly with the corresponding buffer (62, 63). Note that mechanical stress during centrifugation may lead to leakage of small solutes from the aqueous liposome interior. In such cases, other methods for purification from non-entrapped material should be employed, e.g. dialysis or column filtration.

Glycerol density gradient fractionation was shown to be a useful method for obtaining liposomes of reasonable uniform size in large quantities and high concentrations in a single operation (64). Similarly, proteoliposomes, i.e. liposomes bearing covalently attached proteins on their surface, were separated from non-bound protein (IgG) by density gradient centrifugation using either metrizamide or Ficoll 70 (63) or sucrose (59). A typical protocol for the density gradient centrifugation is given below.

Centrifugation through molecular sieves was first used for the separation of liposomes from free material with minimum dilution of the sample (65). This method has also been successfully adapted for kinetic studies of cholate-induced rapid release of inulin from inulin-loaded liposomes (66). In this procedure, liposomes are separated from low molecular weight solutes on minicolumns of Sephadex G-50 made from the barrels of 1 ml or 5 ml plastic syringes. Excess fluid is removed from the Sephadex beads in the first centrifugation step. Thereafter, the liposomal preparation, i.e. a mixture of solute-loaded liposomes and free, non-entrapped material, is applied to the column bed. During the second centrifugation step liposomes are forced through the column into a test-tube while the free solute is retained in the Sephadex. The procedure is applicable to a variety of solutes and 92–100% recovery is achieved for both charged and neutral liposomes (65). Numerous samples can be processed simultaneously within minutes without any dilution of the liposomal preparation and non-entrapped material can be easily recovered from the minicolumn in a small volume of buffer. A typical protocol is given below.

Protocol 7

Separation of REV proteoliposomes from non-bound protein (according to ref. 63)

Equipment and reagents

- Optima TLX ultracentrifuge with swinging bucket rotor (Beckman)
- Metrizamide (2-[3-acetamido-5-*N*-methylacetamido-2,4,6-triiodobenzamido]-2-deoxy-D-glucose), Grade I (Sigma)

Method

1 Mix up to 0.1 ml crude proteoliposome preparation, i.e. a mixture of proteoliposomes and non-bound protein (total lipid between 5–20 mg/ml) with 1.5 ml of 40% (w/v) metrizamide and transfer the sample into a centrifuge tube.

2 Overlay this 40% metrizamide phase carefully with 3 ml of 30% (w/v) metrizamide followed by a layer of 0.5 ml buffer.

3 Centrifuge for 2 h at 150 000 g.

4 Collect the purified proteoliposomes from the buffer/30% metrizamide interface. Unbound protein is concentrated in the lower layer.

5 Remove metrizamide by dialysis before lipid and/or protein determination.

Protocol 8

Separation of low molecular weight solutes from liposomes by centrifugation through a minicolumn (from ref. 65)

Equipment and reagents

- General-purpose centrifuge with swinging bucket rotor
- Barrels of 1 ml or 5 ml plastic syringes
- Sephadex G-50 (20–80 mesh)

Method

1 Swell Sephadex G-50 in appropriate buffer (use the same buffer in which the liposome sample has been prepared).

2 Place a disc cut from a 1/16 inch porous polyethylene sheet or a small ball of cotton wool in the barrel of the syringe to support the gel and fill the syringe with Sephadex.

3 Insert the column into a test-tube so that it is supported at the top of the tube by the finger grips of the syringe.

4 Spin for 3 min at 1000 g to remove excess buffer from the gel.

5 Transfer the syringe with the gel into a new test-tube and apply up to 1 ml of the liposomal preparation to the Sephadex bed.

6 Spin for 10 min at 50 g.

7 Spin for 3 min at 1000 g to expel the liposomal material from the column into the test-tube.

8 Discard the gel or recover non-encapsulated solute from the column by washing with buffer and eluting by centrifugation at 1000 g.

References

1. Avanti Polar Lipids, Inc. (2000). Products Catalog, edn VI, p. 172. Alabaster, AL.
2. Pidgeon, C., Apostel, G., and Markovich, R. (1989). *Anal. Biochem.*, **181**, 28.
3. Papahadjopoulos, D. and Watkins, J. C. (1967). *Biochim. Biophys. Acta*, **135**, 639.
4. Gast, K., Zirwer, D., Ladhoff, A.-M., Schreiber, J., Koelsch, R., Kretschmer, K., and J. Lasch (1982). *Biochim. Biophys. Acta*, **686**, 99.
5. Kirby, C. J. and Gregoriadis, G. (1984). *Biotechnology*, **2**, 979.
6. Szoka, Jr., F. and Papahadjopoulos, D. (1978). *Proc. Natl. Acad. Sci. USA*, **75**, 4194.
7. Duezguenes, N., Wilschut, J., Hong, K., Fraley, R., Perry, C., Friend, D. S., *et al.* (1983). *Biochim. Biophys. Acta*, **732**, 289.
8. Schurtenberger, P., Mazer, N., Waldvogel, S., and Känzig, W. (1984). *Biochim. Biophys. Acta*, **775**, 111.
9. Milsmann, M. H. W., Schwendener, R. A., and Weder, H. G. (1978). *Biochim. Biophys. Acta*, **512**, 147.
10. Brunner, J., Skrabal, P., and Hauser, H. (1976). *Biochim. Biophys. Acta*, **455**, 322.
11. Holloway, P. W. (1973). *Anal. Biochem.*, **53**, 304.
12. Ueno, M., Tanford, Ch., and Reynolds, J. (1984). *Biochemistry*, **23**, 3070.

13. Rhoden, V. and Goldin, S. M. (1979). *Biochemistry*, **18**, 4173.

14. Peschka, R., Purmann, Th., and Schubert, R. (1998). *Int. J. Pharm.*, **162**, 177.

15. Lasic, D. D., Martin, F. J., Neugebauer, J. M., and Kratohvil, J. P. (1989). *J. Colloid Interface Sci.*, **133**, 539.

16. Nozaki, Y., Lasic, D. D., Tanford, Ch., and Reynolds, J. A. (1982). *Science*, **217**, 367.

17. Levy, D., Bluzat, A., Seigneuret, M., and Rigaud, J. L. (1990). *Biochim. Biophys. Acta*, **1025**, 179.

18. Ollivon, M., Eidelman, O., Blumenthal, R., and Walter, A. (1988). *Biochemistry*, **27**, 1695.

19. Fischer, T. H. and Lasic, D. D. (1984). *Mol. Cryst. Liq. Cryst. Lett.*, **102**, 141.

20. Brunner, S., Skrabal, P., and Hauser, H. (1976). *Biochim. Biophys. Acta*, **455**, 322.

21. Hamilton, R. L. and Guo, L. S. (1984). In *Liposome technology* (ed. G. Gregoriadis), Vol. 1, p. 37, CRC Press, Boca Raton.

22. Lelkes, P. I. (1984). In *Liposome technology* (ed. G. Gregoriadis), Vol. 1, p. 51. CRC Press, Boca Raton.

23. Purmann, T., Mentrup, E., and Kreuter, J. (1993). *Eur. J. Pharm. Biopharm.*, **39**, 45.

24. Barenholz, Y., Amselem, S., and Lichtenberg, D. (1979). *FEBS Lett.*, **99**, 210.

25. Hamilton, R. L., Goerke, J., Guo, L. S., and Williams, J. (1980). *Lipid Res.*, **21**, 981.

26. Mentrup, E. and Stricker, H. (1990). *Pharm. Ind.*, **52**, 343.

27. Brandl, M., Bachmann, D., Drechsler, M., and Bauer, K. H. (1990). *Drug Dev. Ind. Pharm.*, **16**, 2167.

28. Brandl, M., Bachmann, D., Drechsler, M., and Bauer, K. H. (1993). In *Liposome technology*, 2nd edn (ed. G. Gregoriadis), Vol. I, p. 49. CRC Press, Boca Raton.

29. Dürr, M., Hager, J., and Löhr, J. P. (1994). *Eur. J. Pharm. Biopharm.*, **40**, 147.

30. Bachmann, D. (1994). Diss. rer. nat., Fakultät f. Chemie u. Pharmazie, Albert-Ludwigs-Universität, Freiburg.

31. Bachmann, D., Brandl, M., and Gregoriadis, G. (1993). *Int. J. Pharm.*, **91**, 69.

32. Gamble, R. C. (1986). *Eur. Pat. Appl. EP* No. 86300641.7.

33. Sorgi, F. L. and Huang, L. (1996). *Int. J. Pharm.*, **144**, 131.

34. Mayhew, E., Lazo, R., Vail, W. J., King, J., and Green, A. M. (1984). *Biochim. Biophys. Acta*, **775**, 169.

35. Mayhew, E., Conroy, S., King, J., Lazo, R., Nicolopoulus, G., Siciliano, A., and V. J. Vail (1987). In *Methods in enzymology* (eds R. Green and K. J. Widder), Vol. 149, p. 64. Academic Press, New York.

36. Masson, G. (1989). *Progr. Colloid Polym. Sci.*, **79**, 49.

37. Talsma, H., Özer, A. Y., van Bloois, L., and Crommelin, D. J. A. (1989). *Drug Dev. Ind. Pharm.*, **15**, 197.

38. Gregoriadis, G., DaSilva, H., and Florence, A. T. (1990). *Int. J. Pharm.*, **65**, 235.

39. Meyer, J., Whitcomb, L., Collins, D., (1994). *Biochem. Biophys. Res. Commun.*, **199**, 433.

40. Vemuri, S., Yu, C. D., Wangsatornthnakun, V., and Roosdorp, N. (1990). *Drug Dev. Ind. Pharm.*, **16**, 2243.

41. Mayhew, E., Nikolopoulos, G., and Siciliano, A. (1985). *Am. Biotechnol. Lab.*, **3**, 36.

42. Vuillemard, J. C. (1991). *J. Microencapsulation*, **8**, 547.

43. Berger, N. (1999). Diss. rer. nat. Fakultät f. Chemie u. Pharmazie, Albert-Ludwigs-Universität, Freiburg.

44. Kriftner, R. W. (1992). In *Liposome dermatics* (ed. O. Braun-Falco, H. C. Korting, and H. I. Maybach), p. 91. Springer–Verlag, Berlin.

45. Lelkes, P. I. (1990). In *Liposomes: a practical approach*, 1st edn (ed. R. R. C. New), p. 49. IRL Press, Oxford.

46. Goldbach, P., Brochart, H., Wehrle, P., and Stamm, A. (1995). *Int. J. Pharm.*, **117**, 225.

47. Liu, D., Mori, A., and Huang, L. (1992). *Biochim. Biophys. Acta*, **1104**, 95.

48. Liu, D. and Huang, L. (1992). *J. Liposome Res.*, **2**, 57.

49. Berger, N., Sachse, A., Bender, J., Schubert, R., and Brandl, M. (2001). *Int. J. Pharm.*, **223**, 55.

50. Bender, J. (2000). Diss. rer. nat. Fakultät f. Chemie u. Pharmazie, Albert-Ludwigs-Universität, Freiburg.

51. Barnadas-Rodriguez, R. and Sabes, M. (2001). *Int. J. Pharm.*, **213**, 175.

52. Diederichs, J. E. and Müller, R. H. (1993). *Proc. Int. Symp. Control. Rel. Bioact. Mater.*, **20**, 482.

53. Kabalnov, A. S. and Shchukin, E. D. (1992). *Adv. Colloid Interface Sci.*, **38**, 69.

54. Brandl, M. (1998). In *Emulsions and nanosuspensions* (ed. R. H. Müller, S. Benita, and B. Böhm), p. 267. Medpharm Scientific Publishers, Stuttgart.

55. Karau, C. (1995). Diss. rer. nat., Fakultät f. Chemie u. Pharmazie, Eberhard-Karls-Universität, Tübingen.

56. Manosroi, A. and Bauer, K. H. (1989). *Drug Dev. Ind. Pharm.*, **15**, 2531.

57. Brandl, M., Becker, D., and Bauer, K. H. (1989). *Drug Dev. Ind. Pharm.*, **15**, 655.

58. Weissig, V., Lasch, J., Klibanov, A. L., and Torchilin, V. (1986). *FEBS Lett.*, **202**, 86.

59. Niedermann, G., Weissig, V., Sternberg, B., and Lasch, J. (1991). *Biochim. Biophys. Acta*, **1070**, 401.

60. Ames, B. N. (1966). In *Methods in enzymology* (eds S. P. Colorick and N. O. Kaplan), Vol. 8, p. 115. Academic Press, New York.

61. Barenholz, Y., Gibbes, D., Litman, B. J., Goll, J., Thompson, T. E., and Carlson, F. D. (1977). *Biochemistry*, **16**, 2806.

62. Weissig, V., Lasch, J., and Gregoriadis, G. (1989). *Biochim. Biophys. Acta*, **1003**, 5.

63. Weissig, V. and Gregoriadis, G. (1993). In *Liposome technology*, 2nd edn (ed. G. Gregoriadis), Vol. III, p. 231. CRC Press, Boca Raton.

64. Goormaghtigh, E. and Scarborough, G. A. (1993). In *Liposome technology*, 2nd edn (ed. G. Gregoriadis), Vol. I, p. 315. CRC Press, Boca Raton.

65. Fry, D. W., White, C., and Goldman, D. (1978). *Anal. Biochem.*, **90**, 809.

66. Lasch, J. and Schubert, R. (1993). In *Liposome technology*, 2nd edn (ed. G. Gregoriadis), Vol. II, p. 233. CRC Press, Boca Raton.

Chapter 2
Characterization of liposomes[1]

Nicolaas Jan Zuidam
Present address: Unilever Research and Development Vlaardingen,
The Netherlands.

Remco de Vrueh
OctoPlus Technologies, Leiden, The Netherlands.

Daan J. A. Crommelin
OctoPlus Technologies, Leiden, The Netherlands; and Department of
Pharmaceutics, Utrecht Institute for Pharmaceutical Sciences,
Utrecht University, The Netherlands.

1 Introduction

The chemical and physical characteristics of liposomes determine their *in vivo*
and *in vitro* behaviour (1, 2). Thus, the availability of analytical methods to establish these characteristics is essential. Extensive work was performed over the last
thirty years on characterization of liposomes and up until now FDA approved
four parenteral liposome drug products. But, no formal guidelines for liposome
characterization have been defined yet (for reviews see refs 3 and 4, and references listed therein). Quality control of liposomal dispersions is complicated by
the supermolecular nature of the systems to be analysed. The various components are held together by relatively weak interactions to form lipid vesicles of
the desired size and lamellarity. Moreover, all chemical analyses require dissolution, solubilization, or extraction of the liposomal components, which must be
complete, non-selective, and enable analysis and quantification of each of the
components. Table 1 lists various quality control characteristics of a liposomal
formulation that should be assessed during the different phases of its development from research product to commercial product.

The methods presented in this chapter to establish these characteristics are
divided into two parts:

(a) Analytical methods to assay liposomal components.

(b) Methods to examine physical properties of intact liposomes.

---

[1] Major parts of the text and figures of this chapter were taken from Chapter 3 'Characterization
of liposomes', by R. R. C. New, 1st edn of this book.

Table 1 Summary of quality control assays of liposomal formulations

Basic characterization assays	Methodology
pH	pH meter
Osmolarity	Osmometer
Trapped volume	Measure of intra-liposomal aqueous phase
Phospholipid concentration [PL]	Lipid phosphorus content (modified Bartlett method), HPLC, enzymatic assay
Phospholipid composition	TLC (combined with the Bartlett method), HPLC
Phospholipid acyl chain composition	GC
Cholesterol concentration	Enzymatic assay, HPLC
Active compound concentration	....
Residual organic solvents and heavy metals	NMR, GC, pharmacopeial protocols
Active compound/phospholipid ratio	Determination of active compound and phospholipid concentrations
$[H]^+$ or ion gradient before and after remote loading	Fluorescent indicators, ESR indicators, $[^{31}P]NMR$, $[^{19}F]NMR$, intra-liposomal ion concentration

Chemical stability

Phospholipid hydrolysis	(HP)TLC, HPLC
Non-esterified fatty acid concentration	HPLC or enzymatic assay
Phospholipid acyl chain autoxidation	Conjugated dienes, lipid peroxides, TBA reactive species, and fatty acid composition (GC)
Cholesterol autoxidation	TLC, HPLC
Antioxidant degradation	TLC, HPLC
Active compound degradation	....

Physical characterization

Appearance	Pharmacopeial protocols (visual inspection)
Vesicle size distribution	
Submicron range	Dynamic light scattering (DLS), static light scattering (SLS), microscopy, gel exclusion chromatography, turbidimetry
Micron range	Coulter counter, light microscopy, laser diffraction, SLS, and light obscuration
Electrical surface potential and surface pH	Use of membrane-bound electrical field probes and pH-sensitive probes
Zeta potential	Electrophoretic mobility
Thermotropic behaviour, phase transition, and phase separation	DSC, NMR, fluorescence methods, FTIR, Raman spectroscopy, ESR, specific turbidity
Percentage of free drug	Gel exclusion chromatography, ion exchange chromatography, precipitation by polyelectrolyte, (ultra)centrifugation

Microbiological assays

Sterility	Pharmacopeial protocols
Pyrogenicity (endotoxin level)	Pharmacopeial protocols

2 Chemical analysis of liposomal components

2.1 Spectrophotometric quantification of phospholipids

2.1.1 The Bartlett assay

The principle of the Bartlett assay (5) is based on the colorimetric determination of inorganic phosphate. The phospholipid content of liposomes can be determined after destruction of the phospholipid with perchloric acid to inorganic phosphate. The inorganic phosphate is converted to phospho-molybdic acid by the addition of ammonium molybdate, which is reduced to a blue-coloured complex by 4-amino-2-naphthyl-4-sulfonic acid during heating. This compound can be determined colorimetrically at 830 nm. Here, a Bartlett assay modified by Barenholz and co-workers is presented (3).

Protocol 1

The Bartlett assay for determination of inorganic phosphate

Equipment and reagents

- 10–15 ml tubes[a]
- Boiling stones
- Marbles
- 180 °C heating block
- Cuvettes
- Spectrophotometer
- 0.65 mM phosphorus standard solution (Sigma)
- 70% perchloric acid

- 4-Amino-2-naphthyl-4-sulfonic acid reagent: weigh out 0.8 g Fiske and Subbarow Reducer (Sigma) and dissolve in 5 ml of double-distilled water. It is stable for a few months at 4 °C in the dark. Precipitation in this solution might occur, but may not be a problem when using the supernatant.
- 5% (w/w) ammonium molybdate solution: dissolve 5 g ammonium molybdate in 100 ml double-distilled water

Method

1. Add 0, 25, 50, 100, 125 µl phosphorus standard solution and an appropriate amount of the samples in triplicate (containing about 30 nmol phospholipids) in separate 10–15 ml tubes.[b,c,d]

2. Add one or two boiling stones in each tube.

3. Add 0.4 ml of 70% perchloric acid.

4. Cover the tubes with marbles and incubate them for 30 min at 180 °C in a pre-equilibrated heating block.[e]

5. Cool the tubes to ambient temperature.

Protocol 1 continued

6 Add to each tube 1.2 ml water, 0.2 ml of 5% (w/w) ammonium molybdate solution, and 50 μl amino-naphthyl-sulfonic acid reagent.

7 Vortex each tube and place the tubes in boiling water for 7 min.

8 Cool the tubes to ambient temperature, and measure the absorbance of the standards and samples at 830 nm within about 1 h.

9 Plot the absorbance against the phosphate concentration to check the linearity of the standard curve and calculate the concentration of the (phospho)lipid in a sample from the absorbance by reference to the standard curve.

[a] A problem may occur when the tubes themselves contain phosphate. Use borosilicate glass tubes that have been washed well and have not been used for any other purposes.

[b] Be sure that standards and samples are treated in the same way and with the same solutions.

[c] The presence of inorganic phosphate in buffers will interfere with phospholipid quantification. This interference can be overcome by using a Bligh and Dyer-extraction (see Section 4.1), or by using another assay such as the Stewart assay (see Section 2.1.2).

[d] The range of sensitivity can be changed by a factor of five by choosing other sample and reagent volumes (see ref. 3 for further information).

[e] The temperature of the heating block should be very closely controlled, so as not to exceed 200 °C, because then perchloric acid will evaporate resulting in a blue colouring of the samples at the final stage of the assay and also not to go below 180 °C to ensure total formation of inorganic phosphate.

2.1.2 The Stewart assay

In the Stewart assay for phospholipids (6), the ability of phospholipids to form a complex with ammonium ferrothiocyanate in organic solution is utilized. The advantage of this method is that the presence of inorganic phosphate does not interfere with the assay (cf. Bartlett assay). A simple conversion factor is used to translate absorbance values into milligrams of phospholipid. Since this factor differs for phospholipids with different head groups, this method is not applicable to samples where mixtures of unknown phospholipids may be present. This method is especially unresponsive to phosphatidylglycerol. In liposomes which contain only phosphatidylcholine and phosphatidylglycerol, the Stewart assay could be used as a specific test for the former, and the proportion of phosphatidylglycerol could be inferred after carrying out a Bartlett phosphate assay (see Section 2.1.1) on the sample, which would measure total phospholipid.

Protocol 2

The Stewart assay for determination of phospholipids

Equipment and reagents

- 10 ml centrifuge tubes
- Bench centrifuge
- Cuvettes
- 0.1 M ammonium ferrothiocyanate solution: dissolve 27.03 g of ferric chloride hexahydrate and 30.4 g of ammonium thiocyanate in double-distilled water, and make up to 1 litre. The solution is stable at room temperature for several months.

- Spectrophotometer
- Preparation of standard and sample solutions: make up 10 ml of solution of phospholipid in chloroform at a concentration of 0.1 mg/ml. Prepare samples at approximately the same concentration.

Method

1   Pipette reagents and standard into 10 ml centrifuge tubes as follows:

Tube no.	Standard (ml)	Chloroform (ml)	Ferrothiocyanate (ml)
0	0.0	2.0	2.0
1	0.1	1.9	2.0
2	0.2	1.8	2.0
3	0.4	1.6	2.0
4	0.6	1.4	2.0
5	0.8	1.2	2.0
6	1.0	1.0	2.0

Prepare duplicates of each tube. Perform the same procedure with the test samples.

2   Vortex contents of each tube vigorously for 15 sec.

3   Spin each tube for 5 min at 1000 r.p.m. (approx 300 g) in a bench centrifuge, and remove the lower layer using a Pasteur pipette.

4   Read the optical density of it at 485 nm for samples and standards.

5   Find the concentration in the test sample solutions by comparing with the standard curve.

2.2 Thin-layer chromatography of lipids

For phospholipids, the most common stationary phase is silica gel, which is moderately hygroscopic, and consists of granules which under normal conditions are surface coated with a layer of tightly-bound water. The mobile phase is usually a mixture of solvents including chloroform. The composition of the mobile phase can be altered in hydrophilicity (e.g. by variation of the quantity of polar solvents, such as methanol in chloroform, or by the addition of water). This alters the partition coefficient of solutes between the two phases. Acids or bases can also be added, which will define the ionic charge on solute molecules, and modulate the extent of their interaction with the stationary phase.

The method described here separates phospholipids principally according to differences in their head group, although acyl chain characteristics have some impact as well (i.e. broadening of spots). The lipids are visualized either by means of specific stains that are sprayed onto the plate, or non-specifically by such methods as charring, or iodine uptake. Using the phosphomolybdate method, quantities of phospholipid down to 1 μg can be detected. In the case of lipids, which absorb strongly in UV light, their presence may be detected without the need for staining, by employing TLC plates containing a fluorescent material (e.g. fluorescein) incorporated into the solid phase. Upon illumination with UV light, a dark spot will be seen on a light background, where the fluorescence of the fluorophore has been quenched by the lipid. Identification of the different lipids is based on the relative distance over which they run compared to that of the solvent front (expressed as the R_f value, which ranges from 0 to 1), and by comparing spot positions to those of standards which are run on the same plate as the test mixture. Identification of lipids gains in reliability when using two TLC protocols with at least two different mobile phases.

TLC provides information about the purity and the concentration of the lipids. If a compound is pure it should run as a single spot in all elution solvents. Synthetic phosphatidylcholines (PCs) usually give more narrow spots than PCs from natural sources, which are composed of a mixture of components. Phospholipids which have undergone extensive oxidation may be observed as a long smear with a tail trailing to the origin, compared with the pure material which runs as one clearly defined spot. Upon hydrolysis extra spots will be observed indicating the presence of lysophospholipids and fatty acids. Quantification can be performed by scanning densitometry, or by scraping the spots followed by phosphate determination. Both techniques are described in full detail below in this section. Examples of elution patterns for different lipids on silica gel are given in Figure 1.

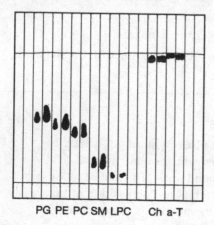

PG PE PC SM LPC   Ch a-T

Figure 1 Thin-layer chromatography of lipids. This figure shows the relative positions of commonly used lipids on a silica gel TLC plate after being run with a solvent such as chloroform/methanol/water (65:25:4, by vol.). Abbreviations: PG, phosphatidylglycerol; PE, phosphatidylethanolamine; PC, phosphatidylcholine; SM, sphingomyelin; LPC, lysophosphatidylcholine; Ch, cholesterol; α-T, α-tocopherol.

Protocol 3

TLC of lipids

Equipment

- TLC tank
- Whatman No. 1 filter paper sheet
- 10 μl microdispenser with disposable tips

Mobile phases[a]

(a) Chloroform/methanol/water (65:25:4, by vol.): mix 65 ml chloroform, 25 ml methanol, and 4 ml double-distilled water thoroughly. Purpose: separation of phospholipids, however no separation between PS, PC, and PI, between LPE and LPC, or between PG and cardiolipin.

(b) Chloroform/methanol/water/25% ammonia (130:60:8:4, by vol.): measure out 65 ml chloroform, 30 ml methanol, 4 ml double-distilled water, and 2 ml ammonium hydroxide, and mix thoroughly. Purpose: separation of PE, PC, PI, LPC, and PA, or PC and PG. However these conditions are not suitable for the separation of LPG and PC.

(c) Chloroform/acetone/methanol/acetic acid/water (6:8:2:2:1, by vol.): measure out 30 ml chloroform, 40 ml acetone, 10 ml methanol, 10 ml glacial acetic acid, 5 ml double-distilled water, and mix thoroughly. Purpose: separation of PC and PG.

(d) Ethyl acetate/cyclohexane (1:1, v/v): mix 50 ml ethyl acetate with 50 ml cyclohexane. Purpose: separation of neutral lipids such as fatty acids, triglycerides, and cholesterol.

Stains

(a) Molybdenum blue spray reagent: 1.3% molybdenum oxide in 4.2 M sulfuric acid (Sigma Chemical Company). Make up according to manufacturer's instructions: add 10 ml of 4.2 M sulfuric acid to 10 ml of the spray reagent. Upon staining, phosphate-containing compounds will stain blue within 15 min.

(b) 50% (v/v) sulfuric acid spray: carefully add 50 ml concentrated sulfuric acid to 50 ml methanol. Mix in a 500 ml glass beaker surrounded by ice. Upon staining, egg yolk, PC, and PG will stain brown, cholesterol will stain red–brown, and α-tocopherol will stain gold–brown.

(c) 0.2% ninhydrin spray reagent in ethanol (Sigma Chemical Company or Merck). Upon staining and heating to 110 °C for a few minutes, phospholipids containing primary amines such as PS and PE will stain red.

(d) Iodine tank. Sprinkle approx. 10 g of solid iodine crystals on the bottom of a glass chromatography tank. Keep the tank closed with a well-fitting lid. Dried plates put into an iodine tank for 5–15 min will show dark brown spots, marking the position of lipids containing double bonds. Saturated compounds such as DPPC will not stain easily.

Protocol 3 continued

A. Sample preparation

Use of one of the following sample preparations:

1   Solid lipids. Dissolve the lipids in chloroform to a concentration of 20 mg/ml. If the solution is cloudy, use chloroform/methanol (2:1, v/v) as the solvent.

2   Lipid solutions. Dilute the lipid solutions with an appropriate solvent to a concentration of 20 mg/ml.

3   Liposomes:

   (a) Either, extract the lipid using acidified Bligh–Dyer procedure as outlined in Section 4.1.

   (b) Or, dry a small volume of the aqueous liposome dispersion containing 2 mg of lipid under nitrogen and redissolve in 50 μl methanol. Then add 50 μl chloroform to give a concentration of 20 mg/ml phospholipid.

B. Assay method

1   Line the inside of a tank with Whatman No. 1 filter paper sheet. Cover the bottom of a TLC tank with approx. 1 cm of the mobile phase, and equilibrate for 1–2 h or until the filter paper is completely soaked with solvent.

2   Draw with a pencil a thin line on a pre-coated silica gel plate[b] (200 × 200 mm) (Sigma, Whatman, or Merck) at about 2.5 cm from the lower edge of the plate—this is the spotting origin. If possible, place the TLC plate on a pre-heated hot plate (50 °C).

3   Spot 10 μl of each standard in separate lanes on the spotting origin line using a 10 μl microdispenser with disposable tips or micropipettes.

4   Carefully place the plate into the equilibrated tank and cover.

5   Allow the solvent to ascend to within 3–4 cm of the top of the plate—about 50 min for polar systems, 30 min for neutral solvents.

6   Remove the plate from the tank and mark the solvent front with the point of a pencil.

7   Air dry the plate for 15 min in a fume hood. Spray the plate with the appropriate stain. Use back–forth and up–down motions across the entire plate, but take care to avoid saturating the plate. Air dry the plate in a fume hood for 10 min, and heat the plate if necessary to visualize the lipids.

C. Quantification of compounds

Quantify the compounds by using one of the methods described below:

1   Scraping of spots. The lipids on the plate can be put into labelled tubes by scraping off the spot. Preparing the plate by spraying with double-distilled water may facilitate the scraping. Quantification of the compounds can be performed by, e.g. phosphate determination (see Section 2.1.1). The presence of silica gel may increase the turbidity of the coloured solution, so scrape off approximately the same quantity of silica gel without the presence of a compound for the blank determination.

Protocol 3 continued

2 Densitometry. The positions of spots that have been visualized by any of the above methods may be recorded by running under a TLC plate scanning densitometer. In cases where a single component is to be quantified, peak heights may be used and compared with a standard curve obtained from standards of a range of concentrations spotted onto the same plate.

[a] If necessary, the mobile phase can be slightly adapted for the separation of the individual components of a sample.

[b] Improved performance may be achieved by reactivating the silica of TLC plates for 3 h at 200 °C.

2.3 HPLC analysis of (phospho)lipids

HPLC analysis of one or a mixture of (phospho)lipids such as phosphatidyl-choline, phosphatidylglycerol, phosphatidylethanolamine, phosphatidylserine, phosphatidic acid, sphingomyelin, cholesterolhemisuccinate, dicetylphosphate, lysophospholipids, and a cationic lipid can be performed on an amino (NH_2) phase column (7, 8). Here a combination of a normal phase and reversed-phase HPLC is used to analyse lipids: the separation is based both on differences in head group and on large differences in acyl chains. The adequate separation of phospholipids and their hydrolysis products (lysophospholipids) makes this method very useful in stability tests of liposome dispersions (9). Compounds such as cholesterol, α-tocopherol, and free fatty acids have a similar retention time as the solvent front, which may interfere with their individual detection. These compounds can be better analysed by using other assays (see ref. 10 and Section 2.4). Interestingly, cationic lipids elute slightly faster from the amino phase column than the solvent front.

Protocol 4

HPCL analysis of (phospho)lipids

Equipment and reagents

- Zorbax NH_2 or a Spherisorb S5NH$_2$ column (25 cm $\times$ 4.6 mm, I.D., 5 μm particle size) with or without an appropriate guard column, in an appropriate HPLC apparatus, with an evaporative light-scattering detector or a high-sensitive refractive index detector[a]

- 0.1 M ammonium acetate solution pH 4.8: weigh out 3.0 g acetic acid (analytical grade) in a flask and add to it 450 ml double-distilled water. Adjust the pH to 4.8 with a dilute ammonium hydroxide solution (~10%). Finally, adjust the volume of the solution to 500 ml.

- Mobile phase: mix acetonitrile, methanol (both HPLC grade), and 0.1 M ammonium acetate solution pH 4.8 together, e.g. a mixture of 52:32:16 or 70:20:4 (by vol.) (see below for optimization of the mobile phase composition). If only neutral phospholipids such as phosphatidylcholine have to be analysed the ammonium acetate solution can be replaced by water.

Protocol 4 continued

A. Preparation of standards and samples

1 Standards: dissolve each (phospho)lipid separately in the mobile phase or, if that turns out to be problematic, in a mixture of methanol/ chloroform (4:1, v/v) (up to 3 mM of lipid). These standards can be stored in screw-capped vials at –20 °C. Dilute these stock solutions to obtain standards at different concentrations for the measurement of the calibration curve.

2 Samples: liposome dispersions or pure lipids can be dissolved in mobile phase, or if precipitation is observed, in methanol or a methanol/ chloroform (9:1, v/v) mixture. Buffer components and salts may interfere with relevant phospholipid peaks in the chromatograms. If so, the samples should be prepared by the Bligh and Dyer-extraction (see Section 4.1) followed by 5–10 × dilution of the lower phase with methanol, or the mobile phase should be adjusted.

B. Assay method

1 Degas the mobile phase by bath sonication, or by bubbling through 100% helium. It is recommended to degas the mobile phase also during operation, if possible. Run the mobile phase at a flow rate of 1.5 ml/min through the column at a constant temperature (e.g. 35 °C) for 30 min (or overnight when a refractive index detector is used).

2 Due to column-to-column variations, the separation of phospholipids on each individual column differs slightly. The composition of the mobile phase which results in the best separation of the (phospho)lipids can easily be found by plotting in a figure the retention times of the (phospho)lipids to be analysed as a function of two or three different acetonitrile/methanol volume ratios, e.g. acetonitrile/methanol/ ammonium acetate buffer (70:20:5, 60:30:5, and 50:40:5, by vol.). This function is almost linear. A decrease or increase in only the relative volume of ammonium acetate of the mobile phase can be used to increase or decrease, respectively, the retention times of all phospholipids without changing their relative retention times.

3 When the mobile phase is optimized, apply in duplicate 20–100 μl (phospho)lipids and four different concentrations of appropriate phospholipids as standards for calibration to the column. Allow about 15–20 min for each run, and apply the next sample when the baseline is stable (that may be after another 30 min when using a refractive index detector).

4 Plot the peak area against the concentration to check the linearity of the standard curve and calculate the concentration of the (phospho)lipid in a sample from the area by comparison with the standard curve.

[a] Three types of detectors are commonly used: evaporative light-scattering detectors, refractive index detectors, and UV detectors. The signal of an evaporative light-scattering detector (e.g. Polymer Labs, Alltech Associates, Inc., Sedere) lacks a (large) solvent peak, and is more sensitive and stable than the signal of a refractive index detector. However, it has the disadvantages that recycling of the mobile phase is not possible and that evaporation of large volumes of the eluens calls for an appropriate recollection system. Moreover, the mobile phase should be volatile and no inorganic buffer systems can be used. The use of an UV detector in stability tests to estimate the amount of unsaturated (phospho)lipids poses problems, because the molar response of phospholipids is changing due to oxidation (see Section 2.6). However, this may be used to monitor the oxidation state of an unsaturated (phospho)lipid. Preliminary results of the first author indicate that the ratio of the peak areas measured at 233 nm and 215 nm can be used as an oxidation index for separated phospholipids species.

More sophisticated analytical techniques provide structural details of regularly used phospholipids not brought to light with the above TLC and HPLC assays. For example, through HPLC/mass spectrometry combinations one can unequivocally assign the position of acyl chains on the glycerol backbone (11).

Another challenge is the quantification of poly(ethylene glycol)-phosphatidyl-ethanolamine (PEG-PE) in (phospho)lipid mixtures. Recently, Vernooij *et al.* (12) published a ^{1}NMR method to determine the relative amounts of PEG-PE in mixtures of PC, PG, and cholesterol. Moreover, an FTIR-based strategy was developed to monitor hydrolysis of PEG-PE containing liposomes. They could demonstrate that hydrolysis of the PEG-PE linker (urethane anchored) is slower than the acyl ester hydrolysis (13).

2.4 HPLC analysis of cholesterol and α-tocopherol

The convenient HPLC method presented here can be used to analyse cholesterol (14), α-tocopherol, and derivatives of both compounds such as a hemisuccinate derivative (see Figure 2). Moreover, the adequate separation of cholesterol and its oxidation products makes this method very useful in stability tests of liposome dispersions (15).

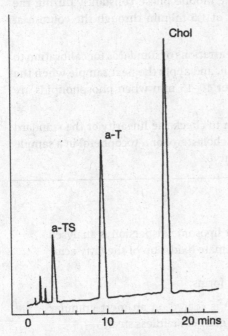

Figure 2 High performance liquid chromatographic separation of cholesterol (Chol), α-tocopherol (α-T), and its hemisuccinate derivative (α-TS) on a reverse-phase (RP18) HPLC column with methanol as eluting solvent. Phospholipids may be removed from the sample mixture by Sep-Pak separation prior to application (see Section 4.2). Individual components can be accurately quantified by comparison of peak heights with those of a range of standards of known concentration.

Protocol 5

HPLC analysis of cholesterol and α-tocopherol

Equipment and reagents

- Non-endcapped Spherisorb S-5 ODS-1 (25 × 0.46 cm I.D.) (C18) reverse-phase HPLC column in an appropriate HPLC apparatus with an UV detector operating at 207 nm in case of cholesterol or at 214 nm in case of α-tocopherol

- Methanol (HPLC grade)

A. Preparation of standards and samples

1 Standards: dissolve about 100 mg cholesterol or α-tocopherol in 250 ml methanol.

2 Samples: liposome dispersions or pure lipids can be dissolved in 100% methanol or a mixture of methanol/chloroform (9:1, v/v).

B. Assay method

1 Degas 100% methanol (HPLC grade) by bath sonication for 15 min or by bubbling through 100% helium. If possible, degas the mobile phase constantly during the assay. Run the mobile phase at a flow rate of 1.5 ml/min through the column at ambient temperature.

2 Apply 20 μl samples, and five different concentrations of standards for calibration to the column. Allow about 15 min for each run, and apply the next sample when the baseline is stable (which might take another 10–15 min when phospholipids are present in the sample).

3 Plot the peak area against the concentration to check the linearity of the standard curve and calculate the concentration of the cholesterol or α-tocopherol in a sample from the area by reference to the standard curve.

2.5 GLC analysis of fatty acids

The fatty acid composition of a phospholipid or liposome dispersion is analysed by GLC. This method is also very suitable to estimate oxidation of the fatty acids (see Section 2.6).

Columns for GLC work come in two different forms:

(a) Packed columns, in which the liquid phase is coated on an inert granular support which is packed into a coiled tube of glass or stainless steel.

(b) 'Capillary' columns, which are much narrower in bore, and longer, made out of a glass or fused silica capillary which contains no packing, but where the liquid phase is coated directly onto the inner surface of the capillary wall itself.

The capillary columns are more popular, as they are more sensitive than packed columns, since the background noise is markedly reduced. Essentially, the same liquid phases which are suitable for separating fatty acids on packed columns can be used on capillary columns with slight differences in operating conditions (oven temperature, etc.).

Cyanosilicone liquid phases (e.g. Silar 10C) are often used for analytical studies of fatty acids, since they can separate the *cis*- and *trans*-isomers of unsaturated fatty acids. For the purpose of investigating changes in composition due to oxidation, however, such resolution is unnecessary, and even counterproductive, since it can make identification of the smaller peaks more difficult, especially if there is overlap between homologues of different chain length. In this case the selection of a phase such as the polyglycols (e.g. Carbowax 20M) is preferable. Using this coating, homologous fatty acids of the same chain length but different number of unsaturated bonds are separated, with the parent saturated fatty acid eluting first followed by the mono-, di-, tri-, etc. unsaturated fatty acids. The important point is that these homologues should run close enough together that they are all off the column before the saturated homologue of the next higher chain length arrives. In the case of mixtures of fatty acids where only even number carbon chains are found, this can easily be achieved (see Figure 3), so that interpretation of the GLC chromatogram can be carried out without the help

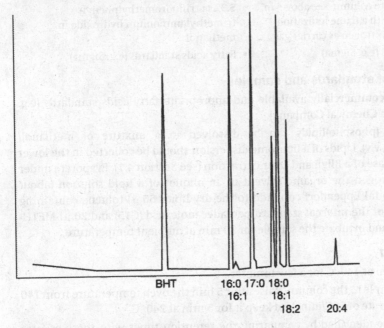

Figure 3 Gas-liquid chromatography of fatty acids of egg phospholipid. Separation of derivatized fatty acid chains from egg lecithin on a Carbowax 20M GLC column. Ideally, the homologues of the same chain length should all have eluted off before the saturated homologue of the next highest chain appears. Note that the antioxidant butylated hydroxytoluene (BHT, included to minimize oxidation during the derivatization procedure) comes off in approximately the C14 position. Natural phospholipids, however, contain no fatty acids shorter than C16. Normal heptadecanoic acid is added to the mixture to aid in the interpretation, since this odd-numbered chain fatty acid is absent in phospholipid mixtures from natural sources.

of additional analytical techniques. Other liquid phases can be employed (e.g. methyl silicone—SP2100, OV1) in which case the members of the homologous series elute in reverse order, e.g. C18:2, C18:1, then C18:0. For precise information of operating conditions for individual columns, we refer to the manufacturer's instructions or to ref. 16 and references therein. A more detailed discussion of GLC (and other techniques) for structural analysis of lipids is given in ref. 3. A protocol from this reference for obtaining derivatized fatty acids from phospholipids is given below. In this protocol, the fatty acids of phospholipids are methylated by the kit METH-PREP II (Alltech, containing 5.3% *m*-trifluoromethylphenyl-trimethylammonium hydroxide in methanol). This method of methylation is fast, can be performed at ambient temperature, and does not need further sample preparation such as extraction.

Protocol 6

GC analysis of fatty acids

Equipment and reagents

- 6FT 10% Silar 10C (Alltech) column (or another appropriate column, see above) in a GLC apparatus with a flame ionization detector (FID) and nitrogen as carrier gas
- Pentadecanoic acid (e.g. Sigma)

- METH-PREP II (Alltech) containing 5.3% *m*-trifluoromethylphenyl-trimethylammonium hydroxide in methanol
- Fatty acids standards (e.g. Sigma)

A. Preparation of standards and samples

1 Standards: use commercially available and appropriate fatty acids standards (e.g. Alltech or Sigma Chemical Company).

2 Samples: pure (phospho)lipids can be dissolved in a mixture of methanol/chloroform (4:1, v/v). Lipids of a liposome dispersion should be collected in the lower (chloroform) phase of a Bligh and Dyer-extraction (see Section 4.1). Evaporate under a stream of nitrogen the organic solvent of an aliquot of a lipid solution (about 1 μmol) in a 0.5 ml Eppendorf cup. Add to the dry lipids 50 μl toluene containing about 0.2 μmol of the internal standard pentadecanoic acid (C15) and 20 μl METH-PREP II. Vortex and incubate the sample for 30 min at ambient temperature.

B. Assay method

1 Stabilize the oven at 140 °C for a few minutes.

2 Apply 1–2 μl sample to the column. Raise after 5 min the oven temperature from 140 up to 240 °C at a rate of 5 °C/min, and keep it for 5 min at 240 °C.[a]

3 Methyl esters are identified by comparing the retention times with those of fatty acid standards. Divide the area or height of the peaks with the one of pentadecanoic acid. Plot these ratios against the concentrations to check the linearity of the standard curves, and calculate the concentrations of fatty acids of each sample from the area or height by comparison with the standard curve.

[a] The analytical conditions such as oven temperature and flow rate of the carrier gas should be optimized for each system.

2.6 Chemical analysis of degradation of liposomal phospholipids

2.6.1 Introduction

In Chapter 5, Section 2, oxidation and chemical hydrolysis of liposomal (phospho)lipids are discussed and measures to prevent or minimize these degradation processes are listed as well. Here methods and assays are presented to estimate the amount of chemical degradation. It is clear that some of the methods described above to characterize the chemical properties of liposomes can be used for this purpose as well.

2.6.2 Oxidation

For the purpose of monitoring phospholipid oxidation, in a simplified form the oxidation process can be considered to develop in three stages:

1. Conjugation of isolated double bonds.
2. Formation of lipid hydroperoxides and cyclic peroxides.
3. Aldehyde production and chain scission.

Most oxidation products are subject to further degradation. At least two separate tests should always be performed to estimate the extent of oxidation. GLC analysis of (remaining) fatty acids (see Section 2.5) is the most quantitative one to estimate the extent of oxidation and is therefore widely used. However, a major problem is that GLC analysis of fatty acids can not estimate the initial oxidation extent of (phospho)lipids; oxidation can only be estimated by comparing the fatty acid concentrations before and after a treatment (e.g. upon preparation or storage). Ideally, GLC analysis of fatty acids should be combined with a method which detects oxidation products of the phospholipids. Four of such methods are presented below. The reader should be warned that these assays might be misleading, especially when a sample is not followed with time, because the oxidation products are subject to further degradation.

i. UV absorbance method (for conjugated dienes and trienes)

The UV absorbance method is based upon the absorbance of conjugated dienes and trienes at 233 and 270 nm, respectively. Phospholipids do not absorb at these wavelengths.

Protocol 7

UV absorbance method for determination of conjugated dienes and trienes

Equipment and reagent

- UV spectrophotometer
- 1 cm quartz cuvettes
- Ethanol, p.a.

Protocol 7 continued

Method

1 Add an aliquot of 0.4 μmol phospholipids to 2 ml ethanol.[a]

2 Scan the UV absorbance spectrum of each sample over the range 200–300 nm on an UV absorption spectrophotometer using 1 cm quartz cuvettes. Use as a blank ethanol (with an aliquot containing only buffer or drug, if necessary). Typical examples of such scans are shown in Figure 4.

3 Measure the absorbance at 233 nm. Correct these values for background deviations by subtracting from each the absorbance at 300 nm.

4 Calculate the concentration of dienes in the sample by dividing the corrected absorbance at 233 through a molar extinction coefficient of 30 000 cm^{-1} L.mol^{-1}. Express the levels of dienes per amount of lipid.[b]

[a] Some materials with strong absorbance between 200–300 nm may interfere with the assay. Interfering water soluble compounds such as water soluble drugs may be separated from the phospholipids by Bligh and Dyer-extraction (see Section 4.1). Interfering lipophilic compounds such as cholesterol (its oxidation can be estimated as described in Section 2.4) may be separated by passage through a Waters Sep-Pak silica gel column (see Section 4.2) or by HPLC (see also Protocol 4, footnote a).

[b] Alternatively, the relative amount of conjugated dienes in a liposome dispersion may be expressed by the oxidation index (17):

$$\text{oxidation index} = \frac{\text{absorbance at 233} - \text{absorbance at 300 nm}}{\text{absorbance at 215} - \text{absorbance at 300 nm}}$$

The absorbance at 215 nm is used as a measure for the amount of phospholipids, and it is not so very sensitive to low levels of oxidation (see Figure 4). A drawback of this method is that it provides no quantitative data.

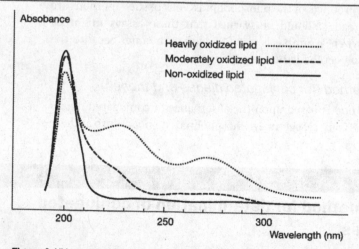

Figure 4 UV spectra of oxidized phosphatidylcholines. Changes in the UV absorbance of lipids are the first sign of the occurrence of radical chain reactions that can lead to oxidation. The presence of conjugated dienes is indicated by the appearance of a peak around 230 nm, while the formation of conjugated trienes (as a result of abstraction of two hydrogen atoms per molecule) gives rise to a new peak at 270–280 nm.

ii. TBA method (for endoperoxides)

Although not a sensitive assay to monitor oxidation, the TBA (= thiobarbituric acid) method is a widely used lipid peroxidation assay. It has been modified in many ways. In general the sample is heated with an aqueous solution of TBA. Under these conditions, the lipid oxidation product malondialdehyde reacts with TBA giving a pink chromophore that can be quantified spectrophotometrically at 533 nm. During the heating step, some labile lipid hydroperoxides can be converted into malondialdehyde, especially when iron ions are present, and will also be measured by this assay (18). Some tests artificially increase the TBA-reactive products in a sample by adding ferric chloride to it. Here, a modified method of Ondrias et al. (19) is given, which will only measure the endoperoxides present in the original sample. Oxidation during the experimental conditions of the test is prevented by the use of butylated hydroxytoluene (BHT).

Protocol 8

TBA method for determination of endoperoxides

Equipment and reagents

- UV spectrophotometer
- 1 cm cuvettes
- TBA-TCA solution: dissolve 2.1 g thiobarbituric acid (TBA) in around 200 ml water. If necessary, the solution can be heated up to 70 °C. Dissolve in another flask 84 g trichloroacetic acid (TCA) and 3.6 ml of 37% HCl in around 200 ml water. Mix both solutions together and adjust the volume to 500 ml. Store the solution in the dark. Precipitation during storage is not a problem when using the supernatant or a filtrate of the solution.

- BHT solution: dissolve 75 mg butylated hydroxytoluene (BHT) in 50 ml ethanol, and store at 4 °C
- 1,1,3,3 Tetraethoxypropane (TEP) stock solution: add 50 μl TEP (44 mg) into a 100 ml flask and adjust the volume to 100 ml with double-distilled water to give a concentration of 2 mM. Prepare weekly, and store refrigerated at 4 °C.
- TEP working solution: take 2.5 ml TEP stock solution and adjust the volume to 100 ml with double-distilled water to give a concentration of 50 μM. Mix well. Prepare fresh each time.

A. Preparation of standards and samples

1 Prepare the standards in 10 ml tubes as follows:

Tube no.	TEP (μl)	Double-distilled water (μl)	TEP (nmol per assay)
0	0	300	0
1	50	250	2.5
2	100	200	5
3	200	100	10
4	300	0	15

Protocol 8 continued

2 Samples: add an aliquot of 3 μmol (2.3 mg) liposomes to a 10 ml tube and adjust the total volume to 300 μl with the hydration medium of the liposomes. Interfering compounds, such as sugars, may be separated by the Bligh and Dyer-extraction (see Section 4.1), drying the lower (chloroform) phase under a stream of nitrogen, and adding 300 μl water.

B. Assay method

1 Add 1.8 ml TBA-TCA solution and 180 μl BHT solution to each tube, and vortex well.

2 Loosely cover all the tubes (e.g. with marbles) and incubate the samples at 80 °C for 15 min.

3 Cool the samples down to room temperature in water.

4 Vortex well and centrifuge for 5 min at 2000 g in a table centrifuge. A dark-red precipitate can be found at the bottom of a tube.

5 Measure the absorbance of the supernatant at 533 nm against the blank. Correct this value by subtracting the background at 600 nm.

6 Calculate the TBA reactivity of a sample as μmol of TEP equivalent per μmol of phospholipid by comparison with a TEP standard curve.

iii. Iodometric method (for hydroperoxides)

This assay is based on the ability of hydroxyperoxide to oxidize iodide to iodine, which can be quantified spectrophotometrically at 353 nm. The assay is sensitive to the presence of oxygen, so it should take place in an inert atmosphere.

Protocol 9

Iodometric method for the determination of hydroperoxides

Equipment and reagents

- UV spectrophotometer
- 1 cm cuvettes
- 10 ml test-tubes
- 7.2 M potassium iodide solution: dissolve 6 g of potassium iodide crystals in 5 ml double-distilled water in a 25 ml glass conical flask, and place it in an ice-bath. Purge with a stream of nitrogen for 15 min.
- Acetic acid/chloroform (3:2, v/v): mix together 12 ml glacial acetic acid and 8 ml chloroform. Degas in a bath sonicator for 10 min, and purge with a stream of nitrogen for 5 min.

- Cadmium acetate solution: dissolve 0.5 g of cadmium acetate in 100 ml distilled water. Caution: cadmium acetate is a suspected carcinogen. Purge with nitrogen for 10 min, then store under nitrogen at 4 °C in a screw-capped bottle.
- Cumene hydroperoxide solution: dissolve 15 ml of 80% cumene hydroperoxide in 100 ml ethanol (degassed by sonication) to give a concentration of 0.8 μmol/ml. Store the stock solution under nitrogen at 4 °C in a screw-capped bottle.

Protocol 9 continued

Method

1. Dry approx. 5 mg of phospholipid[a] in a stream of nitrogen in a 10 ml glass centrifuge tube.

2. Prepare a standard curve by measuring out 250, 200, 150, 100, and 50 μl of the cumene hydroperoxide solution into 10 ml test-tubes.

3. To each of the samples, and to the cumene hydroperoxide standards, add 1 ml acetic acid/chloroform mixture.

4. Add 50 μl of potassium iodide solution to each tube, flush with nitrogen, cap tubes, vortex well, and incubate in the dark for 5 min at room temperature.

5. Add 3 ml of cadmium acetate to each tube, flush with nitrogen, cap tubes, mix well, and spin at 1000 g for 10 min.

6. Read the upper phase at 353 nm, and calculate the amount of hydroperoxide in a sample by comparison with the standard curve obtained with the cumene hydroperoxide samples.

[a] Hydroperoxides originating from cholesterol are also estimated by this assay. If necessary, the cholesterol can be separated from the phospholipid by passage through a Waters Sep-Pak silica gel column (see Section 4.2).

---

iv. FOX assay (for hydroperoxides)

A second method to detect lipid hydroperoxides in liposomes is the ferrous ion oxidation in xylenol orange (FOX) assay developed by Jiang et al. (20). The assay is based on the peroxide-mediated oxidation of Fe^{2+} to Fe^{3+}, which forms a complex in the presence of xylenol orange. This complex can be measured spectrophotometrically (560 nm). Endoperoxides exhibit lower or no reactivity in the assay. An excellent detailed evaluation of the method has been presented by Nourooz-Zadeh (21). Therefore, only a brief description of the method will follow in this chapter. Samples and standards (e.g. hydrogen peroxide, cumene hydroperoxide) are diluted with methanol or triphenylphosphine (TPP). TPP reduces hydroperoxides to their corresponding alcohols, and allows background correction in the assay. After 30 min at room temperature, FOX reagent (butylated hydroxytoluene (BHT), sulfuric acid, xylenol orange, and ammonium iron (II) sulfate hexahydrate, dissolved in methanol) is added. Similar to the TBA method, BHT is added to the reagent to prevent further peroxidation within the assay itself. Finally, after incubation for 30 min at room temperature, the absorbance is measured at 560 nm.

2.6.3 Estimation of hydrolysis levels of liposomal (phospho)lipids

In an aqueous liposome dispersion, liposomal (phospho)lipids (PC) can be hydrolysed to free fatty acids (FFA) and 2-acyl- and 1-acyl-lyso(phospho)lipids (LPC) (see Chapter 5, Section 2.2). The LPCs hydrolyse further to glycero phospho compounds (GPC).

The degree of hydrolysis is often expressed as [LPC] / [PC$_{t=0}$]. However, one should realize that LPC is an intermediate in the hydrolysis reactions (Chapter 5, Figure 3) and this expression of degree of hydrolysis is certainly not correct above 10% levels. Neglecting to take GPC into account can result in an underestimation of the degree of hydrolysis when expressed as LPC/PC levels. Moreover, in some studies the conversion ratio of LPC to GPC was reported to be faster than that of hydrolysis of PC to LPC. An accurate method to measure hydrolysis is to monitor the PC and LPC content in time by HPLC (see Section 2.3) or TLC (see Section 2.2) and GPC by total phosphate analysis of the supernatant (methanol/water phase) after extracting the lipids according to Bligh and Dyer, Section 4.1, and express the degree of hydrolysis as:

$$\% \text{ hydrolysis} = 100\% - [PC] \times 100\% / \{[PC] + [LPC] + [GPC]\}$$

Another advantage of this approach is that it is not necessary to know the absolute phospholipids concentration of the liposomal formulation at $t = 0$ to estimate the level of hydrolysis.

A better, alternative strategy to estimate low hydrolysis levels is the determination of FFA, because then one measures a non-hydrolysable degradation product of hydrolysis. FFA can be quantified by an enzymatic assay described in ref. 10.

3 Physical characterization of liposomes

In Table 1 a list is presented of 'Quality control assays of liposomal formulations'. A number of physical characteristics have to be determined in different stages of research and development of (drug-containing) liposomal dispersions. A number of strategies to obtain information on these physical characteristics are discussed below.

3.1 Determination of percentage capture

It is clearly essential to measure the quantity of material entrapped inside liposomes before studying the behaviour of this entrapped material in physical or biological systems. After removal of non-liposome associated material by the separation techniques during preparation as described in Chapter 1, one may assume that the quantity of material remaining is 100% liposome associated, but that proportion may change rapidly upon storage (see Chapter 5), or when the liposomes are handled subsequently. Therefore, for long-term stability tests and also for the initial stages of development of new liposome formulations, or when designing new methods of preparation, a technique to quantify the fraction of liposome-associated material is needed. This technique should be rapid, require small quantities of sample, and have a 'high-throughput' character.

3.1.1 Leakage through phase separation

Lipophilic compounds may phase separate from liposomal bilayers (see Chapter 5). A simple light microscope is a very suitable tool to identify these crystals or amorphous precipitate in liposomal dispersions. Generally, liposomes are less than 1–2 μm in diameter. The larger ones form Maltese crosses when viewed under a light microscope with two cross-positioned polarizing light filters. The percentage liposome entrapment of lipophilic drugs in a liposome dispersion when phase separation is observed or expected may be estimated by measuring the drug content per mol phospholipid in the supernatant after 10–30 sec centrifugation in a table top centrifuge. It is assumed that only the precipitated material is spun down under those conditions. However, this assumption should be carefully checked, e.g. by monitoring the phospholipid concentration in the supernatant. Another, more laborious option to separate liposomes and precipitate from each other is the use of liposome extrusion through a polycarbonate filter with pore sizes smaller than 0.1 μm. Here, it is assumed that the liposomes can be forced through the filter and the precipitate can not. A drawback of this procedure is that shear forces during extrusion may further promote phase separation of the lipophilic drug.

3.1.2 Leakage via membrane penetration

Leakage of water soluble compounds out of the liposomes might be estimated by ultracentrifugation followed by quantification of the free drug content in the supernatant. However, this method has the potential drawback that both ultracentrifugation and dilution (which is often necessary) might induce leakage. Two other methods are described below to offer alternative options (Protocols 10 and 11).

Protocol 10

Minicolumn centrifugation method (22)

Equipment and reagents

- Sephadex G-50 (Pharmacia)
- 0.9% NaCl
- 1 ml disposable plastic syringes
- Whatman GF/B filter pad
- Bench centrifuge
- 13 × 10 mm centrifuge tube

A. Column preparation[a,b]

1 Allow 10 g of Sephadex G-50 (medium) to swell in 120 ml of 0.9% NaCl in a glass screw-capped bottle for at least 5 h at room temperature. Store at 4 °C until required for use.

2 Remove the plungers from 1 ml disposable plastic syringes (one for each sample) and plug each barrel with a Whatman GF/B filter pad.

3 Rest each barrel in a 13 × 10 mm centrifuge tube.

4 Fill the barrels to the top with hydrated gel, using a Pasteur pipette with the tip removed.

5 Place the tubes containing the columns in a bench centrifuge, and spin at 1000 g for 3 min to remove excess saline solution. After spinning, the gel column should be dry and have come off from the sides of the barrel. The height of the bed should be level with the 0.9 ml mark (see Figure 5).

6 Empty the eluted saline from each collection tube.

B. Processing of samples

1 Apply exactly 0.2 ml of liposome suspension (undiluted) dropwise to the top of the gel bed. Take care not to let the sample trickle down the sides of the column bed.

2 Spin the columns at 1000 g for 3 min in a bench centrifuge to expel the void volume containing the liposomes into the centrifuge tube.

3 Remove eluates from each tube and set aside for assaying.

4 Apply 0.25 ml of saline to each column, spin as previously, and remove eluates from each tube. This sample may or may not contain liposomes, depending upon size, lipid composition, etc. Unentrapped solute should not come out at this stage.[c,d]

5 Load 0.1 ml of saline onto each column. Centrifuge to recover all eluate, containing the unentrapped material. Repeat this step if necessary until all free material has come off the column.

6 Measure the concentration of free or entrapped material in eluates by standard methods.

7 Measure the phosphate concentrations in the manner outlined in Section 2.1.

[a] Larger sizes of column can be used (5–10 ml syringe barrels) capable of handling 1 ml of liposome suspension at a time, so that for small scale 'manufacturing' experiments, this technique can be used as a preparative method for the separation of liposomes from unentrapped solute (see Chapter 1).

[b] A ready-to-use minicolumn is also commercially available from, e.g. Pharmacia.

[c] An advantage of this technique is that the liposomes can be recovered with practically no dilution, since the excess void fluid that would supplement the liposome volume has already been drained off in the previous spin.

[d] This method is based on the assumption that liposomes are not retained by physical interactions with the column material. This should be checked first.

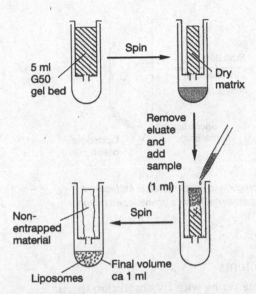

5 ml
G50
gel bed

Spin

Dry
matrix

Remove
eluate
and
add
sample
(1 ml)

Spin

Non-
entrapped
material

Final volume
ca 1 ml

Liposomes

Figure 5 Removal of unentrapped material by minicolumn centrifugation. This method can be used both as a means of purification of liposomes on a small scale, and analysis of a liposomal dispersion to determine percentage entrapment. The method is satisfactory for solutes less than 7 kDa.

Protocol 11

Protamine aggregation[a]

Equipment and reagents

- 10 ml centrifuge tube
- Bench centrifuge
- Normal saline: 0.9% NaCl
- 10 mg/ml protamine solution
- 10% Triton X-100

Method

1. Place 0.1 ml of liposome suspension (20 mg/ml lipids in normal saline) in a 10 ml conical glass centrifuge tube.

2. To the liposome suspension add 0.1 ml of protamine solution (10 mg/ml). Mix it using a micropipette and allow it to stand for 3 min.

3. To the mixture add 3 ml of saline. Spin in a bench centrifuge (using a swing-out rotor) for 20 min at 2000 g at room temperature.

4. Take off the top 2 ml of supernatant, and assay the concentration of free, unentrapped compound by standard methods.

5. Remove the remainder of the supernatant from the tube and discard. Resuspend the pellet in 0.6 ml of 10% Triton X-100. When liposomal material is properly dissolved (after warming, if necessary), make the solution up to a final volume of 3.2 ml with normal saline and assay the concentration of entrapped material by standard methods.

[a] This method (23, 24) and illustrated in Figure 6 may be used for liposomes of any composition (either neutral or negatively charged). However, a preliminary test should be carried out beforehand to check that the liposome entrapped substance does not precipitate itself in the presence of protamine after release from liposomes.

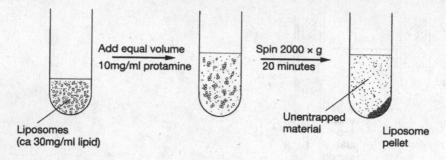

Figure 6 Protamine aggregation method for determination of the percentage entrapment. Liposomes may be precipitated in the presence of protamine, leaving unentrapped material remaining in the supernatant after centrifugation.

3.1.3 Measurement of liposomal contents

Measurement of liposome contents (non-interfering with UV absorption spectra of the bilayer forming (phospho)lipids) can be carried out by the addition of 10 µl of liposomes to 2 ml ethanol, or, if the agent is not soluble in ethanol (e.g. potassium chromate) by mixing of 10 µl of liposomes with 10 µl of 10% Triton X-100 (with warming for 30 min if necessary, for example, for cholesterol-containing liposomes), followed by dilution to 2 ml. Solutions obtained by either method are sufficiently clear for direct spectrophotometric determinations to be made. Radioactive markers are easily measured by addition of liposomes to a scintillation cocktail (see Appendix 1 of the first edition of this book).

3.2 Determination of percentage release

Having prepared a suspension of liposomes containing a known quantity of entrapped solute, with minimal solute remaining in the extra-liposomal buffer, one needs to know at what rate the liposomal contents leak out into the medium. Under normal circumstances, with a well-formulated preparation, leakage will be very slow and the techniques described above will suffice. Where the projected use of a liposome preparation is a pharmaceutical application for drug delivery or targeting, the marker for measuring release in long-term stability tests will naturally be the incorporated pharmacological agent itself. For other applications, however, particularly those in which release is induced deliberately as a result of a biochemical or biophysical change in environment, it may be desirable to use special, 'purpose-designed' markers that simplify measurements and interpretation in such experiments. These are discussed in this section.

3.2.1 Choice of marker

Liposomes are often used as model membrane systems to investigate the effects of biological modulators directly on membrane properties such as fluidity, phase transition, or permeability. Changes in these parameters can give quantitative and qualitative information about membrane interactions. Relatively rapid changes in permeability can be brought about by, for example, calcium-mediated fusion, interaction with polyanions or anaesthetics, passage through the phase transition temperature, ligand-mediated induction of a phase change, or antibody/complement-mediated lysis of antigen-bearing liposomes (see Chapter 9).

In the study of the release of water soluble markers from liposomes, it is advisable to choose the marker to be used with some care. Ideally, one would like to use a molecule:

(a) That does not pass through intact membranes.

(b) That is highly water soluble.

(c) With a very low solubility in organic media.

(d) That does not associate with membranes in any way so as to destabilize or aggregate them.

(e) That can be easily separated from liposomes by conventional methods.

Table 2 presents a list of compounds, classified according to method of detection, which are widely used, and are generally considered to meet the specifications outlined above. Most of these materials can be measured easily after separation from liposomes by the methods already described. However, there are some agents (marked with an a) whose extra-liposomal concentration can be

Table 2 Water soluble markers for liposomal entrapment studies

Detection method	Marker	Molecular weight
Optical density	Sodium chromate	162
	Ponceau red	760
	Arsenazo III[a]	776
	Cytochrome c	13000
	Haemoglobin	64500
Fluorescence	Fluorescein	319
	Carboxyfluorescein[a]	362
	Calcein[a]	620
	Fluorescein dextran	4000–2 million
Enzymatic	Glucose[a]	181
	Isocitrate[a]	258
	Soybean trypsin inhibitor[a]	22000
	Superoxide dismutases[a]	16500, 30000
	Horseradish peroxidase[a]	40000
Radiolabel	[^{14}C]glucose	183
	[^{99m}Tc]DTPA	492
	[^{111}In]bleomycin	1153
	[^{14}C]inulin	5000
	[^{125}I]PVP	10000–360000
	[^{3}H]DNA	Millions

[a] Use of these markers avoids the need for liposome separation procedures.

determined *in situ* without the need for a separation step. These are discussed in the following sections.

3.2.2 Arsenazo III

This method, developed by Weissman and colleagues (25) for the investigation of liposome integrity *in vitro* and *in vivo*, makes use of the fact that the spectral characteristics of the dye, arsenazo III (2,7-bis[2-arsonophenylazol-1,8-dihydroxy-naphthalene-3,6-disulfonic acid) differ in the presence and absence of calcium ions. Calcium binds strongly to the dye and produces a spectral shift from 560 nm to 606/660 nm, that is, a change from red to blue which is clearly distinguishable by eye (see Figure 7). This property of the dye can be used in two ways. In the first, liposomes can be made incorporating the purified calcium-free dye. Under these circumstances, both the entrapped and non-entrapped dye will be coloured red, and will have low absorbance at 660 nm. The liposome suspension can be diluted out so that interference due to scattering is minimized. Upon addition of calcium, the unentrapped dye binds to calcium while the encapsulated dye remains unchanged. Upon addition of Triton X-100, the liposome membrane is disrupted sufficiently to allow calcium ions access to the internal compartment, and all dye molecules present in the sample change their absorbance. The difference in readings before and after Triton X-100 allows the proportion of dye entrapped to be calculated. The determination can be carried out in a more sophisticated

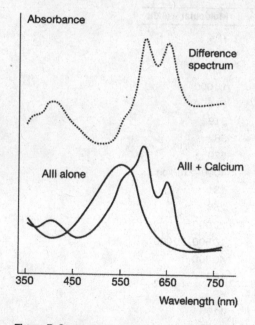

Figure 7 Spectral characteristics of arsenazo III. The addition of calcium ions to the strongly coloured arsenazo III dye induces a spectral shift which permits one to distinguish between dye outside liposomes and that entrapped inside liposomes, without recourse to physical methods of separation, since calcium does not enter into the liposome within the time course of the determination.

way using a double-beam spectrophotometer (or a single beam with the blanks measured sequentially), in which samples treated in various ways are compared as shown in Protocol 12. In this way, allowance is made for any differences in scattering due to lysis of liposomes by detergent.

The problem with this method is the requirement of free calcium ions. A number of liposome compositions are sensitive, to a greater or lesser degree, to the presence of calcium that may make interpretation of the results rather difficult. These objections can be overcome, in part, by carrying out a test in reverse, that is by preparing liposomes containing the dye plus calcium bound to each other in stoichiometric proportions, and measuring the portion released by addition of EGTA, which competes with arsenazo III for calcium ions and converts the complex to the free dye. The scheme of measurements is shown in Protocol 12, part B. Methods for purifying arsenazo III (to remove any free calcium before use) and for quantification are given in ref. 25. This method is a very useful and versatile one. It can be used to monitor processes where normal separation procedures are not feasible, for example fusion between liposomes, or interaction with living cells. Its only drawback is that, because the indicator system is calcium-dependent, membrane processes which themselves rely on interactions with calcium ions are not amenable to rigorous study.

Protocol 12

Arsenazo III method for measurement of percentage release

Equipment and reagents

- Cuvettes
- Double-beam spectrophotometer
- 3 mM (2.3 mg/ml) arzeno III in demiwater (for method A) or 3 mM (2.3 mg/ml) arzeno III and 0.45 mg/ml $CaCl_2$ in demiwater (for method B)
- 100 mM (15 mg/ml) $CaCl_2$ in demiwater (for method A)
- 100 mM (38 mg/ml) EGTA in demiwater (for method B)
- 5% (v/v) Triton X-100 in demiwater
- Calcium-free buffer

A. Assay method for liposomes not affected by calcium ions

1   Prepare liposomes in 3 mM arzeno III (2.3 mg/ml).

2   Dilute liposomes 1:100 in calcium-free buffer before adding to cuvette.

3   Put 2 ml 1:100 diluted arzeno III liposomes both in blank and sample cuvette and set the absorbance at 660 nm to zero.

4   Add 200 μl buffer to the blank cuvette and 200 μl $CaCl_2$ to the sample cuvette, mix, and measure the absorbance at 660 nm (reading 1).

5   Add 100 μl Triton X-100 to both cuvettes, mix, and measure again the absorbance at 660 nm (reading 2).

6   Calculate the % dye entrapped as (reading 2 – reading 1) / reading 2 × 100%.

Protocol 12 continued

B. Assay method for calcium-sensitive liposomes[a]

1 Prepare liposomes in 3 mM arzeno III and 0.45 mg/ml $CaCl_2$.

2 Dilute liposomes 1:100 in calcium-free buffer before adding to cuvette.

3 Put 2 ml 1:100 diluted arzeno III liposomes both in blank and sample cuvette and set the absorbance at 660 nm to zero.

4 Add 200 µl buffer to the blank cuvette and 200 µl EGTA to the sample cuvette, mix, and measure the absorbance at 660 nm (reading 1).

5 Add 100 µl Triton X-100 to both cuvettes, mix, and measure again the absorbance at 660 nm (reading 2).

6 Calculate the % dye entrapped as (reading 2 – reading 1)/reading 2 × 100%.

[a] This method can be used when calcium only causes aggregation. One should check if it does not induce leakage. See also text.

3.2.3 Carboxyfluorescein and calcein

Carboxyfluorescein (CF) is very much less lipophilic than its parent compound fluorescein, and has a much lower tendency to associate with phospholipid membranes. Consequently its use in place of fluorescein as a marker for the aqueous compartment of liposomes is to be recommended. The main property of carboxy-fluorescein, which lends itself to *in situ* determinations of liposome contents is its ability to self-quench (26), that is, at high concentrations, the fluorescence of carboxyfluorescein is very much reduced compared with diluted samples, probably because of intermolecular interactions.

Thus, the basic approach when using this compound is to prepare liposomes containing a highly quenching concentration of CF (usually about 100 mM in 10 mM Tris or HEPES, which is iso-osmolar with physiological saline), and then dilute the suspension approximately 10 000-fold, whereupon the non-entrapped material will fluoresce intensely, while the entrapped CF gives no signal (Figure 8). Upon addition of Triton X-100, the liposomal contents will be released, and, being diluted in the suspending medium, they will also fluoresce, so that the concentration of CF initially inside, as well as outside the liposomes can be deduced. As long as the final concentration of CF in the measuring cuvette is 3–30 µM (when fluorescence is completely unquenched, see Figure 9), the fluorescence readings will be directly proportional to the concentration.

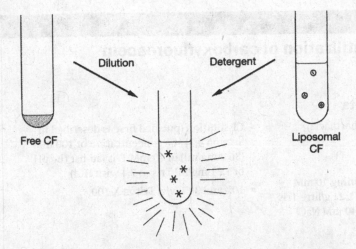

Figure 8 Unquenching of carboxyfluorescein fluorescence. At high concentrations, carboxyfluorescein (CF) fluoresces only weakly because of self-quenching (*top left*). Reducing the concentration of CF by diluting CF solutions results in increased fluorescence (*centre*) as this quenching is reduced. CF which is entrapped inside liposomes at high concentration will give no increase in fluorescence, however, even when the liposome dispersion is diluted, since the concentration of the entrapped liposomal contents remains unchanged (see *right-hand side*). On the other hand, CF, which has leaked out of the liposomes into the extra-liposomal medium, will display enhancement of fluorescence upon dilution of the suspension. This may also be accomplished by lysis of diluted liposomes with detergent. This technique can be used to investigate liposomal leakage and permeability processes over time ranges too short to permit separation of components by physical means.

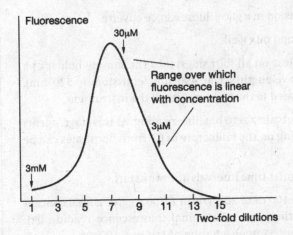

Figure 9 Change in carboxyfluorescein fluorescence with increasing dilution. Self-quenching of carboxyfluorescein is not completely relaxed until the solution has been diluted to 30 μmol concentration. For accurate quantitative work, it is important to carry out determinations at a concentration range below 30 μM. (Data provided by R. R. C. New and R. E. Stringer.)

Protocol 13

Preparation and utilization of carboxyfluorescein liposomes

Equipment and reagents

- Sephadex G-50 column (Pharmacia)
- Spectrofluorimeter
- Fluorescence cuvettes
- Tris-buffered saline containing 10 mM Tris–HCl (adjust the pH of 1.21 g/litre Tris to 7.4 with 1 M HCl) and 140 mM NaCl (8.2 g/litre)

- CF solution (purified first as described in Section 4.3) at a concentration of 100 mM (36.2 mg/ml) in 10 mM Tris (adjust the pH of 1.21 mg/ml Tris to 7.4 with HCl)
- 10% and 20% (v/v) Triton X-100

Method

1 Use the CF solution to prepare liposomes by any of the standard methods.

2 Remove unincorporated dye by passage through a Sephadex G-50 column equilibrated in Tris-buffered saline and pre-saturated with empty liposomal lipids.

3 Determine the concentration of CF in the purified liposomes by dissolving 100 μl in 100 μl of 10% Triton X-100, making the volume up to 2 ml, and measuring the optical density at 470 nm. Compare the reading obtained with a standard curve prepared over the range 0.1–1 mM of CF.

4 On the basis of the measured concentration, dilute the liposomes in Tris-buffered saline to give a final concentration of 2 mM CF.

5 Place 10 μl of the liposome suspension in a glass fluorescence cuvette.

6 Add 2.0 ml of Tris-buffered saline and mix well.

7 Insert the fluorescence cuvette (clear on all four sides) into the sample holder of a spectrofluorimeter (excitation wavelength set at 490 nm, emission at 520 nm). Ensure that the sample is equilibrated to the temperature of the instrument.

8 Measure fluorescence emission to obtain a zero baseline reading. At this stage, agents under study that may have a bearing on the efflux rate of CF from liposomes can be added.

9 Measure the fluorescence (F) at regular time intervals after the start.

10 At the end of the experiment, add 100 μl of 20% Triton X-100 to give a final concentration of 1%. Mix well by pipetting, and take a final fluorescence reading (Ft). Correct for the increase in volume of 5% upon addition of Triton X-100.

[a] It has been reported that CF liposomes are susceptible to leakage in high gravitational fields, so use of the minicolumn centrifugation method for separation should be carefully checked.

Carboxyfluorescein has been used very widely for studying release of entrapped solutes from liposomes in the presence of biological fluids (26), and during the course of these investigations, a number of features have come to light where some caution needs to be exercised in the use of this method. These are as follows:

(a) The fluorescence intensity of CF (in its unquenched state) is pH dependent, increasing by a factor of two over the range pH 6–8, as the proportion of the ionized species of the molecule increases.

(b) Leakage of CF from liposomes is enhanced at low pH, as the molecule becomes more protonated.

(c) Serum components bind CF, and some quenching can occur; in the presence of Triton X-100 this quenching is enhanced, particularly with human serum (26).

With the use of strongly buffered solutions at neutral pH, and the inclusion of appropriate controls, allowances can be made for these potential inaccuracies. In cases where difficulties are still encountered, the use of calcein (also a self-quenching fluorophore; excitation wavelength 491 nm, emission at 511 nm) as an alternative may be considered. The fluorescence of this marker molecule, although at neutral pH similar to CF (both are fluorescein derivatives) is less pH dependent (27). However, its interaction with serum components has not been widely documented and at high dilutions, calcein seems to be more prone to artefacts such as adherence to glassware, etc. Preparation procedures for CF and calcein are given in Section 4.3.

3.2.4 Glucose

Extra-liposomal concentrations of unlabelled glucose can be determined by enzymatic means, making use of the coupled ATP-driven conversion of glucose to 6-phosphogluconate (28). The reaction is catalysed by hexokinase and glucose-6-phosphate dehydrogenase (G-6-PDH) with the reduction of NADP to NADPH, the formation of which can be monitored by an increase in absorbance at 340 nm. One mole of NADPH is formed for every mole of glucose available, so the concentration of extra-liposomal glucose is linearly related to the UV absorbance of NADPH. The procedure to carry out measurements is as follows.

Protocol 14

Preparation and utilization of glucose-containing liposomes

Equipment and reagents

- Spectrophotometer
- Quartz cuvettes
- Tris-buffered saline (TBS): 100 mM Tris, 64 mM NaCl, 3.5 mM $MgCl_2$, 0.15 M $CaCl_2$. Measure out 1.21 g Tris, 0.37 g NaCl, 70 mg $MgCl_2 \cdot 6H_2O$, and 22 mg $CaCl_2 \cdot 2H_2O$. Dissolve in 100 ml of double-distilled water, mix well, and adjust to pH 7.5 with 1 M HCl.
- Stock 10 mM ATP solution: dissolve 100 mg of ATP in 20 ml TBS. Subdivide into 1 ml aliquots and store frozen at –20 °C until required for use.
- Stock 5 mM NADP solution: dissolve 75 mg of NADP in 20 ml TBS. Subdivide into 1 ml aliquots and store frozen at –20 °C until required for use.
- Hexokinase (yeast) solution (Boehringer Mannheim): dissolve 2 mg in 1 ml of distilled water. Remove ammonium sulfate by dialysis overnight in the cold against 2 litres of distilled water. Make up to 15 ml with TBS, subdivide into 1 ml aliquots, and store at 4 °C (do not freeze).
- Glucose-6-phosphate dehydrogenase (yeast) solution (Boehringer Mannheim): dissolve 1 mg in 1 ml of distilled water. Remove ammonium sulfate by dialysis overnight in the cold against 2 litres of distilled water. Make up to 15 ml with TBS, subdivide into 1 ml aliquots, and store at 4 °C (do not freeze).
- Glucose assay reagent (prepare freshly on the day of use): add together 1 ml each of stock ATP, NADP, hexokinase, and G-6-PDH solutions and mix well. This is sufficient for eight assays. In addition, prepare 1 ml of reagent as above, with one of the components (e.g. ATP or NADP) replaced by TBS, to act as a control blank.
- 300 mM glucose solution: dissolve 0.54 g of glucose in 10 ml of distilled water

Method

1. Use the 300 mM glucose solution to prepare liposomes by any of the standard methods at a concentration of approx. 10 mg lipid/ml.

2. Remove unentrapped glucose by the minicolumn method (see Protocol 10).

3. Dilute the liposomes approx. 20-fold by addition of 500 µl of the liposome suspension to 10 ml TBS.

4. For each sample to be studied introduce 500 µl of a glucose assay reagent into a 1.5 ml (quartz) semi-micro cuvette (clear on two sides).

5. To an additional cuvette, introduce 500 µl of control buffer (either TBS or assay reagent minus one component).

6. Make the volume of cuvettes up to 1 ml with 500 µl of buffer. At this stage, additional agents may be added to each mixture to study their effect on the release process.

7. Place both cuvettes in a double-beam spectrophotometer, with the control cuvette in the reference beam.

8 To each cuvette add 100 μl of liposome suspension, and mix well by gently pipetting, then immediately take a reading of the difference in optical density between blank and sample at 340 nm. Set instrument reading to zero at this stage if desired.

9 Incubate the reaction mixture in the cuvettes at room temperature for 30 min, then measure the difference in optical density again at 340 nm as before.

10 Determine the quantity of total glucose separately by adding 25 μl of 50% (v/v) Triton X-100 to 100 μl of liposomes and mixing well (with warming if necessary). Then add 500 μl TBS, mix well, and add 500 μl of assay reagent. Incubate for 10 min at room temperature, then measure the optical density (relative to control) at 340 nm. Make a correction for the increase in volume due to the added Triton X-100.

The main disadvantage of the enzymatic determination of glucose is that it is not instantaneous, so that it is not suitable for use in kinetic studies where release of glucose is fairly rapid. The principal application for this method to date has been the quantification of immune lysis of antigen-bearing liposomes in the presence of antibody and complement (29). Even then, difficulties may be encountered as a result of interference by the presence of high levels of endogenous glucose in animal sera. Most workers routinely dialyse these sera to remove glucose before addition to the assay mixture. It is possible that the use of glucose-6-phosphate instead of glucose as the entrapped agent could overcome this problem. In this case, hexokinase and ATP would no longer be required.

The advantage of the method is that it is inexpensive, requires simple instrumentation, will handle many samples at one time, and is relatively insensitive to small variations in experimental conditions.

3.2.5 Other markers for entrapment and release

Presumably, satisfactory methods analogous to the above could be devised, in which substrates of other enzyme systems—horseradish peroxidase, alkaline phosphatase, esterase—are entrapped inside liposomes or in which chromogenic substances are coupled with NADPH production. Where one wishes to investigate entrapment of larger molecules such as proteins, the enzymes themselves could be used as markers, using the enzymatic activity of the mixture to differentiate between contents and protein outside the liposomes. One would have to bear in mind that the process of entrapment itself could have a deleterious effect on the activity of the enzyme, although this can be allowed for if comparison is made between activity before and after solubilization of liposomes. It is conceivable, however, that this approach could give a misleading picture if the liposome membrane were selectively leaky to small molecules such as the substrates, but not the enzymes themselves, in which case liposomally-entrapped enzymes would contribute to the 'extra-liposomal' reaction.

Such a reservation does not arise in the case of soybean trypsin inhibitor, a protein with a molecular weight of 22 000, which is not an enzyme itself, but is able to inhibit the enzymatic activity of trypsin. Protein concentration is assayed by observing inhibition in the generation of a chromophore resulting from the action of trypsin (30), which itself has no access to the internal contents of liposomes. This general approach of using enzyme inhibitors is of particular interest, not only for large molecules, but for low molecular weight substances as well. The signal arising from leakage of materials from liposomes is amplified as the number of moles of inhibitor released inhibits conversion of a far greater number of moles of substrate.

3.3 Determination of entrapped volume

For intermediate or large unilamellar vesicles (where the membrane thickness is small compared with the diameter), the entrapped volume (litre/mole lipid) is dependent on the radius (R in m) of the vesicles according to the relation:

$$\text{entrapped volume (litre/mol)} = 500/3 \cdot A \cdot N \cdot R$$

where A is the area of the membrane occupied by one lipid (in m^2) and N is the Avogadro constant (6.022×10^{23} mol^{-1}). Typical values for A are 0.52 nm^2 for DPPC, 0.82 nm^2 for DOPC, 0.65 nm^2 for DOPE, and 0.30 nm^2 for cholesterol. However, these values for A depend for example, on the temperature, the presence of other lipids in the bilayer, etc. (see ref. 31). With the formula above one can calculate that the entrapped volume of an unilamellar liposome composed of DPPC and 200 nm in diameter is 5.2 litre/mol $\{= (500/3) \times (0.52 \times 10^{-18}$ $m^2) \times 6.022 \times 10^{23}$ $mol^{-1} \times (100 \times 10^{-9}$ m)$\}$. The entrapped volume of a population of liposomes can often be deduced from measurements of the total quantity of solute entrapped inside liposomes, assuming that the concentration of solute in the aqueous medium inside the liposomes is the same as that in the solution used to start with, and assuming that no solute has leaked out of the liposomes after separation from unentrapped material. In many cases, however, such assumptions may be invalid. For example, in two-phase methods of preparation, water can be lost from the internal compartment during the drying down step to remove organic solvent. On other occasions, water may enter, or be expelled from the liposome as a result of unanticipated osmotic differences.

3.4 Lamellarity

An estimate of the degree of lamellarity can be made simply by measuring the average particle diameter (see next section) and comparing the calculated value for entrapped volume with that obtained by experimental determination as described in the preceding section. If the experimental value is less than that expected from theory, then either the dispersion contains a significant proportion of small vesicles (for which the above simple relation does not hold), or some or all of the vesicles are multilamellar.

3.4.1 Derivatization of the outside leaflet of the bilayer

An alternative way of reaching the same conclusion is to measure the proportion of phospholipid, which is exposed on the outside surface of the vesicles. For large unilamellar vesicles this will be 50% (i.e. the outer leaflet, but not the inner leaflet of the single bilayer membrane). For SUVs the proportion will be even higher, since the lipid distribution is asymmetric, while for MLVs the value will be lower than 50%. The proportion of lipid at the surface can be measured either chemically, or by spectroscopic means. In the first method, a small quantity of phosphatidylethanolamine (PE) is incorporated into the liposome membrane during preparation, which is then derivatized in the intact vesicle by reaction with trinitrobenzene sulfonic acid (TNBS). Only the outer, exposed PEs will react to give trinitrophenylated (TNP-) PE (32). In parallel, aliquots of the same liposome dispersion are disrupted in Triton X-100 before derivatization, in which all the PE molecules present are available for reaction. Both samples are then made up to the same concentration in acidified Triton X-100 to stop further reaction, and the optical density is measured. The derivatized product TNP-PE absorbs more strongly than the reactants. The possible use of TLC in the determination of TNP-PE will improve the outcome of the results (see refs 33 and 34) for detailed information). Unfortunately, interpretation of results obtained with this method is not always so straightforward. This technique assumes that the PE is evenly distributed throughout both leaflets of the bilayer. It can give misleading results when working with populations containing small liposomes, since in membranes of high curvature, the PE may be located in higher concentration on the inner leaflet than on the outer, because of the difference in shape of the PE molecules, and its different packing characteristics.

3.4.2 NMR

The spectroscopic method involves measuring the phosphorus NMR signal of the PC head groups of a population of liposomes before and after addition of manganese ions to the external medium (35). Manganese ions interact with the phosphorus on the outer surface of the bilayer membrane such that the resonance signal is broadened beyond detection; thus the remainder of the peak height is due to phospholipid head groups inside the vesicle, which do not come into contact with manganese ions. Direct comparison of the size of the two signals readily reveals the proportion of phospholipid in the outer leaflet. A serious drawback of this method is that manganese ions might induce fusion of negatively charged liposomes, causing leak in of the manganese ions, and consequently interfere with the assay.

Using the methods outlined above, it is not possible to determine the exact number of lamellae in a liposome population, since one can not tell what is the precise configuration that has been adopted by the internal lamellae. A liposome with all its lamellae concentrated around the outside bilayer will have far fewer bilayers than one in which the lamellae are located in the centre, even though both liposomes have the same weight of internal lipid, since the quantity of lipid required to form each lamella depends upon its diameter. A more detailed discussion of the subject can be found elsewhere (36). Small angle X-ray scattering (SAXS) measurements or electron microscopical observations may help to provide the necessary information.

3.4.3 SAXS

The amplitude and the phase of the X-rays characterize the SAXS pattern of a liposomal sample. The amplitude is directly proportional to the local electron density in a structure, which place can be identified from the phase. Unfortunately, only the intensities are measured in an X-ray diffraction pattern. Information about the phase can only be derived in an indirect way by comparing the experimentally obtained pattern with the theoretical pattern, which has been calculated assuming a certain electron density profile (based on other information). Only liposomes with a number of concentric bilayers at well-defined distances will be recognized as multilamellar vesicles. Multivesicular structures will be recognized as single bilayer structures by SAXS. A major additional advantage of SAXS is that this technique enables one to determine the position of proteins attached to a bilayer. A drawback, however, is the limited availability of intense X-ray sources, like synchrotron radiation. The reader is referred to ref. 37 and references therein for further information about SAXS.

3.4.4 Electron microscopy

Electron microscopy might be another alternative to estimate the lamellarity of liposomes. Negative staining (e.g. phosphotungstic acid and ammonium molybdate) followed by dehydration is often used to visualize the liposomes (38), but sample preparation may induce fusion or aggregation of the liposomes. One way to overcome sample preparation artefacts is the use of the so-called freeze-fracture technique in combination with suitable shadowing (39). A sample is quickly frozen to about –200 °C, and subsequently fractured with a sharp knife in vacuum. The fracture plane falls often in the middle of a membrane, which is one of the weakest regions. Finally, an ultrathin metal layer, e.g. of platinum, is evaporated onto the surface at a fixed angle providing a shadowing structure of the real structure. It is this replica that is investigated with a transmission electron microscopy. Unfortunately, the fracture plane often falls in the middle of the outer membrane, which limits freeze fracture electron microscopy in the estimation of the lamellarity of liposomes. Another method, which is free of fusion or aggregation if properly used, is cryo-electron microscopy (40–42). The sample is frozen so quickly that it is embedded in amorphous ice, which improves the material contrast considerably. Cryo-electron microscopy is a very suitable method to estimate the lamellarity of liposomes. However, this technique is limited to visualize structures smaller than 300–500 nm.

Electron microscopy is rather expensive and might be misleading if sample preparation and data analysis are not carefully performed and evaluated. Artefacts can not only be caused by negative staining as described above, but they can also be a result of osmotic stress or temperature gradients caused by insufficiently rapid cryofixation during the sample preparation procedures. Another drawback of electron microscopy is that quantification of liposome characteristics is laborious. A few hundred vesicles have to be analysed to obtain statistically reliable results, and corrections for observational bias have to be included in data analysis. The reader is referred to the literature mentioned above for further detailed information about it.

3.5 Size determination of liposomes

3.5.1 Introduction

Methods for determining the size of liposomes vary in complexity and degree of sophistication. Undoubtedly, the most precise method is that of electron microscopic examination following a validated protocol, since it permits one to view each individual liposome, and given time and patience, and the skill to avoid numerous artefacts, one can obtain accurate information about the profile of a liposome population over the whole range of sizes. Unfortunately, it can be very time-consuming (more than 400 vesicles should be counted), and requires equipment that may not always be immediately at hand.

In contrast, laser light scattering analysis is simple and rapid to perform, but suffers from the disadvantage of measuring an averaged property of the bulk of the liposomes. Even with the most advanced refinements, it may not pick up or describe in detail small deviations from a mean value or the nature of residual peaks at extremes of the size range. Laser light scattering analysis will provide useful information on size distribution for liposomes up to (roughly speaking) 1 μm. For larger liposomes information on size distribution can be collected with a Coulter counter, through laser diffraction (e.g. Mastersizer™), or through light obscuration techniques (e.g. Accusizer™). In this section we will focus only on the laser light scattering analysis of liposomes.

All methods mentioned above require costly equipment. If only an approximate idea of size range is required, then gel exclusion chromatographic techniques can be recommended, since the only expense incurred is that of buffers and gel materials. The reader is referred to literature elsewhere (3, 43) for further details. If one wishes to compare between different liposome populations of identical composition and concentration, and only relative rather than absolute values are required, then the even simpler method of optical density measurement (i.e. turbidity due to scattering) can be employed (3, 44). This may be useful if one requires a rapid check on whether liposomes are changing in size during sonication, extrusion or microfluidization processes, storage, etc.

3.5.2 Principle of liposome size measurement by photon correlation spectroscopy

Photon correlation spectroscopy (PCS) is the analysis of the time dependence of intensity fluctuations in scattered laser light due to the Brownian motion of particles in solution/suspension (45). Since small particles diffuse more rapidly than large particles, the rate of fluctuation of scattered light intensity varies accordingly (Figure 10). Once the signal has been recorded in terms of a series of photomultiplier bursts over a period of time (Figure 11), a mathematical process called 'correlation' is carried out, in which the similarity is measured between the signal and the signal separated from the first one by a time delay (which is the so-called channel sampling time, see below). In essence this is performed by multiplying the amplitudes of the signal and its time-delayed copy together at different time points to give a correlation function. As the signals become more and more out of phase with each other (i.e. the time separation is increased), their randomness with respect to each other results in a decay of the correlation

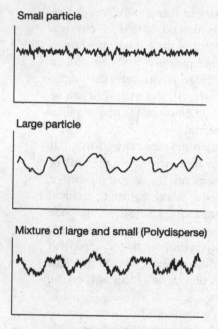

Small particle

Large particle

Mixture of large and small (Polydisperse)

Figure 10 Fluctuations in light intensity in relation to particle size. Fluctuations in light intensity of a beam of laser light passing through a suspension of particles occur because of movement of the particles in the beam as a result of Brownian motion. The movement of large particles in a fluid medium is slower than for small particles, and the fluctuations in light intensity are therefore correspondingly slower.

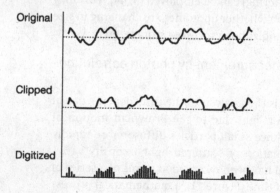

Original

Clipped

Digitized

Figure 11 Processing of signal fluctuations. The signal is processed so that intensity variations with time can be stored and manipulated easily by the computer in the form of a series of digits

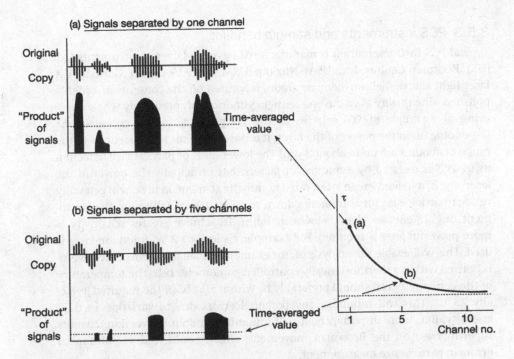

Figure 12 Derivation of correlation curve. The correlation curve (from which the diffusion coefficient is deduced) is a measure of how quickly a signal becomes completely out of phase with itself. This is determined by multiplying the signal with a copy of itself separated from the original by a given period of time (i.e. a set number of channels). The product, expressed as the cumulative area under the curve obtained, is plotted for each time separation against the channel number corresponding to that separation. The result is a curve, which decays exponentially to a mean value at a rate that depends on the rapidity of the signal fluctuations (and hence the particle size). The value to which it decays will depend on the intensity of the signal fluctuations.

function to a constant value (Figure 12). The correlation function at any given time separation is described mathematically as:

$$G(t) = <n>^2 (1 - Be^{-\Gamma t})$$

in which n is the intensity of the signal averaged over many sample times, B is a constant determined by mechanical constraints of the apparatus and the sampling procedure, and Γ, the decay constant, is $2DK^2$, where K is the scattering vector (dependent on the detection angle, etc.) and D is the diffusion coefficient of the particles causing the fluctuation. Having obtained a value for the diffusion coefficient, particle radius can then be determined by inserting D in the Stokes–Einstein equation thus:

$$D = kT / 6\pi\eta R_h$$

where k is the Boltzmann's constant, T is the absolute temperature, η is the solvent viscosity, and R_h is the mean hydrodynamic radius.

3.5.3 PCS instruments and sample handling

Typical PCS instrumentation is manufactured by, e.g. Malvern Instruments Ltd. (UK), Beckman Coulter, Inc. (USA), Nicomp (USA), and ALV-GmbH (Germany). A laser light source (helium–neon or argon) is focused on the contents of a highly polished, fine quality glass cuvette (either cylindrical or, preferably when measuring at an angle of 90° relative to the laser beam, square cross-section). Depending upon the power of the laser, it is possible to measure particles in the range of about 3 nm up to about 3 μm. The lower limit of particle size detection using PCS is dictated by a number of factors, but principally the power of the laser. Use of a helium–neon laser, rated nominally at about 35 mW, will generally restrict particle size measurements down to about 10 nm (although the instrument might generate 'data' below this limit). To achieve greater sensitivity, a more powerful laser is required. For example, typically a 2 W argon ion laser is used. This will enable the analysis of, for example, micellar systems. The cuvette is housed within a thermostatically-controlled goniometer cell. The temperature of the goniometer cell should preferably be within ±0.1 °C of the required (typically 25 °C). This will minimize any potential errors due to variation in fluid viscosity. But, more importantly, it will minimize random convection currents superimposed on the Brownian movement, which could lead to substantial errors in particle size measurement.

The sample under examination can be suspended in a range of dispersion media, the only information required being viscosity and refractive index of the medium. These can be determined using a suitable viscometer and refractometer, respectively, ideally at the temperature at which PCS is being performed. The viscosity of a hydration medium can also be determined using PCS measurements of standard particles (46). To eliminate potential light flare at the surfaces through which the laser beam passes, it is recommended that the sample cell be immersed in a liquid which matches the refractive index of the dispersion fluid. Scattered laser light from the sample is detected by a photomultiplier assembly usually situated at an angle of 90° relative to the laser beam.

The technique of performing PCS analysis requires stringent attention to detail in particular when measuring particles in the lower size range (smaller than 0.1 μm). Ideally, the photon correlation spectrometer should be housed in its own room and mounted on a vibration-free surface. The environment should be dust-free and strong light sources in the vicinity of the photomultiplier assembly should be avoided. If necessary, glass cuvettes can be soaked in chromic acid for 24 h before use and then rinsed thoroughly with 0.22 μm filtered distilled water prior to drying.

Samples for measurement of small sized liposomes should, in general, be constituted in media that have been passed through a suitable 0.22 μm filter. This should normally eliminate problems usually attributable to 'dust'. However, it is generally worthwhile monitoring the 'clarity' of the constitution medium by checking the photon count at the photomultiplier assembly. This enables a rational choice of sample concentration and can give a rapid indication of poor sample preparation. The required count can be achieved by suitable dilution of the sample and/or adjustment of the photomultiplier aperture. When observed from the side, the laser beam should pass cleanly through the sample with no evidence of 'flare' adjacent to the beam within the confines of the cuvette. Large variations of the photo count usually indicate poor sample preparation with the presence of very coarse material in suspension. To avoid interference by very large aggregates that are non-representative of the preparation as a whole, the sample might be passed through a 5 μm pore size (or smaller) membrane filter or might be subject to centrifugation before measurement (providing this does not adversely affect the sub-5 μm liposome population).

The choice and configuration of correlator sample time might be critical in achieving meaningful results. Choosing excessively long sample times can result in only a few channels responding to scattered light. Conversely, excessively short sample times might 'select' only a proportion of the total signal (Figure 13). Nowadays, however, the channel numbers of correlators may be so large (≥1000) that they cover a wide range of sample times.

3.5.4 Data analysis

Data can be presented either as mean particle size (assuming spherical equivalence), or alternatively, a more rigorous analysis can yield details of two or more subpopulations of particles in solution/suspension. Various methods of data

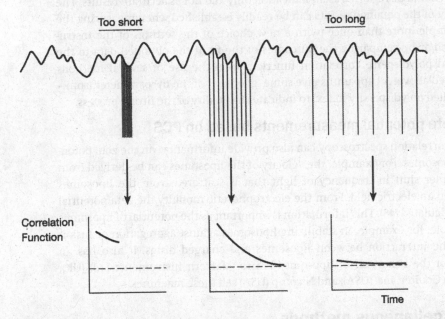

Figure 13 Choice of channel sample time. The choice of channel sample time is important in ensuring that sufficient information is acquired to enable a full plot of the correlation curve to be obtained. Ideally, the channel sample time should correspond roughly to the frequency of signal fluctuations. Although correlation curves can be drawn when the sample time is long or short, values derived for the diffusion coefficient will not be so accurate.

analysis are available depending upon the types of samples being studied. For a theoretical overview, the reader is referred to the literature (45). If the particles are non-spherical (e.g. DNA and DNA–cationic lipid complexes), rotational motions will also attribute to the changes in light scattering. Reasonable results of a monodisperse sample might still be obtained when the data are analysed by a forced homogeneous model (47). Fortunately, we can assume that in general liposomes are spherical. Many situations may be found where the sample is either very polydisperse, skewed, bi- or multi-modal and therefore can not be described adequately by simple mean values. The correlation function is now the sum of the contributions of each fraction present. In these instances, the measurements should ideally be done with different values for both the scattering angle and the correlator sample time. The obtained data can be fitted to the polydisperse correlation function using different methods. One method is to use the Taylor series expansion, with or without assuming a certain distribution (e.g. a Gaussian shape). A more recent method is to use the inverse Laplace transformation. The reader is referred to the literature (45) for further information about this strategy. A problem for the proper fitting of a polydisperse correlation function is caused by the fact that large particles scatter much more than small particles (intensity $\propto R_h^6$). Therefore, the results may be misleading, especially when the measurements are performed at a constant value for the scattering angle and/or correlator sample time. In those cases, results of the measurements of highly polydisperse samples should be regarded as an indication only and not as accurate results. The reliability of the obtained results can be readily established when measuring the same sample more than once (with a new choice of the settings of the instrument) and/or by comparing the outcomes of the fit of the obtained data to the measured polydisperse correlation function upon the use of several methods mentioned above. All apparatus give some 'goodness of the fit' parameter (sometimes called polydispersity index) to indicate the quality of the fitting process.

3.6 Zeta potential measurements based on PCS

Photon correlation spectroscopy can also provide information on the zeta potential of liposomes. For example, the velocity of the liposomes can be derived from the Doppler shift in frequency of light that is scattered from the liposomes moving in an electric field. From the electrophoretic mobility the zeta potential can be calculated (48). This information is important as the potential of liposomes plays a role, for example, in stabilizing liposomes against aggregation or fusion and in the interaction between liposomes and charged drugs. It also has an impact on the behaviour of liposomes *in vivo*. Malvern Instruments Ltd. (UK), Beckman Coulter, Inc. (USA), and Nicomp (USA) sell these machines.

4 Miscellaneous methods

4.1 Bligh and Dyer-extraction

The Bligh and Dyer-extraction (49) enables one to separate between various components of the formulation and is described below.

Protocol 15

Bligh and Dyer-extraction

Equipment and reagent

- Eppendorf cup
- Bench centrifuge
- 0.1 M HCl

Method

1 Add 100 μl lipid dispersion to an Eppendorf cup.

2 Add 125 μl chloroform and 250 μl methanol.

3 Vortex until a clear solution is obtained.

4 Add 125 μl of 0.1 M HCl and 125 μl chloroform.

5 Vortex and centrifuge at 2700 g for 15 min to obtain two clear phases: the upper phase consists of methanol and water and the lower phase consists of practically 100% chloroform.

The Bligh and Dyer-extraction might be simplified by adding 225 μl lipid colloids in an aqueous dispersion, 250 μl methanol, and 250 μl chloroform together at once in an Eppendorf cup. In general, lipophilic constituents are extracted into the chloroform-rich lower phase and hydrophilic constituents are extracted in the aqueous methanolic upper phase. However, some hydrophilic compounds such as carbohydrates (especially polysaccharides), many proteins, and nucleic acid may precipitate during the extraction procedure, either to the bottom during the monophasic step of the extraction process or at the interphase in the final two phases stage. Partitioning of certain lipids, especially free fatty acids, can be controlled with the pH of the system. In general, the 0.1 M HCl is necessary to acidify charged lipids, else a 'pancake' between the phases might be seen when, for example, phosphatidylglycerol is present. Alternatively, 0.2–1.0 M sodium bicarbonate can be used to extract, for example, fatty acids in the upper phase. In all biphasic extraction procedures, separation between the lipophilic and hydrophilic constituents may be improved by the use of well-defined pH. For example, when the drug in the formulation is an amphipathic weak base, the use of acidic conditions will improve the separation of drug from lipid. In the biphasic extraction procedure, the acidic condition does not present any problems since most of the acid is extracted into the more polar phase and its traces can be removed by a rewash with a synthetic polar phase (methanol/water in a ratio of 250:225, v/v). The chloroform-rich phase can be concentrated or even evaporated to dryness. In general, when the volume of the liposome dispersion is too large the extraction can be preceded by a lyophilization step.

4.2 Sep-Pak minicolumn extraction

This method is useful for separation of lipid components and is taken from the previous edition of this book.

Protocol 16

Sep-Pak minicolumn extraction

Equipment and reagent

- 1 ml disposable plastic syringe
- Sep-Pak C18 minicolumn (Waters)
- Silica gel Sep-Pak minicolumn (Waters)

- 10 ml glass syringe
- Aqueous elution medium: mix 40 ml methanol with 20 ml of 0.1 M HCl

Method

1 Draw up 0.1 ml of liposomes into a 1 ml disposable plastic syringe.

2 Fix a syringe onto the inlet port of a Waters Sep-Pak C18 minicolumn, and introduce the liposomes onto the minicolumn. Make sure all the material is on the column.

3 Replace the empty 1 ml syringe with a 10 ml glass syringe containing 10 ml of the aqueous elution medium,[a] and flush the column through with the contents of the syringe. Keep the syringe and column pointing vertically downwards each time elution is performed. Collect aqueous eluate in beaker. Lipids will remain on the column.

4 Separation of cholesterol and α-tocopherol from phospholipids. Attach a 10 ml glass syringe containing chloroform to the inlet port of the minicolumn. Allow 0.5 ml of chloroform to enter the column, and discard the eluate. Then fix the outlet port of the C18 column to the inlet port of a silica gel Sep-Pak minicolumn using a short male-to-male luer adaptor. Flush both columns with the remainder of the chloroform in the syringe. Disconnect the two columns, and pass a further 10 ml of chloroform through the second column. Retain the eluate, which will contain cholesterol and α-tocopherol, while phospholipids will remain on the silica column.

5 Remove phospholipids from the silica column by flushing with 20 ml methanol.

[a] Acid or alkali may be employed in the aqueous elution medium in cases where separation is difficult because of ionic interactions between solute and lipids.

4.3 Preparation of carboxyfluorescein and calcein solutions

Protocol 17

Preparation of carboxyfluorescein solution[a]

Equipment and reagents

- 1 litre conical flasks
- Activated charcoal
- Water-bath
- Buchner funnel
- Whatman filter paper No. 50
- Desiccator
- Silica gel TLC
- Sephadex LH20 hydrophobic column (2.5 × 40 cm)

- Carboxyfluorescein (acid form from e.g. Eastman Kodak)
- 6 M NaOH
- 6 M HCl
- 10 mM Tris–HCl buffer pH 7.5
- Chloroform/methanol/water (65:25:4, by vol.)

A. Recrystallization (for removal of polar contaminants)

1 Dissolve 35 g of carboxyfluorescein in 200 ml ethanol in a conical flask.

2 Add 2 g of activated charcoal, and boil for several minutes in a water-bath.

3 Filter the mixture through a Buchner funnel (using Whatman filter paper No. 50), and collect the filtrate in a 1 litre conical flask.

4 Add cold distilled water slowly with stirring until the solution is no longer clear (about 400 ml will be required).

5 Cool slowly to +4 °C, then leave overnight in a freezer at –20 °C.

6 The following day, collect the precipitated carboxyfluorescein in a Buchner funnel (using Whatman filter paper No. 50) and wash thoroughly with ice-cold distilled water.

7 Dry the solid carboxyfluorescein in the funnel, then in a desiccator.

B. Column chromatography (for removal of hydrophobic contaminants)

1 Place 30 g of carboxyfluorescein in a 100 ml beaker, and add 40 ml of 6 M NaOH. With stirring, adjust to pH 7.5 by slow dropwise addition of 6 M HCl. Take care not to overshoot. Warm the solution to 50 °C if necessary to achieve complete dissolution. Concentration of the resultant solution will be approx. 2 M.

2 Apply 10 ml of concentrated carboxyfluorescein solution to the top of a Sephadex LH20 hydrophobic column (2.5 × 40 cm).

3 Elute the sample with 10 mM Tris–HCl buffer pH 7.5 and collect it in 2 ml fractions.[b]

4 Monitor the purity of fractions by silica gel TLC, using a solvent system composed of chloroform/methanol/water (65:25:4, by vol.).

Protocol 17 continued

5   Pool the fractions containing pure carboxyfluorescein, and adjust to the desired concentration in Tris–HCl buffer.[c,d] Store in the dark at 4 °C until required for use. It is stable for many months.

[a] The method for carboxyfluorescein purification described here is adapted from Weinstein *et al.* (26) and taken from the first edition of this book.

[b] The first peak to elute off the column is a non-fluorescent polar contaminant, closely followed by carboxyfluorescein itself. Hydrophobic impurities are retained on the top of the column as a brownish non-fluorescent residue.

[c] The most suitable concentration for use in standard liposome experiments is that which is iso-osmolar with physiological buffers (275 mOsm), which works out at about 100 mM carboxyfluorescein in 10 mM Tris–HCl buffer. The concentration of the solution eluted off the column may be determined by measuring its optical density at 492 nm and relating that to its molar extinction coefficient at 492 nm, which is around 75 000 M^{-1} cm^{-1}. An alternative method is to measure the osmolarity directly using an osmometer, and then adjust the solution to 275 mOsm by addition of 10 mM Tris–HCl buffer.

[d] Several workers have reported that good purification can be achieved using the column chromatography alone, and that the recrystallization step can be omitted. It should be noted, however, that even after purification, most commercially-derived CF is a mixture of two isomers (5- and 6-carboxyfluorescein). Preparations using mixtures of both these isomers give good results in the types of application described here.

The same basic methods as described above may be used for the purification of calcein, if necessary. However, calcein is commercially available in a rather pure form (e.g. from Sigma) and may be used without purification.

Protocol 18

Preparation of calcein solution

Equipment and reagents

- pH meter
- 50 ml beaker
- Osmometer

- Calcein (e.g. from Sigma)
- 4 M NaOH

Method

1   Weigh 938 mg calcein (MW = 938) in a 50 ml beaker.

2   Add 10 ml of demiwater.

3   Adjust the pH from about 2.2 to 7.4 with 4 M NaOH. Allow some time to make sure calcein is completely dissolved.

4   Measure the osmolarity with an osmometer and adjust the osmolarity to 275–300 mOsm by addition of demiwater. The final volume is about 20 ml and the final concentration of calcein is about 50 mM.

References

1. Crommelin, D. J. A. and Schreier, H. (1994). In *Colloidal drug delivery systems* (ed. J. Kreuter), p. 73. Marcel Dekker, New York.

2. Barenholz, Y. and Crommelin, D. J. A. (1994). In *Encyclopedia of pharmaceutical technology* (ed. J. Swarbrick), p. 1. Marcel Dekker, New York.

3. Barenholz, Y. and Amselem, S. (1993). In *Liposome technology*, 2nd edn (ed. G. Gregoriadis), Vol. I, p. 527. CRC Press, Boca Raton, FL.

4. Barenholz, Y. (ed.) (1993) in Quality Control of Liposomes. Special issue of *Chem. Phys. Lipids*, **64**.

5. Bartlett, G. R. (1959). *J. Biol. Chem.*, **234**, 446.

6. Stewart, J. C. M. (1959). *Anal. Biochem.*, **104**, 10.

7. Grit, M., Crommelin, D. J. A., and Lang, J. K. (1991). *J. Chromatogr.*, **585**, 239.

8. Jääskeläinen, I. and Urtti, A. (1994). *J. Pharm. Biomed. Anal.*, **12**, 977.

9. Grit, M. and Crommelin, D. J. A (1993). *Chem. Phys. Lipids*, **64**, 3.

10. Samuni, A. M., Lipman, A., and Barenholz, Y. (2000). *Chem. Phys. Lipids*, **105**, 121.

11. Vernooij, E. A. A. M., Kettenes-van den Bosch, J. J., and Crommelin, D. J. A. (1998). *Rapid Commun. Mass Spectrom.*, **12**, 83.

12. Vernooij, E. A. A. M., Gentry, C. A., Herron, J. N., Crommelin, D. J. A., and Kettenes-Van den Bosch, J. J. (1999). *Pharm. Res.*, **16**, 1658.

13. Vernooij, E. A. A. M. (2000). *Thesis*, Utrecht University.

14. Lang, J. K. (1990). *J. Chromatogr.*, **507**, 157.

15. Lang, J. K. and Vigo-Pelfrey, C. (1993). *Chem. Phys. Lipids*, **64**, 19.

16. Mangold, H. K. (ed.) (1984). In *CRC handbook of chromatography. Lipids*, Vol. I. CRC Press, Boca Raton, FL.

17. Klein, R. A. (1970). *Biochim. Biophys. Acta*, **210**, 486.

18. Gutteridge, J. M. C. and Quinlan, G. J. (1983). *J. Appl. Biochem.*, **5**, 293.

19. Ondrias, K., Misik, V., Gergel, D., and Stasko, A. (1989). *Biochim. Biophys. Acta*, **1003**, 238.

20. Jiang, Z-Y., Hunt, J. V., and Wolff, S. P. (1992). *Anal. Biochem.*, **202**, 384.

21. Nourooz-Zadeh, J. (1999). In *Methods in enzymology*, Vol. 300, p. 58.

22. Fry, D. W., White, C., and Goldman, D. J. (1978). *Anal. Biochem.*, **90**, 809.

23. Rosier, R. N., Gunter, T. E., Tucker, D. A., and Gunter, K. K. (1979). *Anal. Biochem.*, **96**, 384.

24. Gunter, K. K., Gunter, T. E., Jarkowski, A., and Rosier, R. N. (1982). *Anal. Biochem.*, **120**, 113.

25. Weissman, G., Collin, T., Evers, A., and Dunham, P. (1976). *Proc. Nat. Acad. Sci. USA*, **73**, 510.

26. Weinstein, J. N., Ralston, E., Leserman, L. D., Klausner, R. D., Dragsten, P., Henkart, P., et al. (1984). In *Liposome technology* (ed. G. Gregoriadis), Vol. 3, p. 183. CRC Press, Boca Raton.

27. Allen, T. (1984). In *Liposome technology* (ed. G. Gregoriadis), Vol. 3, p. 177. CRC Press, Boca Raton.

28. Kinsky, C. S. (1974). In *Methods in enzymology*, Vol. 32, p. 501.

29. Alving, C. R., Shichijo, S., and Mattsby-Baltzer, I. (1984). In *Liposome technology* (ed. G. Gregoriadis), Vol. 2, p. 157. CRC Press, Boca Raton.

30. Schlieren, H., Rudolph, S., Finkelstein, M., Coleman, P., and Weissman, G. (1987). *Biochim. Biophys. Acta*, **542**, 137.

31. Lis, L. J., McAlister, M., Fuller, N., and Rand, R. P. (1982). *Biophys. J.*, **37**, 657.

32. Barenholz, Y., Gibbes, D., Litman, B. J., Goll, J., Thompson, T. E., and Carlson, F. D. (1977). *Biochemistry*, **16**, 2806.

33. Goren, D., Gabizon, A., and Barenholz, Y. (1990). *Biochim. Biophys. Acta*, **1029**, 285.

34. Amselem, S., Cohen, R., and Barenholz, Y. (1993). *Chem. Phys. Lipids*, **64**, 219.

35. Hope, M. J., Bally, M. B., Webb, G., and Cullis, P. R. (1985). *Biochim. Biophys. Acta*, **812**, 55.

36. Pidgeon, C., Hunt, A. H., and Dittrich, K. (1986). *Pharm. Res.*, **3**, 23.

37. Bouwstra, J. A., Gooris, G. S., Bras, W., and Talsma, H. (1993). *Chem. Phys. Lipids*, **64**, 83.

38. Sommerville, J. and Scheer, U. (1987). In *Electron microscopy in molecular biology: a practical approach*. Oxford University Press, Oxford.

39. Hope, M. J., Wong, K. F., and Cullis, P. R. (1989). *J. Electron Microsc. Techn.*, **13**, 277.

40. Frederik, P. M., Burger, K. N. J., Stuart, M. C. A., and Verkleij, A. J. (1991). *Biochim. Biophys. Acta*, **1062**, 133.

41. Frederik, P. M., Stuart, M. C. A., Bomans, P. H. H., Busing, W. M., Burger, K. N. J., and Verkleij, A. J. (1991). *J. Microsc.*, **161**, 253.

42. Almgren, M., Edwards, K., and Karlsson, G. (2000). *Colloids Surf. A: Physicochem. Eng. Aspects*, **174**, 3.

43. Lesieur, S., Grabielle-Madelmont, C., Paternostre, M., and Ollivon, M. (1993). *Chem. Phys. Lipids*, **64**, 57.

44. Zuidam, N. J., Gouw, H. K. M. E., Barenholz, Y., and Crommelin, D. J. A. (1995). *Biochim. Biophys. Acta*, **1240**, 101.

45. Ostrowsky, N. (1993). *Chem. Phys. Lipids*, **64**, 45.

46. De Smidt, J. H. and Crommelin, D. J. A. (1991). *Int. J. Pharm.*, **77**, 261.

47. Langowki, J., Kermer, W., and Kapp, U. (1992). In *Methods in enzymology*, Vol. 211, p. 430.

48. Cevc, G. (1993). *Chem. Phys. Lipids*, **64**, 163.

49. Bligh, E. J. and Dyer, W. J. (1959). *Can. J. Biochem. Physiol.*, **37**, 911.

Chapter 3
Physical methods of study: differential scanning calorimetry

Kevin M. G. Taylor
School of Pharmacy, University of London, 29–39 Brunswick Square, London, UK.

Duncan Q. M. Craig
The School of Pharmacy, The Queen's University of Belfast, 97 Lisburn Road, Belfast, UK.

1 Introduction

Thermal methods, and in particular differential scanning calorimetry (DSC), are well established within the liposome field, and are most frequently used to measure the phase behaviour of the phospholipid bilayers, from which information on phospholipid conformation, bilayer fluidity, drug–liposome interactions, and rate of drug release may be derived. In addition, knowledge of the transition behaviour of phospholipids is essential for the rational development of manufacturing protocols. There is also a growing interest in the use of thermal methods for the examination of freeze-dried liposomes, particularly in terms of characterizing the glass transitional behaviour of these systems.

Scanning thermal analysis involves measuring the response of a sample to an applied heating or cooling signal, from which information about the structure, phase behaviour, and reaction kinetics may be obtained. The term thermal analysis covers a wide range of instruments and approaches, of which three will be outlined here, namely DSC, high sensitivity DSC (HSDSC), and modulated temperature DSC (MTDSC). This chapter will outline the principles underlying these techniques, together with information on the practicalities associated with such studies, as well as discussing the relevance of such information to liposome characterization.

2 Overview of techniques

2.1 Differential scanning calorimetry

Differential scanning calorimetry (DSC) involves applying a linear heating or cooling (or isothermal) signal to a sample and reference, and then measuring the temperature and energy associated with thermal events such as melting, crystallization, or lipid phase transitions. For more information on the principles and practicalities of the technique, the texts by Charsley and Warrington (1), Wunderlich (2), Haines (3), and Ford and Timmins (4) are recommended.

DSC was developed from differential thermal analysis (DTA) which measures the temperature (rather than heat flow) difference between the sample and reference. DSC has effectively superseded DTA in all but a limited number of specialist applications such as pyrolysis studies. There are two types of DSC instrument: power compensation and heat flux, as shown in Figure 1. The power compensation approach, patented by Perkin-Elmer Ltd., involves the application of heating signals to a sample and a reference via two separate furnaces in the DSC cell. When the sample undergoes a thermal event such as an exothermic crystallization or an endothermic melting (or lipid phase transition), power (heat per unit time) is supplied by one or other furnace in order to maintain thermal equilibrium, as given by:

$$P = dQ/dt = I^2R \qquad [1]$$

where P is power, dQ/dt is the heating rate, I is the current supplied to the heater, and R is the resistance of that heater. Consequently, both the temperature at which the thermal event takes place and the energy associated with the transition may be measured. Heat flux DSC uses a single furnace which supplies heat to both the sample and reference, and the differential temperature is measured. This is then converted to heat flow via:

$$\Delta Q = (T_S - T_R)R_T \qquad [2]$$

where ΔQ is the heat differential, T_S and T_R are the sample and reference temperature respectively, and R_T is the thermal resistance of the cell. A typical DSC response showing a glass transition (discussed later), crystallization exo-

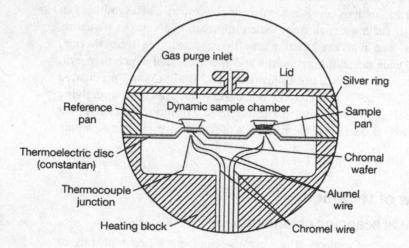

Figure 1 Schematic representation of (a) a heat flux and (b) a power compensation DSC cell. Adapted from ref. 3.

therm and melting endotherm is shown in Figure 2. With appropriate calibration, the temperature associated with the event may be read off the abscissa, with the ordinate indicating the power associated with the measurement. The practice of not giving an ordinate scale on published DSC traces is not recommended.

Almost invariably, thermal events take place over a range of temperatures rather than at a single defined point. This may be due to crystal imperfections, impurities, or molecular weight polydispersity in the sample which broaden the measured range. In addition, thermal lag effects as the sample undergoes the transition and then returns to equilibrium with the heating programme will also cause broadening. This range presents the difficulty of the choice of parameter to take as, for example, the melting point (T_m). Inspection of the melting curve shown in Figure 2 shows that the onset of the event may be chosen, as may the extrapolated onset (taken by back-extrapolating the leading edge of the curve to the baseline). In addition, the peak may be taken, which may be the method of choice for complex systems, or those with extended onsets where it is not possible to identify the commencement of the event with confidence. Given the possibilities available, the most appropriate recommendation is to state which point is being chosen in order to avoid apparent discrepancies between data sets.

Inspection of Equations 1 and 2 indicates that as power is being measured, it should be possible to obtain the energy associated with the event. This is achieved by measuring the area under the peak of the sample, as the integral of power against temperature at a known scanning rate is directly proportional to the energy of the transition. The area is compared to that of a standard which undergoes an event with a known specific enthalpy; the melting (heat of fusion) of indium is commonly used.

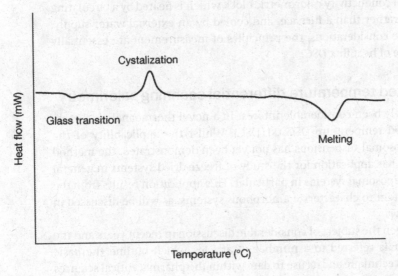

Figure 2 Schematic representation of DSC trace for quench cooled polyethylene terephthalate, showing the glass transition, crystallization, and melting responses.

2.2 High sensitivity differential scanning calorimetry

While conventional DSC is the standard method for measuring liposomal phase transitions, there are several advantages to using a related technique, high sensitivity DSC (HSDSC), which operates on a similar principle but which is more suited to the analysis of certain liquid samples. The essential differences between HSDSC and DSC are first, the higher sensitivity of the former, due to the employment of a more sensitive thermocouple: HSDSC can measure baseline changes of approximately 1 μW, which represents an approximately tenfold increase in sensitivity compared to conventional DSC. Secondly, the sample size may be considerably increased as the sample vessel has a volume of approximately 1 cm^3. Both these factors serve to increase the sensitivity of the technique to low energy transitions. Our experience has been that, in addition to the above, the technique is considerably easier to use than conventional DSC for measuring liposomal transitions; loading and encapsulation of sample are more straightforward and the reproducibility is superior. There are, however, some disadvantages. The scanning rates used are extremely low compared to conventional DSC (1–2 °C/min is a typical range), while the measurable temperature range is more limited (e.g. the Setaram DSC III has a range of –20 to 120 °C). In addition, the increased baseline sensitivity renders the technique more prone to noise and artefacts, and as yet there is no universally accepted aqueous-based chemical calibration standard for the instrument. Given that the technique is designed to measure small transitions in aqueous systems such as protein solutions, the limitations regarding temperature range and scanning speed have not proved to be prohibitive.

The equipment mentioned above consists of sample and reference vessels with lids which form a seal via the inclusion of Viton O-rings. The vessels fit into the high thermal conductivity calorimetric block which is heated by a circulating fluid (n-decane) rather than a furnace, and cooled by an external water supply. Other than these considerations, the principles of measurement are essentially identical to those of heat flux DSC.

2.3 Modulated temperature differential scanning calorimetry

There has recently been considerable interest in a novel thermoanalytical technique, modulated temperature DSC (MTDSC). Whilst the applicability of the technique to liposomal suspensions has not yet been demonstrated, the method almost certainly has application for the study of freeze-dried systems in general and lyophilized liposomal systems in particular. This application results from the ability of the system to characterize amorphous systems, as will be discussed in more detail below.

MTDSC has been the subject of considerable discussion in recent years and the interested reader is referred to a number of articles which outline the basic principles of the technique and its use to date within the pharmaceutical sciences (5–9). The field has been somewhat complicated by the availability of several instruments which may be classified under the MTDSC term but operate in ways which the manufacturers argue are distinct. In this discussion, the TA Instruments model, modulated DSC (MDSC), will be described; the extent to which the comments are applicable to the other models is not yet clear.

MTDSC involves the superimposition of a sinusoidal heating signal onto the underlying temperature programme. In essence, therefore, the sample undergoes the same average temperature programme as that generated using conventional DSC, hence no information is lost. In addition, the response to the oscillation is measured. This may be most easily visualized via:

$$\frac{dQ}{dt} = Cp \frac{dT}{dt} + f(t,T) \qquad [3]$$

where dQ/dt is the total heat flow (Js^{-1} or W), Cp is the heat capacity (JK^{-1}), dT/dt is the underlying heating rate, and $f(t,T)$ represents a function of temperature and time. This equation essentially describes the measured heat flow in terms of a component related to the heat capacity of the material and to kinetic events. When using conventional DSC, these two components are measured at any one temperature and hence are not considered separately. Modulated DSC allows the operator to split the signal into the constituent components as follows. The average total heat flow (dQ/dt) is measured via Fourier transformation of the heat flow signal. The Cp component is calculated via:

$$A_{MHF}/A_{MHR} \cdot K = Cp \qquad [4]$$

where A_{MHF} and A_{MHR} are the amplitudes of the maximum heat flow and maximum heating rate respectively, and K is a constant. In other words, Cp is calculated from the response to the oscillation. As the heating rate dT/dt is known, then the first two of the three components of Equation 3 have been identified, hence the third (kinetic) component may be found by subtraction. The heat capacity and kinetic components are termed "reversing" and "non-reversing" respectively by the manufacturer (TA Instruments).

The significance of these deconvoluted components may be explained as follows. The heat capacity indicates the energy required to raise the sample temperature by a unit amount. One reason why this parameter is of significance is that the value is altered when a material undergoes a glass transition (T_g). This transition represents a change in molecular mobility rather than a phase change such as melting or crystallization and is a property associated with amorphous (disordered) materials. Such materials undergo a dramatic change in molecular mobility over a narrow temperature range which results in marked alterations in a number of practically significant properties. In particular, the mechanical properties of a material change above and below T_g, with the systems becoming considerably more fluid as the sample is heated through the transition. Other properties such as the propensity of the sample to crystallize, the extent of water uptake, and the chemical stability may all change above or below this value, hence there is considerable interest in developing ways in which to measure T_g, particularly in terms of understanding and choosing the most appropriate processing and storage conditions. The most common method is conventional DSC, whereby the transition is seen as a shift in the baseline. However, such measurements are often problematic, as the baseline shift tends to be small and may also be obscured by other events such as relaxation endotherms which arise due to stress relaxation processes and give the glass transition a similar appearance to that of a melting response. MTDSC allows the Cp to be measured in isolation from other kinetic events such as the aforementioned relaxation process, hence the technique has attracted considerable interest as a means of detecting and characterizing glass transitions.

One type of product for which the measurement of T_g is particularly important is freeze-dried materials. These are very often amorphous in nature, hence it is necessary to measure the T_g of both the frozen system in order to choose the most appropriate drying temperature and the final product in order to ascertain suitable storage conditions. If, for example, the product is stored above T_g then the system may undergo collapse whereby the porous structure collapses under its own weight, while storage below T_g maintains the sample in a more rigid form. More details of both the glassy state (10, 11) and freeze-drying (12–14) may be found in a number of texts. However, it may be seen that the ability to measure T_g with greater clarity and reliability is of great interest and consequently, MTDSC is receiving considerable attention as a novel approach to characterizing such systems.

3 Practical aspects of making DSC measurements

3.1 Choice of pans

To obtain reliable measurements, a number of factors should be taken into account. The choice of pans may be extremely important and should always be stated. For most applications with solid samples, non-hermetically sealed aluminium pans are generally used. These pans do not prevent the escape of residual solvent but, due to the pan being crimped around the sample, do allow good thermal contact to be established between the pan and the material, thereby reducing thermal lags. A practical recommendation is to exercise care if evidence of thermal decomposition is seen after or during (or indeed prior to) melting. This is often observed as a series of rapidly altering deviations from the baseline. While this may provide a worthwhile study area in its own right, the decomposition products may coat the furnace, necessitating extensive cleaning.

Hermetically sealed pans are essential for volatile liquid samples and are invariably necessary for studies involving liposome suspensions or when investigating systems in which it is essential to retain the volatile component. These pans tend to have a larger volume to permit encapsulation of sufficient liquid to allow a measurable response to be obtained. It should, however, be borne in mind that the seal of the pans will be broken at higher temperatures due to the increase in vapour pressure from the volatile components. Our experience suggests that for a sample containing 2% (w/w) water or more, consideration must be given to the possibility of seal failure above around 120 °C. The temperature at which the seal breaks varies according to the pan type and the material under study. We have found it useful to run thermogravimetric analysis studies (TGA) on equivalent samples, whereby the weight of a sample is measured as a function of temperature, in order to establish the temperature at which the seal becomes compromised prior to using the DSC. This may be helpful not only to avoid artefacts but also to prevent damage to the DSC via rupture of the pan. Pin-holed pans have become increasingly widely used. These have a small hole drilled in the lid of the pan in order to allow escape of volatile components in a controlled and reproducible manner. Finally, open pans which have no lid may be used. These are useful for certain applications such as the study of hydrates, as the dehydration event is seen considerably more clearly under these conditions due to the loss process occurring over a narrow temperature range. The difficulty associated with this approach is that thermal contact between the pan and sample tends to be poor, increasing the possibility of thermal lags within the material, while the baseline also tends to be inferior using this approach. The most important recommendation, however, is to state clearly which pans are being used. Hill *et al.* (15) showed a difference in the measured glass transition of lactose of 35 °C depending on the pan type used, even though prior to the experiment the sample was identical in all cases.

3.2 Sample size

The sample size should be considered and stated: the choice will depend on the size of thermal response to be measured and the availability of the sample. In general, sample sizes in the region of 5–10 mg are used for solid samples. If too small a sample is used, the thermal event will not be distinguished from the baseline (this is particularly pertinent for glass transition measurements). If too large a sample is used, thermal lags may be set up, depending on the thermal conductivity of the material and the scanning rate used. A further consideration is the amount of material that may be physically placed within the pan. Systems such as freeze-dried materials may present some problems in this respect, as these products are highly porous and thus occupy a large volume per mg sample.

3.3 Calibration

A very important consideration is the calibration of the instrument, which again should always be described in methodologies. There are essentially four calibration approaches: baseline, temperature, enthalpy, and heat capacity. Baseline calibration is performed in order to account for differences in the thermal properties of the sample and reference systems and is performed by running a baseline with two empty pans. Any bowing of the baseline may be corrected in this manner. Temperature and enthalpy calibration may be performed using one or more of a range of recommended standards: indium is usually used for pharmaceutical systems. It is, however, preferable to use more than one standard such that the two points used reflect the temperature range under study for a

Table 1 Calibration materials for DSC and DTA

Material	Thermal event[a]	Temperature (°C)	Enthalpy (J/g)
Cyclohexane	t	−83	
	m	7	
1,2-Dichloroethane	m	−32	
Phenyl ether	m	30	
Biphenyl	m	69.3	120.41
o-Terphenyl	m	58	
Polystyrene	T_g	105	
Potassium nitrate	t	128	
Indium	m	156.6	28.71
Tin	m	231.9	56.06
Potassium perchlorate	t	300	
Zinc	m	419.4	111.18
Silver sulfate	t	430	
Quartz	t	573	
Potassium sulfate	t	583	
Potassium chromate	t	665	
Barium carbonate	t	810	
Strontium carbonate	t	925	

[a] The thermal events are as follows: t = crystal transition, m = melting, T_g = glass transition temperature.
Source: ref. 3.

particular sample. Examples of calibration standards are given in Table 1. Finally, if the heat capacity of a sample is required, it is essential to calibrate adequately using a standard such as sapphire. This is not usually a major consideration for liposomal suspensions but may be important for glass transition measurements.

3.4 Scanning rate

The scanning rate used may have a profound effect on the data obtained. In general, rates of between 2 °C/min and 20 °C/min are used for pharmaceutical systems. Faster rates tend to be advantageous for studying small transitions as the sensitivity is improved. However, there is a concomitant decrease in resolution, hence two thermal events which take place over a similar temperature range may not be resolved. In addition, it is necessary to consider whether the sample is following the temperature programme: DSC systems are controlled by thermocouples adjacent to the sample but may not reflect the temperature experienced by that sample if very fast scanning rates are used. Slower scanning rates are preferable for improved resolution but are inappropriate for studying very small heat flow changes. In addition, the signal-to-noise ratio may be inferior. It should also be borne in mind that slower rates will increase the time spent by the sample at temperatures close to thermal events such as melting, hence changes associated with maintaining a sample at a given temperature over a period of time must be considered. There is also the issue of throughput of samples which is faster using higher scanning rates. It should also be noted that the system should be recalibrated if the scanning rate is changed. Finally, it should be pointed out that when studying the melting of binary systems, the choice of heating rate may be highly important in determining the appearance of the higher melting substance. Lloyd et al. (16) have demonstrated that lower scan rates may result in dissolution of the higher T_m component in the melt of the lower one. It is also important to consider the purge gas used. In general, nitrogen is used for most purposes. However, as an alternative, helium may be used if a higher thermal conductivity is required when, for example, performing rapid scans.

3.5 Conditions required for liposomal studies

The parameters derived from DSC analysis of liposomal suspensions include the onset temperature of the transition (T_o) and the temperature at the peak (T_m), frequently denoted T_c when referring to the gel to liquid-crystalline phase transition. The half-height width of the transition peak ($\Delta T_{1/2}$ or HHW) and the enthalpy of the process (ΔH) can also be derived.

The practicalities outlined above are pertinent to all DSC studies. However, there are a number of additional considerations for the analysis of liposomal suspensions. Some of those practical issues are outlined here, although it should be emphasized that the recommendations are derived from our personal experience, using particular formulations, rather than representing generally accepted practice. However, in the absence of clearly defined existing guidelines on making such measurements, it is hoped that the discussion will be helpful to newcomers to the field. Much of the information below is derived from the work of Parmar (17) and Castile (18).

For the reasons outlined above, it is essential to encapsulate liposomal suspensions in hermetically sealed pans. We have found the use of a microsyringe helpful in this respect in order to ensure adequate coverage of the base of the pan and to avoid spillage on the pan rim which may compromise the seal. In addition, it is necessary to ensure that encapsulation within the pan takes place as quickly as possible after sample loading to minimize evaporation of the sample. Similarly, it is recognized that pre-storage conditions may alter the phase behaviour of certain phospholipids (19, 20), hence it is essential to consider and standardize this variable. The volume used in our studies was between 5–10 μl (i.e. approx. 5–10 mg). There appears to be little consensus in the literature regarding the optimal concentration of phospholipid in the suspension, with systems ranging from 0.04–0.66% (w/w) (21) to up to 50% (w/w) (22) described. Our own studies on DPPC liposomes showed that for both the pre- and main phospholipid transitions a concentration of 100 mg/ml (10%, w/v) was optimal. These studies involved measuring coefficients of variation for enthalpy and peak temperature at concentrations of 25 mg/ml, 50 mg/ml, and 100 mg/ml, hence it is quite conceivable that increasing the concentration further would have resulted in even more favourable reproducibility. However, it is also important to consider the cost of the phospholipids as the preparation of several batches of highly concentrated suspensions may be prohibitively expensive.

The effect of scanning rate has also been investigated (5 °C/min and 10 °C/min) (17). There appeared to be some advantages in using the faster rate, with improved reproducibility and sensitivity found. The latter is particularly important if the transitions under observation are small, as the improved signal-to-noise ratio may aid identification and quantification of the minor peaks. Finally, we have investigated the choice of reference, with comparison made between the use of an empty pan and one containing an equivalent amount of water. There appears to be some advantage in terms of reproducibility of using water as the reference; one would also theoretically expect a more favourable baseline using water due the similarities of the thermal properties of the sample and reference compared to the use of empty reference pans.

In summary, therefore, a suitable starting point for studying liposomal suspensions using DSC would be to use hermetic pans, a sample size of 5–10 mg, a concentration of 100 mg/ml, a scanning rate of 10 °C/min, and the use of water (or buffer) in the reference pan. Clearly, the optimal conditions will be sample dependent but it is hoped that the above will provide a starting point, from which further optimization studies may be developed.

Protocol 1

DSC study of liposomes

Equipment

This protocol is adapted from the methods described in refs 17 and 18, and uses a Perkin-Elmer DSC7 instrument. Similar protocols may be used with alternative DSC models but conditions need to be adapted according to the manufacturer's recommendations and the properties of the particular system under investigation.

Method

1 Prepare liposomes using standard methods.

2 Allow the instrument to warm up for 1 h, prior to calibration and sample measurement.

3 Calibrate the instrument for temperature and enthalpy using indium.

4 Place the liposome sample (10 μl of a 100 mg/ml preparation) dropwise into the aluminium DSC pan using a microsyringe, and calculate the weight of sample.

5 Place an aluminium lid on the pan using forceps and hermetically seal the ensemble.

6 Prepare a reference pan containing 10 μl of ultra pure water in the same manner.

7 Place the pans into the instrument whilst applying an external nitrogen purge.

8 Using the instrument's software perform a scan at 5 °C/min over the temperature range of interest, and collect data.

3.6 Practicalities of HSDSC measurements

Our experience with this technique for the measurement of liposomal systems has been that clear and reproducible results are obtainable at a range of concentrations, giving a total lipid content of 5–8 mg. In addition, we are able to discern features and analyse the shape of the transitions with far greater confidence than is possible using conventional DSC, while the simplicity of loading has considerably improved our throughput, despite the slower scan speeds used. We have found that great care must be taken in cleaning the cells as the presence of trace contaminants may significantly alter the results. We use a biological detergent and a fine bristle brush, followed by thorough rinsing in distilled water. The cell is then washed out with acetone and industrial methylated spirit. Solid samples are more difficult to remove and the use of tweezers may be necessary.

The reference vessel is filled with vehicle to as near as possible an identical mass as is in the sample vessel. It is essential to check the outside of the vessel and the O-ring to ensure that there are no spilt drops of liquid. The lid is then screwed down, the vessels loaded and allowed to equilibrate until the heat flow between sample and reference is constant (30 min is usually sufficient). For liposomal samples, the runs usually consist of linear heating at 1–2 °C/min, although it should be pointed out that HSDSC may be used isothermally for kinetic studies or alternatively may be run in stepwise isothermal mode, whereby the sample is held at a particular temperature for a predetermined time period and then automatically ramped up to a higher temperature at which point the process is repeated.

Protocol 2

HSDSC study of liposomes

Equipment

This protocol is adapted from the methods described in refs 18, 23, and 24, and uses a Seteram Instruments Micro DSC III. Similar protocols may be used with alternative HSDSC models but conditions need to be adapted according to the manufacturer's recommendations and the properties of the particular system under investigation.

Method

1   Prepare liposomes using standard methods.

2   Clean cells thoroughly using ultra pure water and rinse with acetone.

3   When completely dry, weigh sample cell and reference cell (not lids) using the cell holder.

4   Add 0.8 ml of sample (approx. 5 mg of active sample should be present) to the sample cell and weigh to calculate the weight of sample added.

5   Add reference material to the reference cell (containing exactly the same formulation as sample but without active material). Ensure the total weight of the reference cell is exactly the same (to four decimal places) as the sample cell.

Protocol 2 continued

6   Replace O-ring on lids and screw tightly onto cells.

7   Place the sample and reference cells into the DSC furnace, and cover as required.

8   Wait until the heat flow stabilizes (normally after approx. 5 min). If a stabilized value of ± 0.0008 mW is not achieved, check cells for dirt or broken O-ring.

9   Using the instrument's software perform a scan with a run speed not exceeding 1 °C/min over the temperature range of interest, and collect data.

3.7 Practicalities of MTDSC measurements

MTDSC represents a change in the software rather than hardware of the conventional DSC approach, hence all the considerations outlined earlier are applicable here. The basic parameter requirements for simple T_g measurement are now reasonably well established. Here, the basics of measuring practicalities will be outlined. Further information can be found in Craig and Royall (25).

All the considerations outlined for conventional DSC with regard to sample mass, scanning rate, etc. are applicable to MTDSC. However, there are three further parameters to consider: the frequency, the amplitude, and the calibration. The frequency is in some respects the most problematic, as if too rapid an oscillation is used then the sample will be unable to follow the temperature programme and the heat flow signal will become distorted. This may be checked by examination of the raw signal. However, there are problems associated with using a low frequency. One of the requirements of the deconvolution programme is that there must be at least four (and preferably six) oscillations through a transition in order to avoid artefact generation. Consequently if, for example, a transition has a width of 4 °C and a period of 30 sec is used, then four oscillations will require 2 min. Consequently the maximum underlying heating rate that may be used is 2 °C/min. If a 60 sec period is used, then that heating rate becomes 1 °C/min. In other words, using slow periods necessitates the use of slow underlying heating rates, while rapid frequencies may result in the sample not following the signal. Herein lies one of the main disadvantages of MTDSC; it is necessary to use slow underlying heating rates in order to ensure that an adequate number of cycles is present through a transition.

The choice of amplitude is also important, with higher amplitudes resulting in greater sensitivity (as predicted by Equation 4), hence for small glass transitions a large amplitude may be desirable. There are, however, two important riders to this. First, if too large an amplitude is used, the sample may not follow the temperature programme, as was the case for rapid oscillations. Secondly, larger amplitudes will result in the sample actually being cooled for part of the cycle on a heating run. This may not be a problem for T_g measurements, as these responses are reversible. However, it is always advisable to know whether the programme is 'heat (or cool) only' or not. This may be predicted by:

$$A_{MHR} = \frac{H_R \cdot P}{2\pi \cdot 60}$$ [5]

which gives the heating rate amplitude (A_{MHR}) required for any underlying heating rate (H_R) and period (P) which will ensure a zero or positive overall heating rate.

Finally, it is essential to adequately calibrate the instrument. Baseline and heat flow (temperature, enthalpy) calibration are essentially identical to that used for conventional DSC, while a number of options are available for Cp calibration. Inspection of Equations 3 and 4 indicates that the value of Cp is used in the deconvolution process, hence it is essential to calibrate for this value using a standard such as sapphire in order to obtain meaningful quantitative data not just for Cp but also for the enthalpies associated with the reversing and non-reversing components.

As an initial set of conditions, we recommend the following. A sample size of 5–10 mg is usually adequate, with an underlying heating rate of 2 °C/min, an amplitude of 0.2 °C, and a modulation frequency of 30–50 sec. It is important to ensure that the sample is following the temperature programme and is also undergoing sufficient cycling, so it is helpful to check the raw data.

Protocol 3

MTDSC study of freeze-dried liposomes

Equipment

This protocol is adapted from the method described in ref. 26 and uses a TA Instruments 2920 MDSC. Similar protocols may be used with alternative MTDSC models but conditions need to be adapted according to the manufacturer's recommendations and the properties of the particular system under investigation.

Method

1 Prepare liposomes using standard methods, with films hydrated with an aqueous phase containing 10% cryoprotectant (e.g. sucrose, trehalose) to yield a lipid content of 60 mM. Add 1 mM EDTA to prevent aggregation. Extrude through polycarbonate membrane filters to yield vesicles having a mean diameter of approx. 0.1 μm, and freeze-dry using an appropriate protocol.

2 Calibrate the MTDSC instrument for temperature using indium and gallium, for heat flow using indium, and for heat capacity using sapphire.

3 Punch out 2–2.5 mg samples of freeze-dried material and transfer to hermetically sealed aluminium pans under a dry nitrogen environment to prevent water sorption.

4 Scan the sample under heat only conditions using an average heating rate of 2 °C/min, a period of 30 sec, and a temperature amplitude of 0.159 °C.

5 Identify the glass transition from the reversing heat flow signal, using the mid-point of the step change in heat capacity as the T_g.

4 Application of DSC and related techniques to the study of liposomes

4.1 Phase transition behaviour of liposomes

Hydrated phospholipids may exist in one or more mesomorphic forms. Analysis of the phase transitions between these forms is necessary because the state/fluidity of the bilayers is an important determinant of *in vitro* and *in vivo* liposomal stability and drug release profiles.

The phospholipids most commonly employed in the production of liposomes are the phosphatidylcholines. Early DTA studies showed that diacylphosphatidylcholines recrystallize from organic solvents as monohydrates (27). The water, associated with the monohydrate, may be removed by heating samples in open DTA pans, resulting in an endothermic peak, many degrees below the phospholipid melting point. An endothermic peak corresponding to the melting of ice is not observed until the water content of phospholipids reaches 25% (w/w).

Our understanding of the phase transition behaviour of fully hydrated phospholipids is largely derived from DSC and more recently HSDSC studies. A typical DSC trace for a diacylphosphatidylcholine is shown in Figure 3. Pure, synthetic, long chained phospholipids can undergo a number of transitions at defined temperatures. Following prolonged incubation at low temperatures, fully hydrated, long chain phosphatidylcholines, such as DPPC, are in the ordered, condensed crystalline subgel (L_c) state, in which the hydrocarbon chains are in the fully extended, all *trans* conformation, and the polar head groups are relatively immobile at the water interface (19, 29, 30). On heating, L_c state phospholipids undergo a subtransition to the $L_{\beta'}$ state, in which there is increased head group mobility and water penetration into the interfacial region of the bilayer (29–31). The subtransition usually occurs approximately 30 °C below the temperature of the main gel to liquid-crystalline phase transition (20), although DPPC has a subtransition at 21 °C, approximately 20 °C below the temperature of main phase transition (32). Subtransitions can be subdivided into:

(a) Type I "solid–solid" transitions between subgel and gel phase. These are exhibited by saturated phosphatidylcholines with C_{16} to C_{18} chains (20, 33) and dipalmitoylphosphatidylglycerol (34), and are characterized by a small change in rotameric disordering of hydrocarbon chains.

(b) Type II transitions occur in saturated phosphatidylethanolamines and involve more rotameric disordering, and more melting of the subgel phase into the liquid-crystalline phase (20, 35).

Head group interactions are also important: the inclusion of small amounts of the opposite stereoisomer or cholesterol eliminate the subtransition (33). DPPC exhibits a sub-subtransition with a T_m of approximately 6.8 °C (36), without a prolonged period of incubation at low temperature.

On heating, $L_{\beta'}$ gel state phospholipids undergo the pretransition to the "rippled" gel ($P_{\beta'}$) state. The pretransition usually occurs between 5–10 °C below

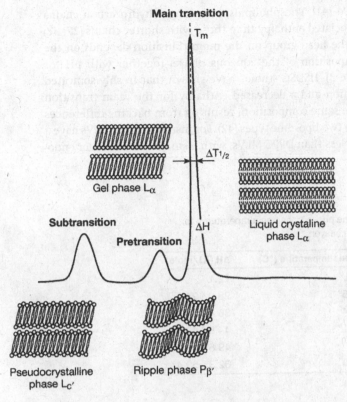

Figure 3 A typical DSC trace of a diacylphosphatidylcholine. Reproduced with permission from ref. 28.

the main transition, with a smaller enthalpy, and may be due to rotation of the polar head groups or co-operative movement of the hydrocarbon chains, prior to melting (21). The pretransition of DMPC and DPPC has been explained in terms of structural changes in the lamellar lattice (37), with the bilayer reorganizing from a one-dimensional lamellar to a two-dimensional monoclinic lattice consisting of lipid lamellae distorted by periodic "ripples" (38). Phosphatidylethanolamines to not exhibit detectable pretransitions (39).

Heating $P_{\beta'}$ state phospholipids results in co-operative "melting" of the hydrocarbon chains (the main gel to liquid-crystalline phase transition) to give the L_c state. The orientation of the carbon–carbon single bonds changes from *trans* to a situation where *gauche* configurations are present. The intermolecular distance between molecules is approximately 2 nm, consequently rotation in one molecule, impacts on adjacent molecules, such that this transition is a co-operative event (40). The temperature of the main phase transition (T_c) is largely determined by the polar head group together with the length and degree of unsaturation of the hydrocarbon chains. For phospholipids having the same head group and degree of hydration, increasing saturation in the hydrocarbon chains increases the T_c (39), with *trans*-unsaturated chains having a higher T_c than those which are *cis*-unsaturated (41). Phospholipids with longer hydrocarbon chains have a higher T_c and associated enthalpy than those with shorter chains (27, 32) (Table 2). The effect of the head group on the main transition depends on the ionic strength and composition of the aqueous phase, together with pH for charged lipids (32) (Table 3). HSDSC studies have shown that freshly sonicated SUVs have no pretransition and a decreased enthalpy for the main transition compared to MLVs of the same composition, resulting from packing differences within the bilayers of the two liposome types (42). For instance, DPPC SUVs have a T_c of approximately 4 °C less than DPPC MLVs, with a smaller and broader endotherm (43).

Table 2 Gel to liquid-crystalline phase transition temperatures for 1,2 diacylphosphatidylcholine bilayers

Lipid[c]	Transition temperature (°C)	ΔH (kJ/mole)
DLPC (C_{12})	0,[a] −1.1[b]	12.1[b]
DMPC (C_{14})	23,[a] 23.5[b]	28.0,[a] 24.7[b]
DPPC (C_{16})	41,[a] 41.4[b]	36.4,[a] 34.7[b]
DSPC (C_{18})	58,[a] 55.1[b]	44.8,[a] 42.3[b]
DAPC (C_{20})	61.8[b]	49.8[b]
DBPC (C_{22})	75,[a] 74.0[b]	62.3,[a] 59.4[b]

[a] Source: ref. 46.

[b] Source: ref. 29.

[c] DLPC = dilaurylphosphatidylcholine, DMPC = dimyristoylphosphatidylcholine, DPPC = dipalmitoylphosphatidylcholine, DSPC = distearylphosphatidylcholine, DAPC = diarachidylphosphatidylcholine, DBPC = dibehenylphosphatidylcholine.

Table 3 Effect of head group on the main transition of dipalmitoyphospholipids[a]

Head group	pH	T_c (°C)	ΔH (kJ/mole)
Choline	7.4	41.4	34.7
Ethanolamine	7.4	64	35.6
Glycerol	1.1	57	37.2
	7.0	41	31.4
Phosphatidic acid	6.5	67	21.8
	9.1	58	12.1
Phosphatidylserine	2.0	67	33.9
	7.0	54	37.7
	12.0	43.1	23.9
Sphigomyelin	7.4	41.3	28.5
	13.0	32	33.5

[a] Source: ref. 29.

4.1 Phase transitions of multi-component systems

4.2.1 Phospholipid blends

Many liposomal formulations employ a mixture of phospholipids. DSC studies show that the main phase transition of mixtures of phospholipids, with different hydrocarbon chains, occurs over a broader temperature range than for pure phospholipids, with asymmetric transitions occurring when compositions other than equimolar are present (44). When the hydrocarbon chains differ by only two carbon atoms, ideal mixing of phases occurs (44, 45), whilst a difference of four carbon atoms results in a system significantly moved from ideality, suggesting that regions of gel phase immiscibility occur (44, 46, 47). A mixture of phospholipids, in which the hydrocarbon chains differ by six carbon atoms or more gives non-ideal mixing, with monotectic behaviour observed (44). Equimolar mixtures of phosphatidylcholines have been reported not to exhibit subtransitions, although the individual constituents do (33).

Naturally occurring phospholipids, such as those derived from egg or soya are mixtures of components having different length hydrocarbon chains. Egg phosphatidylcholine comprises predominantly C_{16} and C_{18} chain phospholipids (48) and exhibits a relatively broad but fairly well defined transition, at –5 to –15 °C (49).

4.2.2 Phospholipid–cholesterol mixtures

Cholesterol is often included in liposome formulations to modify bilayer fluidity (50), allowing control of the rate of release of entrapped hydrophilic materials and enhancing *in vitro* and *in vivo* stability. Inclusion of cholesterol in C_{14} to C_{20} phosphatidylcholine bilayers, at between 2–6 mole%, eliminates the phospholipid pretransition (51, 52). Cholesterol also produces a decrease in the T_c as the DSC endotherm broadens and the enthalpy of transition decreases (40, 53). The main transition endotherm for DMPC and DPPC liposomes containing between 1–25 mole% cholesterol can be deconvoluted into two or possibly three peaks (52, 54), indicative of phase separation into cholesterol-rich and cholesterol-poor regions within the bilayer. A distinct transition is not detectable by DSC when phospholipid bilayers contain 50 mole% cholesterol (52, 55).

4.2.3 Long circulating liposomes

In vivo, liposomes are rapidly removed from the systemic circulation by cells of the mononuclear phagocyte system. Long circulating (Stealth™) liposome formulations may be prepared by inclusion of PEGylated lipids in liposome bilayers or by coating vesicle surfaces with block co-polymers. When increasing concentrations of PEG-750, PEG-2000, and PEG-5000 are included in DSPC liposomes, the main transition enthalpy progressively decreases and is abolished at concentrations greater than 60%, indicating the formation of micelles (56). Inclusion of PEG-PE conjugates, with PEG ≥ 5000 in DPPC liposomes, results in a shoulder on the main transition endotherm (57), indicative of phase separation within bilayers at a high temperature. This may explain why PEG $\geq$ 5000 in certain formulations is unsuitable for long-circulating liposomes (58), since phase separation would result in less sterically stabilized liposomes. Changes in the endotherm with increasing concentration of PEG-PE conjugates correlate with a decrease in vesicle size, indicative of solubilization of the liposomes into mixed micelles (57). DSC studies of the interactions between POE block co-polymers and DPPC liposomes demonstrated a minimal main transition temperature and enthalpy of transition at 1 mole% polymer content, which corresponded with a maximal HHW value, indicating incorporation of the co-polymer into the bilayer (59). Ringsdorf *et al.* (60) used DSC to detect the presence of hydrophobically modified co-polymers of poly-(*N*-isopropylacrylamide) within the bilayers of both DMPC and DSPC SUVs.

In our studies, HSDSC has proved useful for exploring the nature and extent of the interaction between the POE-POP-POE block co-polmers and DMPC and DPPC liposomes (23). Figure 4a, 4b, and 4c respectively show typical HSDSC scans of DMPC liposomes alone, DMPC liposomes following addition of 0.2% (w/v) poloxamer P407, and for DMPC liposomes in which the phospholipid film was hydrated (i.e. incorporated during liposome manufacture) with 0.2% (w/v) P407. Whilst neither the temperature of the pre- and main phospholipid phase transitions, nor the enthalpy of the main transition were changed, the presence of poloxamer significantly reduced the pretransition enthalpy of DMPC MLVs, indicating that, as for hydrophobic materials, the pretransition is the more sensitive parameter for detecting the presence of small quantities of the poloxamer surfactant molecules in phospholipid bilayers. The pretransition enthalpy was significantly lower when the poloxamer was included at the hydration stage rather than added after MLV manufacture, showing that interaction of P407 with liposomal bilayers is enhanced by its inclusion in the hydrating medium.

4.3 Phospholipid–drug interactions

DSC is a very sensitive means of investigating alterations in bilayer packing, with the presence in the bilayer of entities interfering with chain packing causing a reduction in the temperature of the main transition. In most cases, the inclusion of a material in a phospholipid bilayer has a more pronounced effect on the pretransition than the main transition (22, 61). The pretransition can thus be used as a sensitive indicator of the presence and level of impurities or incorporated materials in the bilayer. For instance, we have found the temperature and enthalpy of the pretransition of DPPC liposomes to be much better indicators of the extent of incorporation of the corticosteroid beclomethasone dipropionate than changes in the main transition endotherm (Table 4).

The influence of an additive on the main transition is influenced by its position in the bilayer, especially in the C_1–C_{10} region (62), with alterations in the thermal profile related to the polarity of the additive. Cations interact electrostatically with phospholipid head groups. Monovalent cations do not significantly alter the

Table 4 Transition temperature and enthalpy values ($\pm$ sd) of DPPC liposomes (100 mg/ml) containing beclomethasone dipropionate (BDP)

BDP conc. (mole %)	Pretransition Temperature (°C)	Enthalpy (J/g)	Main transition Temperature (°C)	Enthalpy (J/g)
0	35.41 ± 0.19	6.45 ± 0.34	40.09 ± 0.20	44.97 ± 2.00
0.5	33.70 ± 0.32	3.01 ± 0.57	39.35 ± 0.20	45.17 ± 1.75
1	31.45 ± 0.08	2.05 ± 0.45	39.29 ± 0.17	53.14 ± 4.50
2.5	31.77 ± 0.24	1.40 ± 0.21	38.92 ± 0.16	48.11 ± 2.71
5	31.48 ± 0.56	1.81 ± 0.31	39.85 ± 0.13	47.48 ± 2.41

transition behaviour, but more pronounced effects are evident with di- and trivalent cations (62). These cause rearrangements of the head group (63), giving a reduction in the original transition peak and the appearance of a new peak at a higher temperature, with the original peak completely replaced at very high solute concentrations.

Papahadjopoulos *et al.* (64) proposed that proteins can be classified into one of three categories dependent on their effects on the main phospholipid transition. Category 1 proteins are hydrophilic and adsorbed onto liposomal surfaces, by simple electrostatic interactions, exerting a greater effect on charged, rather than zwitterionic phospholipids. Category 2 proteins are adsorbed onto the surface, with some penetration into the bilayer, whilst Category 3 proteins penetrate into the core of the bilayer. This classification has been largely verified experimentally, using HSDSC (28), although with modification since no hydrophilic protein was found to bind to DPPG liposomes by electrostatic interactions alone. It has thus been proposed that HSDSC can be used to predict protein localization within liposomes (28).

DSC can be used to measure the incorporation of hydrophobic drugs in liposomal formulations. For instance, the entrapment of steroids has been quantified by determining the decrease in the temperature of the onset of the transition (T_o) (65), although measurement of the peak temperature (T_m) has been reported to be preferable to T_o in quantifying shifts in the transition temperature (22). DSC traces of liposomes in the presence of incorporated hydrophobic materials generally show a broadening of the main transition endotherm, quantified by HHW, giving a measure of the co-operativity of the transition (22, 62, 66). This has been employed to maximize the incorporation of hydrocortisone palmitate in DPPC liposomes (22). Although the temperature of the main phase transition was independent of steroid content, the HHW increased to a maximum at 13.2 mole%, indicating maximum drug incorporation, i.e. bilayer saturation. Arrowsmith *et al.* (61) studied the incorporation of cortisone esters in DPPC liposomes (Figure 5). The HHW and the temperature of the main transition were employed as measures of the extent of liposome–steroid interaction. Interaction increased with increasing steroid concentration and increasing ester chain length. Saturation of the bilayer occurred with 11.25 mole% cortisone palmitate.

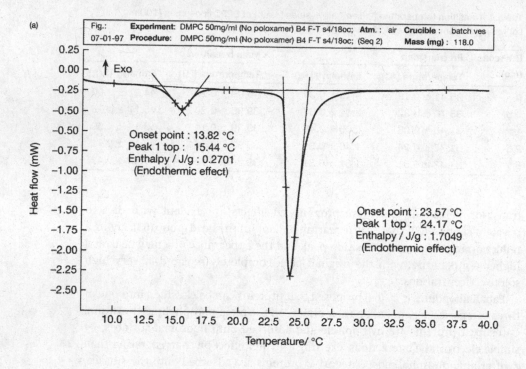

(a)

Fig.: 07-01-97 **Experiment:** DMPC 50mg/ml (No poloxamer) B4 F-T s4/18oc; **Atm.:** air **Crucible:** batch ves
Procedure: DMPC 50mg/ml (No poloxamer) B4 F-T s4/18oc; (Seq 2) **Mass (mg):** 118.0

Onset point : 13.82 °C
Peak 1 top : 15.44 °C
Enthalpy / J/g : 0.2701
(Endothermic effect)

Onset point : 23.57 °C
Peak 1 top : 24.17 °C
Enthalpy / J/g : 1.7049
(Endothermic effect)

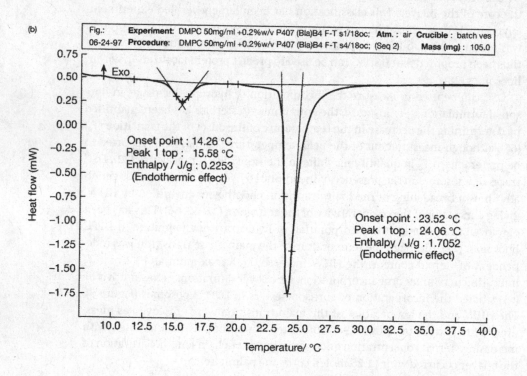

(b)

Fig.: 06-24-97 **Experiment:** DMPC 50mg/ml +0.2%w/v P407 (Bla)B4 F-T s1/18oc; **Atm.:** air **Crucible:** batch ves
Procedure: DMPC 50mg/ml +0.2%w/v P407 (Bla)B4 F-T s4/18oc; (Seq 2) **Mass (mg):** 105.0

Onset point : 14.26 °C
Peak 1 top : 15.58 °C
Enthalpy / J/g : 0.2253
(Endothermic effect)

Onset point : 23.52 °C
Peak 1 top : 24.06 °C
Enthalpy / J/g : 1.7052
(Endothermic effect)

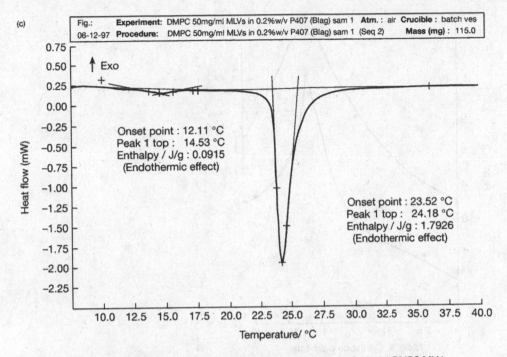

(c)

Fig.: 06-12-97 | **Experiment:** DMPC 50mg/ml MLVs in 0.2%w/v P407 (Blag) sam 1 | **Atm.:** air | **Crucible:** batch ves
Procedure: DMPC 50mg/ml MLVs in 0.2%w/v P407 (Blag) sam 1 (Seq 2) | **Mass (mg):** 115.0

Onset point : 12.11 °C
Peak 1 top : 14.53 °C
Enthalpy / J/g : 0.0915
(Endothermic effect)

Onset point : 23.52 °C
Peak 1 top : 24.18 °C
Enthalpy / J/g : 1.7926
(Endothermic effect)

Figure 4 Typical HSDSC scans of (a) DMPC MLVs incubated at 18 °C for 24 h, (b) DMPC MLVs following the addition of 0.2% (w/v) poloxamer surfactant P407 and incubated at 18 °C for 24 h, (c) DMPC MLVs hydrated in 0.2% (w/v) P407 then incubated at 18 °C for 24 h. Reproduced with permission from ref. 23.

4.4 DSC studies of liposomes as model membranes

DSC has been used to study the interaction between drugs and liposomes as models of biological membranes. For instance, DSC measurements of the interaction of antibiotics with DPPC liposomes have been used to predict their likely interaction with bacterial cell membranes (67, 68). Likewise, the effects of local anaesthetics on the thermal behaviour of DPPC liposomes has been studied (69) as anaesthetics may exert their action by modifying the fluidity of nerve cell membranes (70). However, studies with non-volatile general anaesthetics and steroids have shown that there is not a correlation between therapeutic potency and changes in the phase behaviour of liposomes (71, 72).

4.5 MTDSC of freeze-dried liposomes

To overcome the chemical and physical instability associated with long-term storage of liposome preparations, they may be freeze-dried, and subsequently reconstituted prior to administration. However, the sensitivity of the bilayers to the freezing and drying processes requires that a cryoprotectant, usually a disaccharide, is included. MTDSC allows the measurement of the T_g of the disaccharide, the onset temperature of the devitrification process (T_{dev}), and the

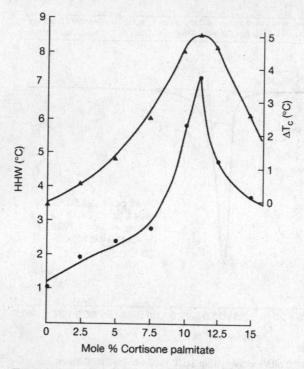

Figure 5 The relationship between the onset of the main phase transition (T_c), the half-height width (HHW) of DSC endotherms, and the incorporation of cortisone palmitate into DPPC liposomes: ● = HHW; ▲ =ΔT_c. Reproduced with permission from ref. 61.

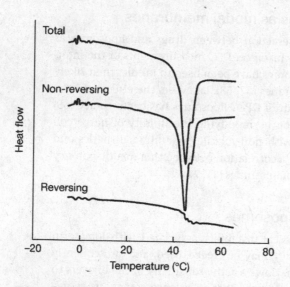

Figure 6 MTDSC scan of freeze-dried liposomes with an extra-liposomal medium containing 10% glucose and 10 mM HEPES pH 7.4, with a residual moisture content of 0.2%. Reproduced with permission from ref. 26.

softening or collapse temperature of the freeze-dried cake (T_s) (73). These parameters may be useful, since T_g gives a measure of the water content of the sugar glass, increasing as water content decreases. T_s relates to the stability of the freeze-dried cake. If the sample temperature exceeds T_s during primary drying, the cake will collapse. The relationship between the devitrification process, occurring at T_{dev} and the stability of frozen liposomes is as yet unclear. Conventional DSC is of limited use for investigating these processes, since the relevant thermal events may occur in the same temperature range (26). For instance, DPPC liposomes freeze-dried from a 10% glucose solution to a residual water content of 0.2% had a $T_{g,onset}$ of 41 °C and an onset temperature for the main bilayer transition of 40 to 41 °C. Using MTDSC, the underlying glass transition can still be resolved in these samples, even in the presence of the large bilayer transition endotherm (26) (Figure 6).

Acknowledgements

We would like to thank Jonathan Castile, Simon Gaisford, Lazeena Khatri, Rina Parmar, Paul Royall, and Mark Saunders for their comments and contributions to this chapter.

References

1. Charsley, E. L. and Warrington, S. B. (ed.) (1992). *Thermal analysis – techniques and applications*. Royal Society of Chemistry, Cambridge.
2. Wunderlich, B. (1990). *Thermal analysis*. Academic Press, London.
3. Haines, P. J. (1995). *Thermal methods of analysis*. Blackie Academic and Professional, Glasgow.
4. Ford, J. and Timmins, P. (1989). *Pharmaceutical thermal analysis: techniques and applications*. Ellis Horwood, Chichester.
5. Reading, M., Elliott, D., and Hill, V. J. (1993). *J. Therm. Anal.*, **40**, 949.
6. Reading, M. (1993). *Trends Poly. Sci.*, **1**, 248.
7. Coleman, N. J. and Craig, D. Q. M. (1996). *Int. J. Pharm.*, **135**, 13.
8. Boller, A., Jin, Y., and Wunderlich, B. (1994). *J. Therm. Anal.*, **42**, 307.
9. Royall, P. G., Craig, D. Q. M., and Doherty, C. (1998). *Pharm. Res.*, **15**, 1117.
10. Craig, D. Q. M., Royall, P. G., Kett, V. L., and Hopton, M. L. (1999). *Int. J. Pharm.*, **179**, 179.
11. Hancock, B. C. and Zografi, G. (1997). *J. Pharm. Sci.*, **86**, 1.
12. Franks, F. (1990). *Cryo-Lett.*, **11**, 93.
13. Nail, S. L. and Gatlin, L. A. (1993). In *Pharmaceutical dosage forms: parenteral medications* (ed. K. E. Avis, H. A. Lieberman, and L. Lachman), p. 163. Marcel Dekker, New York.
14. Pikal, M. J. (1993). In *Formulation and delivery of proteins and peptides* (ed. J. L. Cleland and R. Langer). ACS Symposium series 567, American Chemical Society, Washington.
15. Hill, V. L., Craig, D. Q. M., and Feely, L. C. (1998). *Int. J. Pharm.*, **161**, 95.
16. Lloyd, G. R., Craig, D. Q. M., and Smith, A. (1997). *J. Pharm. Sci.*, **86**, 991.
17. Parmar, R. (1997). *The interaction of a model steroid with phospholipid structures*. PhD Thesis, University of London.
18. Castile, J. D. (1998). *The interaction of multilamellar and freeze-thawed liposomes with poloxamer surfactants*. PhD Thesis, University of London.

19. Fuldner, H. H. (1981). *Biochemistry*, **20**, 3707.
20. Chen, S. C., Sturtevant, J. M., and Gaffney, B. J. (1980). *Proc. Natl. Acad. Sci. USA*, **77**, 5060.
21. Hinz, H.-J. and Sturtevant, J. M. (1972). *J. Biol. Chem.*, **247**, 6071.
22. Fildes, F. J. T. and Oliver, J. E. (1978). *J. Pharm. Pharmacol.*, **30**, 337.
23. Castile, J. D., Taylor, K. M. G., and Buckton, G. (1999). *Int. J. Pharm.*, **182**, 101.
24. Castile, J. D., Taylor, K. M. G., and Buckton, G. (2001). *Int. J. Pharm.*, **221**, 197.
25. Craig, D. Q. M. and Royall, P. G. (1998). *Pharm. Res.*, **15**, 1152.
26. van Winden, E. C. A., Talsma, H., and Crommelin, D. J. A. (1998). *J. Pharm. Sci.*, **87**, 231.
27. Chapman, D., Williams, R. M., and Ladbrooke, B. D. (1967). *Chem. Phys. Lipids*, **1**, 445.
28. Lo, Y.-L. and Rahman, Y.-E. (1995). *J. Pharm. Sci.*, **84**, 805.
29. Cameron, D. G. and Mantsch, H. H. (1982). *Biophys. J.*, **38**, 175.
30. Lewis, B. A., Dasgupta, S. K., and Griffin, R. G. (1984). *Biochemistry*, **23**, 1988.
31. Ruocco, M. J. and Shipley, G. G. (1982). *Biochim. Biophys. Acta*, **684**, 59.
32. Biltonen, R. L. and Lichtenberg, D. (1993). *Chem. Phys. Lipids*, **64**, 129.
33. Finegold, L. and Singer, M. A. (1984). *Chem. Phys. Lipids*, **35**, 291.
34. Blaurock, A. E. (1986). *Biochemistry*, **25**, 299.
35. Wilkinson, D. A. and Nagle, J. F. (1984). *Biochemistry*, **23**, 1538.
36. Slater, J. L. and Huang, C. (1987). *Biophys. J.*, **52**, 667.
37. Janiak, M. J., Small, D. M., and Shipley, G. G. (1976). *Biochemistry*, **15**, 4575.
38. Lubensky, T. C. and Mackintosh, F. C. (1993). *Phys. Rev. Lett.*, **71**, 1565.
39. Ladbrooke, B. D., Williams, R. M., and Chapman, D. (1969). *Biochim. Biophys. Acta*, **150**, 333.
40. Nagle, J. F. (1980). *Annu. Rev. Phys. Chem.*, **31**, 157.
41. Chapman, D., Byrne, P., and Shipley, G. G. (1966). *Proc. Roy. Soc. A*, **290**, 115.
42. Suurkuusk, J., Lentz, B., Barenholz, Y., Biltonen, R. L., and Thompson, T. E. (1976). *Biochemistry*, **15**, 1393.
43. Melchior, D. L. and Stein, J. M. (1976). *Annu. Rev. Biophys. Bioeng.*, **5**, 205.
44. Mabrey, S. and Sturtevant, J. M. (1976). *Proc. Natl. Acad. Sci. USA*, **73**, 3862.
45. Chapman, D., Urbina, J., and Keough., K. M. (1974). *J. Biol. Chem.*, **249**, 2512.
46. van Dijck, P. W. M., Kaper, A. J., Oonk, H. A. J., and de Gier, J. (1977). *Biochim. Biophys. Acta*, **470**, 58.
47. Matubayasi, N., Shigematsu, T., Ichara, T., Kamaya, H., and Ueda, I. (1986). *J. Membr. Biol.*, **90**, 37.
48. Tattrie, N. H., Bennett, J. R., and Cyr, R. (1968). *Can. J. Biochem.*, **46**, 819.
49. Ladbrooke, B. D. and Chapman, D. (1969). *Chem. Phys. Lipids*, **3**, 304.
50. Kirby, C., Clarke, J., and Gregoriadis, G. (1980). *Biochem. J.*, **186**, 591.
51. Malcomson, R. J., Higinbotham, J., Beswick, P. H., Privat, P. O., and Saunier, L. (1997). *J. Membr. Sci.*, **123**, 243.
52. McMullen, T. P. W., Lewis, R. N. A. H., and McElhaney, R. N. (1993). *Biochemistry*, **32**, 522.
53. Oldfield, E. and Chapman, D. (1972). *FEBS Lett.*, **23**, 285.
54. Mabrey, S., Matteo, P. L., and Sturtevant, J. M. (1978). *Biochemistry*, **17**, 2464.
55. Mabrey, S., Matteo, P. L., and Sturtevant, J. M. (1977). *Biophys. J.*, **17**, 82a.
56. Kenworthy, A. N., Simon, S. A., and McIntosh, T. J. (1995). *Biophys. J.*, **68**, 1903.
57. Bedu-Addo, F. K., Tang, P., Xu, Y., and Huang, L. (1996). *Pharm. Res.*, **13**, 710.
58. Maruyama, K., Yuda, T., Okamoto, C., Ishikura, C., Kojima, S., and Iwatsuru, M. (1991). *Chem. Pharm. Bull.*, **39**, 1620.
59. Baemark, T. R., Pedersen, S., Jorgensen, K., and Mouritsen, O. G. (1997). *Biophys. J.*, **73**, 1479.
60. Ringsdorf, H., Sackmann, E., Simon, J., and Winnik, F. M. (1993). *Biochim. Biophys. Acta*, **1153**, 335.

61. Arrowsmith, M., Hadgraft, J., and Kellaway, I. W. (1983). *Int. J. Pharm.*, **16**, 305.

62. Jain, M. K. and Wu, N. M. (1977). *J. Membr. Biol.*, **34**, 157.

63. Trauble, H. and Eibl, H. (1974). *Proc. Natl. Acad. Sci. USA*, **71**, 214.

64. Papahadjopoulos, D., Moscarello, M., Eylar, E. H., and Isac, T. (1975). *Biochim. Biophys. Acta*, **401**, 317.

65. Shaw, I. H., Knight, C. G., and Dingle, J. T. (1976). *Biochem. J.*, **158**, 473.

66. Jain, M. K., Wu, N. M., and Wray, L. V. (1975). *Nature*, **255**, 494.

67. Pache, W. and Chapman, D. (1972). *Biochim. Biophys. Acta*, **255**, 348.

68. Pache, W., Chapman, D., and Hillaby, R. (1972). *Biochim. Biophys. Acta*, **255**, 358.

69. Lee, A. G. (1976). *Biochim. Biophys. Acta*, **448**, 34.

70. Lee, A. G. (1976). *Biochemistry*, **15**, 2948.

71. Pringle, M. J. and Miller, K. W. (1978). *Biochem. Biophys. Res. Commun.*, **85**, 1192.

72. O'Leary, T. J., Ross, P. D., and Levin, I. W. (1984). *Biochemistry*, **23**, 4636.

73. van Winden, E. C. A., Zhang, W., and Crommelin, D. J. A. (1997). *Pharm. Res.*, **14**, 1151.

Chapter 4
Fluorescence methods in liposome research

Nejat Düzgüneş
Department of Microbiology, University of the Pacific School of Dentistry, 2155 Webster Street, San Francisco, CA 94115, USA.

Luis A. Bagatolli
MEMPHYS – Center for Biomembrane Physics, Department of Physics, University of Southern Denmark, Campujev 55, DK-5230 Odense M, Denmark.

Paul Meers
The Liposome Company, 1 Research Way, Princeton, NJ 08540, USA.

Yu-Kyuong Oh
Department of Microbiology, Pochon CHA University, 198-1 Donggyo-ri, Pochon, Kyonggi-do, South Korea.

Robert M. Straubinger
Department of Pharmaceutical Sciences, University at Buffalo, State University of New York, Amherst, NY 14260–1200, USA.

1 Fluorescence assays for liposome fusion

Liposomes of certain compositions can undergo fusion in the presence of the appropriate ionic conditions and pH, or fusion-inducing proteins or peptides (1–4). Thus the molecular requirements for membrane fusion can be explored systematically, using assays that monitor either the intermixing of membrane components or the coalescence of internal aqueous contents of liposomes. In this section we describe widely used fluorescence assays that monitor the kinetics of the fusion process.

1.1 The terbium/dipicolinic acid assay for intermixing of aqueous contents

The interaction of Tb and dipicolinic acid (DPA) results in the formation of the fluorescent $[Tb(DPA)_3]^{3-}$ chelation complex. Fluorescence is generated via internal energy transfer from DPA to the Tb, whose fluorescence intensity then increases by four orders of magnitude. The reactants are initially encapsulated in different populations of phospholipid vesicles, and membrane fusion results in an increase in fluorescence (5, 6). Contents that are released into the external medium are prevented from interacting by the inclusion of a low concentration of EDTA in the medium. Divalent cations which may be used to induce fusion further inhibit the interaction.

Protocol 1

The Tb/dipicolinic acid assay for intermixing of aqueous contents of liposomes

Equipment and reagents

- Three 1 × 20 cm Bio-Rad columns and buffer reservoirs
- Wescor Vapor Pressure Osmometer (Logan, Utah)
- Fluorometer (SLM4000, SLM8000, Spex Fluorolog 2, Perkin-Elmer MPF43, or equivalent)
- High-pass (>530 nm) cut-off filter (e.g. Corning 3–68)
- Four polystyrene 15 ml culture tubes
- Micro stir-bars that will fit in a cuvette

- Buffer A:[a] 100 mM NaCl, 1 mM EDTA, 10 mM TES pH 7.4
- Buffer B: 100 mM NaCl, 10 mM TES pH 7.4
- Sephadex G-75 or G-50 (Pharmacia)
- 2 mM Na dipicolinate (Sigma), 10 mM TES pH 7.4 (for assay calibration)[b]
- 10% (w/v) Na cholate (Calbiochem) or 16 mM $C_{12}E_8$ (octaethyleneglycol-dodecyl ether; Calbiochem)

For large unilamellar liposomes:

- 2.5 mM $TbCl_3$ (Alfa, Danvers, Massachusetts), 50 mM Na citrate, 10 mM TES pH 7.4 (Tb vesicles)[c]
- 50 mM Na dipicolinate (Sigma), 20 mM NaCl, 10 mM TES pH 7.4 (DPA vesicles)[b]

- A 1:1 mixture of the above reagents (Tb/DPA vesicles)

For small unilamellar liposomes:[d]

- 15 mM $TbCl_3$, 150 mM Na citrate, 10 mM TES pH 7.4 (Tb vesicles)[c]
- 150 mM Na dipicolinate, 10 mM TES pH 7.4 (DPA vesicles)[b]

- A 1:1 mixture of the above reagents (Tb/DPA vesicles)

Method

1 Check the osmolality of the solutions, and adjust with NaCl to the desired osmolality if necessary. Prepare the Tb vesicles, DPA vesicles, and Tb/DPA vesicles, according to Protocol 2 or 3.

---

2 Equilibrate the Sephadex G-75 or G-50 columns with buffer A. Pass each vesicle preparation through a separate column to remove the unencapsulated material, using elution buffer A. Discard the first 4 ml after the liposomes are loaded on the gel, and collect the next 3 ml in the culture tube. Flush argon gas over the liposome suspensions for 10 s, tightly cap the tubes, seal with Parafilm, and store in ice.

3 To be used in the calibration of the fluorescence assay, place 1 ml of the already chromatographed Tb vesicles on a Sephadex column equilibrated with buffer B, and proceed as in step 2. This step will eliminate the EDTA in the medium outside the Tb vesicles, producing the 'Tb minus EDTA vesicles'. EDTA would otherwise interfere with the formation of the Tb/DPA complex when the vesicles are lysed to obtain 100% fluorescence.

4 Determine the lipid concentration of the liposomes in each of the culture tubes by inorganic phosphate analysis (see Protocol 4).

5 Place an aliquot (e.g. 25 μM) of the 'Tb minus EDTA vesicles' (equivalent to the amount of Tb vesicles used in the actual assay) in a fluorometer cuvette containing the appropriate volume of buffer B, allowing for the volumes of the subsequent ingredients (to bring the final volume to 1 ml). From the 2 mM DPA stock add 10 μl to the cuvette (final DPA concentration 20 μM), and add 50 μl from either of the detergent stocks (final concentrations: 0.5% (w/v) Na cholate, or 0.8 mM $C_{12}E_8$).[e]

6 Set the excitation wavelength at 276–278 nm, and the emission wavelength to 545 nm, using intermediate slit widths. Place the high-pass cut-off filter before the emission monochromator, to minimize any contributions from light scattering. Crossed polarizers can also been used to minimize light scattering contributions. We have used SLM 4000, SLM 8000, Spex Fluorolog, and Perkin-Elmer MPF43 fluorometers for our experiments. However, other instruments with similar light intensity and sensitivity can be used to perform these assays.

7 Prepare a 1:1 mixture of the Tb vesicles and the DPA vesicles as a stock solution in a culture tube at a final lipid concentration that is 10-fold higher (e.g. 500 μM) than that used for the actual assay (e.g. 50 μM). Add 0.1 ml of the stock solution into 0.9 ml of buffer B, thus diluting the EDTA concentration to 0.1 mM. For a fluorometer with a strip-chart recorder, set the low fluorescence of this suspension to 0% F_{max}, using the offset function of the fluorometer. Make necessary adjustments to the 100% level using the gain function. Repeat the calibration procedure after a set of measurements to ensure that the lamp intensity has not changed.

8 For a fluorometer with computerized data acquisition, calibrate (or normalize) the assay, subtract the initial level of fluorescence [I(0)] from the data set, and divide the resulting data set by the numerical (fluorescence intensity) difference between the fluorescence intensity of the calibration vesicles [I(∞)] and the new 0% level. Multiply the result by 100 to obtain percentage values. The extent of fusion, F(t), as a percentage of maximal fluorescence, may also be calculated from:

$$F(t) = 100 \times [I(t) - I(0)] / [I(\infty) - I(0)]$$

where the fluorescence intensity at time t is I(t).

Protocol 1 continued

9   As an alternative method to calibrate the assay, use 50 μM of the Tb/DPA vesicles to set the 100% value. These vesicles correspond to the fusion product of all the Tb vesicles and DPA vesicles in the fusion assay, assuming that they have the same size distribution and are used at the same lipid concentration as the combination of the Tb and DPA vesicle populations (25 μM of each). Wait approx. 0.5 h after transferring the Tb/DPA vesicles from 0 °C (storage temperature) to room temperature for the fluorescence to equilibrate.

[a] EDTA is included in the buffer to prevent Tb^{3+} binding to the vesicle membrane as the citrate is diluted during gel filtration.

[b] Preparation of the Na dipicolinate solution adjusted to neutral pH is time-consuming, since solvation is a lengthy process and titration can often overcompensate the pH.

[c] The concentrations of the encapsulated reagents have been chosen to achieve iso-osmolality with 100 mM NaCl + 10 mM TES, the eventual medium in which the liposomes will be suspended. If experiments will be carried out in media of higher salt concentrations (for example 150 mM NaCl), the osmolality of the encapsulation solutions should be increased by adding more NaCl. The presence of citrate is essential to chelate the Tb^{3+} which would normally interact with and precipitate negatively charged phospholipids.

[d] Because SUV are not osmotically active, higher concentrations of Tb citrate and Na dipicolinate can be encapsulated. Since the internal volume of SUV is small, higher concentrations of reagents must be used to achieve an appropriate fluorescence signal/noise ratio.

[e] The free DPA is sufficient to chelate all the Tb^{3+}; higher concentrations of DPA should not be used to avoid inner filter effects.

Protocol 2

Preparation of large unilamellar liposomes by reverse-phase evaporation

Equipment and reagents

- Rotary evaporator (Büchi) with attached vacuum gauge and tubing connected to an argon tank
- Bath-type sonicator (Laboratory Supply Co., Hicksville, NY)
- Vortex mixer
- A high pressure extrusion device (Lipex Biomembranes, Vancouver, Canada) or a syringe extrusion apparatus (Avestin or Avanti Polar Lipids)

- Argon tank with tubing connected to a Pasteur pipette, clamped onto a stand
- A high quality glass tube of approx. 1 cm diameter, with a 'screw-cap' with a Teflon lining at the top. A larger tube with a fitting appropriate for a rotary evaporator.
- Teflon tape
- Reagents of fusion assay to be encapsulated (see other protocols)

Method

1   Place a phospholipid mixture (total lipid 10–20 μmol) in chloroform in a glass tube, and dry in vacuum in a rotary evaporator.

Protocol 2 continued

2   Wash a few ml of diethyl ether with a similar volume of distilled or purified water in a tightly capped glass tube by gentle shaking, and allow it to settle.

3   Take 1 ml of the ether (the top layer) and add it to the dried phospholipid film, using a glass pipette or syringe, and make sure the lipid dissolves.

4   Add 0.34 ml the buffer to be encapsulated to the phospholipid solution, let a stream of argon gas over the mixture using a Pasteur pipette, and seal the tube with Teflon tape and a screw-cap. Sonicate the mixture in the sonicator for 2–5 min. A stable emulsion should result at this point.

5   After opening the screw-cap, seal the tube again with Teflon tape and place inside the larger glass tube that fits onto a rotary evaporator. Include about 1 ml of water in the outer tube, both to maintain thermal contact and to minimize the evaporation of the aqueous solution in the inner tube. Immerse the outer tube in the water-bath of the rotary evaporator, maintained at 30 °C.

6   Evaporate the ether in controlled vacuum (approx. 350 mmHg) under constant supervision. Purge occasionally with argon gas attached to the evaporator to maintain the vacuum level and to prevent excessive bubbling. When a gel is formed, allow the vacuum to build up.

7   Remove the inner glass tube and vortex vigorously for 5–10 sec to break up the gel. Place the tube again in the outer tube and resume rotary evaporation. Repeat this step once or twice, until an aqueous opalescent suspension is formed.

8   Add an additional 0.66 ml of the encapsulation buffer to the suspension and rotary evaporate for an additional 20 min to remove any residual ether.

9   Using a high pressure or syringe extruder, pass the liposome suspension several times through polycarbonate membranes of 0.1 μm pore diameter (Poretics, Pleasanton, CA) to achieve a uniform size distribution.

Protocol 3

Preparation of small unilamellar liposomes

Equipment and reagents

- Rotary evaporator (Büchi) with attached vacuum gauge and tubing connected to an argon tank
- Bath-type sonicator (Laboratory Supply Co., Hicksville, NY)
- Vacuum pump or vacuum oven
- Argon tank with tubing connected to a Pasteur pipette, clamped onto a stand
- Vortex mixer

- A high quality glass tube of approx. 1 cm diameter, with a 'screw-cap' with a Teflon lining at the top. A larger tube with a fitting appropriate for a rotary evaporator.
- Teflon tape
- Ultracentrifuge
- Reagents of fusion assay to be encapsulated (see other protocols)

Protocol 3 continued

Method

1 Dispense 10 μmol of a phospholipid mixture in chloroform into the glass tube, seal Teflon tape over the top of the tube, place the tube in the larger glass tube, and dry in a rotary evaporator. When the film is dry, purge with argon to reduce the vacuum. Further evaporate any chloroform by placing the tube in a vacuum jar or vacuum oven, and keep under high vacuum for at least 2 h.

2 Hydrate the dried film with the buffer to be encapsulated, purge the tube with argon gas, seal with Teflon tape, and close the 'screw-cap' tightly. Vortex the mixture for 10 min at room temperature, or at a temperature above the gel to liquid-crystalline phase transition of the lipid mixture.

3 Sonicate the multilamellar suspension in a bath-type sonicator for 0.5–1 h. Ensure that the water in the bath is breaking up due to the sonication, and that the top of the liposome suspension is close to the level of the water in the water-bath and is being agitated, with an aerosol forming occasionally in the argon layer above. Prevent overheating of the bath, preferably keeping it at room temperature by either circulating water through the bath or adding ice and readjusting the level of the water. For lipids with high transition temperatures, maintain the bath a few degrees above this temperature.

4 Centrifuge the resulting opalescent suspension at 100 000 g for 1 h, preferably in a swinging bucket rotor, to pellet any remaining large liposomes. Use the supernatant as the small unilamellar liposome preparation.

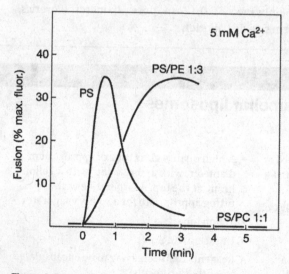

Figure 1 Fusion of large unilamellar liposomes of different composition, induced by calcium ions, monitored by the Tb/DPA assay. PS, phosphatidylserine; PE, phosphatidylethanolamine; PC, phosphatidylcholine (reproduced from ref. 17, with permission).

The Tb/DPA assay has been used in a large variety of liposome fusion systems. These include investigations on the effect of monovalent, divalent, and trivalent cations (7–12), temperature (13–15), osmotic pressure (13), and phospholipid composition (7, 16, 17) on membrane fusion (Figure 1). Other studies utilizing this assay have investigated the role of α-tocopherol (18), cholesterol (19), polyamines (20), lectins (21, 22), and synexin (annexin VII) (23–25) in modulating membrane fusion.

Protocol 4

Phosphate assay to determine the phospholipid concentration of liposomes used for fusion assays[a]

Equipment and reagents

- Test-tubes, 18 mm diameter
- Heating block with inserts for the test-tubes, set at 160–170 °C
- Oxford pipettor
- Vortex mixer
- Boiling water-bath (e.g. a round electric 'fryer')
- Metal tube rack that fits in the water-bath (i.e. round or square)
- H_2O_2 indicator strips (EM Quant Peroxide Test, EM Science, Gibbstown, NJ)
- 10 N H_2SO_4: add 100 ml concentrated H_2SO_4 into water to make up 360 ml of solution, placed in a polypropylene dispenser jar

- 9% H_2O_2: dilute 3 ml of 30% H_2O_2 with distilled or purified water to 10 ml final volume
- 0.22% ammonium molybdate in 0.25 N H_2SO_4: add 25 ml of 10 N H_2SO_4 to distilled or purified water, add 2.2 g ammonium molybdate, bring up to 1 litre with water; place in Oxford pipettor
- ANSA (Fiske) reagent (prepare a 15% $NaHSO_3$ solution): add 250 mg aminonaphthol sulfonic acid and 500 mg Na_2SO_3 to the $NaHSO_3$ solution, bringing the volume up to 100 ml; heat on a stir-plate gently to dissolve all ingredients
- Ascorbate (alternate to ANSA): dissolve 15 g ascorbic acid in 100 ml distilled or purified water; store in the cold

Method

1 Place the samples to be tested in triplicate tubes at an estimated amount of less than 0.1 µmol inorganic phosphate. Place phosphate standards in triplicate (for example (0.01, 0.05, 0.075, 0.1 µmol inorganic phosphate). Add 0.4 ml of 10 N H_2SO_4, and heat for 30 min on the heating block.

2 Cool the tubes and add 0.1 ml H_2O_2 using a pipettor or repeater pipette (e.g. Pipetman or Eppendorf). Heat for 30 min on the heating block. Test fumes for absence of H_2O_2 using the indicator strips.

3 Cool the tubes, add 4.6 ml of 0.22% ammonium molybdate reagent, and mix with the vortex mixer.

4 Add 0.2 ml of ANSA (or Fiske) reagent, and mix with the vortex mixer. Alternatively, 0.1 ml ascorbate can also be used for this step.

Protocol 4 continued

5 Incubate in boiling water for 7–10 min. Cool.

6 Wearing latex or other protective gloves, transfer the contents to spectrophoto-meter cuvettes, or preferably use a spectrophotometer with a sipper accessory (to avoid excessive handling of acid-containing tubes). Read at 812 nm or, if the solution is too concentrated, at 660 nm.

7 From the standard curve, determine the phosphate content of the sample you added to the tubes.

[a] Modified from ref. 26 by T. D. Heath and D. Alford.

1.2 The aminonaphthalene trisulfonic acid/p-xylylene bis(pyridinium) bromide (ANTS/DPX) assay for aqueous contents mixing

Since the protonation of DPA around pH 5 interferes with the formation of the Tb/DPA complex, studies on low pH-induced liposome fusion necessitated the development of assays that were not affected appreciably by low pH. The ANTS/DPX assay is based on the collisional quenching of ANTS fluorescence by DPX, each initially encapsulated in different populations of liposomes (27). Fusion results in the interaction of ANTS and DPX within the confines of the two liposomes, and the quenching of ANTS fluorescence. If liposome contents are released and diluted into the medium, essentially no fluorescence quenching occurs, since high concentrations of DPX are required for this process.

Protocol 5

The ANTS/DPX fusion assay

Equipment and reagents

- Equipment to prepare large unilamellar liposomes (see Protocol 2)
- Wescor Vapor Pressure Osmometer (Logan, Utah)
- Sephadex G-75 or G-50 (Pharmacia) columns
- Three 1 × 20 cm Bio-Rad columns and buffer reservoirs
- Fluorometer (SLM4000, SLM8000, Spex Fluorolog 2, Perkin-Elmer MPF43, LS-50, or equivalent)

- 25 mM aminonaphthalene trisulfonic acid (ANTS; Molecular Probes), 40 mM NaCl, 10 mM TES pH 7.4 (ANTS vesicles[a])
- 90 mM p-xylylene bis(pyridinium) bromide (DPX, Molecular Probes), 10 mM TES pH 7.4 (DPX vesicles[a])
- A 1:1 mixture of the above solutions (ANTS/DPX vesicles[a])
- Buffer C: 100 mM NaCl, 0.1 mM EDTA, 10 mM TES pH 7.4

Protocol 5 continued

Method

1 Prepare three large unilamellar liposome[b] populations encapsulating the different solutions listed above.

2 Chromatograph the liposomes on separate Sephadex G-75 or G-50 columns equilibrated with buffer C. Discard the first 4 ml measured from the point where the liposomes are allowed to partition into the gel. Then collect the next 3 ml in the polystyrene culture tube. Flush with argon, close tightly, seal with Parafilm, and store in ice until use.

3 Determine the phosphate concentrations of each of the liposome preparations, as described in Protocol 4.

4 Set the excitation monochromator to 360 nm, and the emission monochromator to 530 nm, with relatively wide slit widths (10–20 nm). It is desirable to place a high-pass filter (e.g. Corning 3–68) to eliminate any potential effects of light scattering.

5 Set the fluorescence of 25 μM ANTS vesicles in the appropriate amount of buffer (1–2 ml, depending on the fluorometer, with 'flea' or 'castle' stir-bars) to 100%. Set the fluorescence of 50 mM ANTS/DPX vesicles to 0%, since they represent the theoretical fusion product of all the ANTS vesicles and all the DPX vesicles (also 25 μM) used in the assay.

6 Initiate fusion by adding an appropriate fusogen (e.g. divalent cations, protons, fusogenic peptides). Fusion is monitored as the decrease in fluorescence.

[a] These solutions are appropriate for use with 100 mM NaCl in the external medium. For assays involving physiological concentrations of NaCl (e.g. 150 mM), the NaCl concentration in the ANTS solution should be increased to 90 mM, and that in the DPX solution to 50 mM NaCl. Adjusting the pH of the solutions can change their osmolality; therefore adjust the pH first, measure the osmolality, and then add the appropriate amount of NaCl to bring the osmolality to that of the eventual external medium. Keep solutions containing ANTS in the dark, as with all fluorophores, and store all solutions at 4 °C.

[b] Attempts to use the ANTS/DPX assay for the fusion of small unilamellar liposomes have not produced reliable results, presumably because ANTS binds excessively to such vesicles, although it does not bind appreciably to large unilamellar liposomes. Nevertheless, some studies have utilized this assay with small liposomes (31, 45)

The ANTS/DPX assay was first utilized in studies of low pH- or calcium-induced fusion of liposomes (27, 28) (Figure 2). The assay has also been used to study the induction of membrane fusion by poly(ethylene glycol) (29), phospholipase C (30, 31), and certain peptides (32).

1.3 The NBD/rhodamine resonance energy transfer assay for lipid mixing

When the emission band of one fluorophore, the energy donor, overlaps with the excitation band of another, the energy acceptor, the excited state energy of

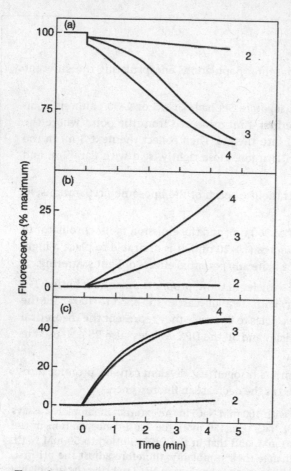

Figure 2 Calcium-induced fusion of oleic acid/phosphatidylethanolamine liposomes monitored by the ANTS/DPX assay (A). The leakage of aqueous contents measured by ANTS/DPX dissociation (B), and lipid mixing assessed by the NBD/rhodamine lipid dilution assay (C) are also shown (reproduced from ref. 28, with permission).

the donor generated by an absorbed photon is transferred non-radiatively to the acceptor, in a process termed resonance energy transfer (RET). The rate and efficiency of energy transfer depend on:

(a) The overlap of the emission spectrum of the donor and the absorption spectrum of the acceptor.

(b) The inverse sixth power of the distance between the two fluorophores.

Numerous pairs of fluorophores have been used for detecting lipid mixing during membrane fusion (33). The assays depend on the dilution of a donor/acceptor pair from 'labelled' liposomes to 'unlabelled' liposomes as a result of lipid mixing during membrane fusion. The efficiency of energy transfer is then decreased. Low concentrations of probes, usually less than 1 mole% of total lipid, are used for RET assays, minimizing the extent of membrane perturbation. We focus here on a RET pair that has been used extensively by a number of laboratories (34): N-(7-nitrobenz-2-oxa-1,3-diazol-4-yl) phosphatidylethanolamine (N-NBD-PE) and N-(lissamine rhodamine B sulfonyl) PE (N-Rh-PE). These probes do not exchange between membranes to any significant extent, and since the fluorophores are attached to the head groups of PE they do not cause appreciable perturbation of bilayer packing.

Protocol 6

The N-NBD-PE/N-Rh-PE RET assay for intermixing of lipids during membrane fusion

Equipment and reagents

- Fluorometer
- N-(7-nitrobenz-2-oxa-1,3-diazol-4-yl) phosphatidylethanolamine (Avanti Polar Lipids or Molecular Probes)
- N-(lissamine rhodamine B sulfonyl) phosphatidylethanolamine (Avanti Polar Lipids or Molecular Probes)

- Appropriate phospholipids and or cholesterol for liposome formation (Avanti Polar Lipids)
- Buffer C: 100 mM NaCl, 0.1 mM EDTA, 10 mM TES pH 7.4

Method

1. Prepare large or small unilamellar liposomes according to Protocols 2 or 3, respectively, using 0.8 mole% of each of the fluorophores in the initial chloroform mixture ('labelled liposomes').

2. Prepare liposomes of the same lipid composition, but without the fluorophores ('unlabelled liposomes').

3. Prepare liposomes as in step 1, but with 0.08 mole% of each fluorophore ('calibration liposomes', or 'mock fused liposomes').

4. After determining the phosphate concentration of each of the liposome preparations (Protocol 4), mix aliquots from the labelled and unlabelled liposomes at a ratio of 1:9 (for a liposome suspension at 50 μM total lipid concentration, this would be 5 μM labelled liposomes and 45 μM unlabelled liposomes) in 2 ml buffer C.

5. Set the excitation monochromator to 460 nm, and the excitation monochromator to 530 nm, and set 100% (or 'maximal') fluorescence using 50 μM calibration liposomes. Set the residual fluorescence of the mixture of labelled and unlabelled liposomes as 0% fluorescence. In essence, the percentage of lipid mixing as a function of time is given by:

$$M(t) = 100 \times [I(t) - I(0)] / [I(\infty) - I(0)]$$

where $I(t)$ is the fluorescence intensity at time t, $I(0)$ is the residual fluorescence, and $I(\infty)$ is the maximal fluorescence.

Protocol 6 continued

6 Introduce the fusogen of interest and monitor continuously the fluorescence. Fusion of the liposomes results in an increase in NBD fluorescence as the probes dilute into the unlabelled liposomes.

7 Alternatively, lyse the labelled liposomes (the same amount to be used in the assay) with an appropriate detergent to set the 100% fluorescence. However, it is necessary to ascertain if the detergent, such as Triton X-100, affects the quantum yield of NBD. Commercial preparations of Triton X-100 require a correction factor of 1.4–1.5. Some purified preparations of this detergent are claimed to have no inhibitory effect on the fluorescence.

When utilizing RET pairs it is important to establish that no lipid mixing takes place under conditions where no fusion is expected, or where the liposomes are expected to aggregate but do not fuse (35). Under some conditions, lipid mixing can be observed in the absence of contents mixing, which has usually been interpreted as arising from 'semi-fusion', the intermixing of the outer monolayers of interacting liposomes, in the absence of any direct communication of the aqueous interiors (36).

The N-NBD-PE/N-Rh-PE RET assay has been used to study low pH-induced fusion of liposomes with each other (28) or with cells expressing influenza haemagglutinin (37), the role of cholesterol in fusion (19), clathrin-induced fusion of liposomes (38), anion-induced fusion of cationic liposomes (39) (Figure 3), and

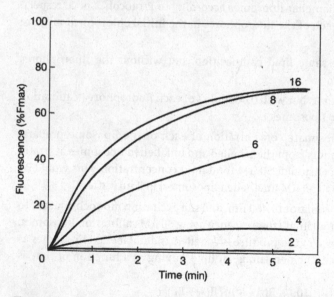

Figure 3 Anion-induced fusion of cationic *N*-[2,3-(dioleyl)propyl]-*N,N,N*-trimethylammonium (DOTMA):PE (1:1) liposomes, monitored by the NBD/rhodamine lipid dilution assay. EDTA at the indicated concentrations (mM) was added to a suspension of labelled and unlabelled liposomes (reproduced from ref. 39, with permission).

fusion of cationic liposomes with anionic liposomes (39). The assay has also been utilized to investigate fusion induced by myelin basic protein (40), the fusion of non-phospholipid vesicles with phospholipid liposomes (41), and divalent cation-induced fusion of liposomes (35, 36, 42, 43). The assay is particularly useful in studying the fusion of liposomes with biological membranes, such as vesicles derived from bacteria (44) and neutrophil plasma membranes in the presence of annexin I (45).

1.4 A fluorescence assay for intermixing of inner monolayers

The interaction of ions, proteins, and other fusogens with the outer monolayer of liposomes containing fluorescent probes can potentially alter the fluorescence intensity of the probes, for example by inducing lateral phase separation. Thus, it would be useful to be able to monitor the intermixing of the inner monolayer whose fluorescence would be unaffected by ion or protein binding to the liposome surface. This can be accomplished by reducing the fluorophores exposed on the outer monolayer of the liposome using dithionate, resulting in the elimination of fluorescence emanating from outer monolayer fluorophores. N-NBD-phosphatidylserine (PS) was found be more suitable for these experiments than N-NBD-PE, since it is less prone to transbilayer movement following reduction (46).

Protocol 7

Fluorescence assay for inner monolayer mixing

Equipment and reagents

- Bio-Gel A-30 spin columns (0.8 ml) (Bio-Rad)
- N-NBD-PS (Avanti Polar Lipids)
- N-NBD-PE (Avanti Polar Lipids)
- DiI(5)C18 (1,1'-dioctadecyl-3,3,3',3'-tetramethylindodicarbocyanine perchlorate) (Molecular Probes)

- Appropriate phospholipids and cholesterol for liposome preparation
- Sodium dithionate: stock solution of 200 mM sodium dithionate, 100 mM Tris pH 10, made shortly before use
- Buffer C (see Protocol 6)

Method

1. Prepare liposomes containing 0.75 mole% each of N-NBD-PS and either N-Rh-PE or diI(5)C18 (20 mM total phospholipid) in buffer C.

2. Mix the liposome suspension and dithionate stock so that the final dithionate concentration is 80–100 mM, and the phospholipid concentration is 10 mM. Incubate for 30–45 min on ice.

3. Remove the dithionate by centrifuging 100 μl aliquots through the spin columns.

4. Proceed as in Protocol 6 to measure inner monolayer mixing.

2 Fluorescence assays for liposome permeability

During the fusion of many types of liposomes, the aqueous contents may be released into the medium. In some cases this process is very slow compared to fusion, in others it is rapid and extensive. Interaction of toxins or peptides with liposomes may also result in the release of internal contents, resulting from either disruption of bilayer integrity or channel formation.

2.1 Release of carboxyfluorescein or calcein

The release of aqueous contents of liposomes may be monitored by encapsulating carboxyfluorescein (47, 48) or calcein (49) (Eastman/Kodak or Molecular Probes) at self-quenching concentrations. Impurities in some commercial preparations of carboxyfluorescein or calcein may be eliminated by chromatographing a concentrated solution in water on Sephadex LH-20 (50). The leakage of these fluorophores into the external medium results in the relief of self-quenching and an increase in the fluorescence. In the case of large unilamellar vesicles, encapsulate 50 mM carboxyfluorescein or calcein (Na salt) with 10 mM TES pH 7.4, and separate the unencapsulated material by gel permeation on Sephadex, using buffer C as the elution buffer, as described above. For small unilamellar liposomes, larger concentrations of carboxyfluorescein or calcein can be used (100 mM), since these liposomes are not osmotically active. The maximal fluorescence (100%) is established by lysing the vesicles with 0.1% (w/v) Triton X-100 or 0.8 mM $C_{12}E_8$. The extent of release, R(t), as a percentage of maximal fluorescence, may also be calculated from:

$$R(t) = 100 \times [I(t) - I(0)] / [I(\infty) - I(0)]$$

where the fluorescence intensity at time t is I(t), the initial residual fluorescence of the liposomes is I(0), and the fluorescence achieved by lysing the liposomes with detergent is I(∞).

This assay has been used to monitor:

(a) The release of aqueous contents that may accompany membrane fusion (5, 7).

(b) The intracellular delivery of liposome contents (51, 52).

(c) The channel-forming properties of bacterial and other toxins (53, 54).

(d) Leakage of contents in immobilized liposome chromatography (55).

(e) Membrane destabilization by viral proteins (56).

(f) The stability of liposomes containing arhaeal bolaform lipids (57).

(g) The pH sensitivity of liposomes (52, 58).

(h) Immune complex-mediated lysis of liposomes (59).

2.2 Release of the Tb/DPA complex

In addition to their use in calibrating the Tb/DPA assay, the Tb/DPA vesicles can be used to measure the leakage of aqueous contents. If the medium contains quenchers of the Tb/DPA reaction (for example, Ca^{2+} and EDTA) the entry of the external medium into the vesicles can also be monitored. Maximum (100%) fluorescence can be set by lysing the liposomes with detergent, and the extent of release as a function of time can be expressed by the equation in Section 2.1.

This assay has been used in correcting the Tb/DPA fusion signal for released or dissociated Tb/DPA complex (8, 9), and monitoring the release of aqueous contents during the fusion of glycolipid-containing liposomes in the presence of lectins (22).

2.3 The release of ANTS/DPX

The ANTS/DPX vesicles can be used to measure the release of aqueous contents of vesicles during fusion, or for investigating the effect of proteins or peptides on membrane permeability (60). The assay is calibrated to maximal (100%) fluorescence by lysing the vesicles with 0.1% (w/v) Triton X-100 or 0.8 mM $C_{12}E_8$. The extent of release as a function of time can be calculated according to the formula in Section 2.1.

The release of ANTS/DPX has been used in numerous systems, including the interaction with liposomes of surfactant-associated proteins (61, 62), the erythrocyte protein 4.1 (63), peptides derived from viral fusion proteins (64, 65), synthetic amphipathic peptides (66), antimicrobial peptides (defensins) (67), and dynorphin (68) (Figure 4).

3 Fluorescent detection of protein binding to phospholipid membranes

Peripheral and integral membrane proteins are important intracellular and extracellular mediators of structure and signalling within the cell. The association of such proteins with cellular membranes, where biochemical reactions can occur essentially in two-dimensional space, has major consequences for cellular function. Therefore, it has been of interest to study the physical factors that control the association of these proteins with phospholipid membranes. Fluorescent methods of detection have been particularly useful in such studies because of their high sensitivity and ease of use. The combination of several fluorescent techniques applied to a particular protein and liposome composition can often elucidate much about these interactions. Methods of detection can be categorized based on the types of fluorophores used and the mechanism of change in fluorescence that is used to detect binding.

We will discuss these methods in terms of a class of proteins called the annexins, which are a prototype for peripheral proteins that bind to phospholipid membranes in a Ca^{2+}-dependent manner, with highest avidity for anionic surfaces (69). Ca^{2+} ions are liganded by both the characteristic annexin fold structure and phospholipid head groups, and thus act as a bridging structure. Other molecular contacts between the annexin surface and the membrane also stabil-

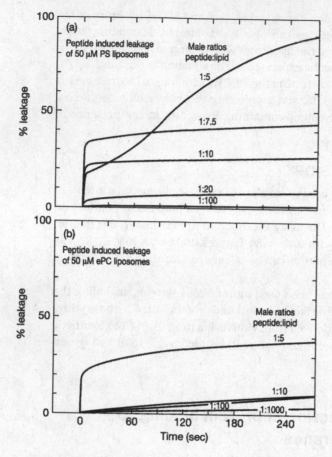

Figure 4 Dynorphin A (1–17)-induced leakage of ANTS/DPX from liposomes (reproduced from ref. 68, with permission).

ize the membrane-bound structure. In most cases, the annexins bind to phospholipid membranes without significant penetration into the hydrophobic interior, although binding appears to involve limited hydrophobic interactions.

3.1 Detection via membrane-associated fluorophores

Monomers of pyrene incorporated into the *sn*-2 acyl chain of phospholipids can associate in the excited state into complexes referred to as excimers. Excimers have excitation and emission spectra distinct from monomers. Excimer formation depends on the effective concentration of monomers and their rate of diffusion.

When pyrene-phospholipid probes are incorporated into liposome membranes, a certain rate of excimer formation exists which depends on the overall two-dimensional concentration of the probes (70). Proteins interacting with membranes can modify the monomer-excimer equilibrium (71–73). The method is outlined in Protocol 8. Many methods have been introduced to prepare model phospholipid membranes for the study of protein association. One of the more convenient methods, compatible with many lipid compositions, is described in Protocol 9. Primarily unilamellar vesicles are prepared by this method. When a zwitterionic phospholipid, phosphatidylcholine (PC), labelled with pyrene is incorporated at 5 mole% into liposomes composed of phosphatidylserine (an anionic phospholipid) (see Protocol 9), Ca^{2+}-dependent binding of annexin V results in an increase in the monomer fluorescence in the range of 10–15% (74). The maximal increase in this range is presumably due to a limiting decrease in probe lateral mobility that decreases the rate of excimer formation. The extent of the change is dependent on the annexin-to-phospholipid ratio.

Protocol 8

Measurement of changes in pyrene monomer fluorescence intensity as a result of protein binding[a]

Reagents

- Brain phosphatidylserine (Avanti Polar Lipids)
- 1-Hexadecanoyl-2-(1-pyrenedecanoyl)-sn-glycero-3-phosphocholine (Molecular Probes)[b]

Method

1 Prepare liposomes containing the appropriate mole percentage of an sn-2 acyl chain derivative of phosphatidylcholine. For studying binding of annexins to phosphatidylserine liposomes, include 5 mole% of 1-hexadecanoyl-2-(1-pyrenedecanoyl)-sn-glycero-3-phosphocholine in the preparation.

2 A typical lipid concentration is of 1–10 μM in a stirred fluorometer cuvette maintained at 25 °C. Maximal fluorescence change is observed in the range of 0.02–0.1 mole protein/external phospholipid for annexin binding.

3 Add Ca^{2+} from a concentrated solution by injection through a port into the stirred cuvette.

4 Record continuously the fluorescence at 377 nm, with the excitation monochromator set at 344 nm, and note the maximal increase.

[a] Adapted from ref. 74.

[b] Pyrene probes are particularly sensitive to quenching by oxygen, because of their long lifetimes. Therefore, changes in the oxygenation of the sample must be avoided during experiments with these probes.

Protocol 9

Preparation of extruded liposomes

Equipment and reagents

- Extrusion device (Northern Lipids, Inc.)
- Rotary evaporator
- Polycarbonate membranes (Whatman/Nuclepore)
- Appropriate phospholipids
- Aqueous buffer: e.g. 150 mM NaCl, 10 mM HEPES pH 7.4

Method

1. Dry a thin film of phospholipid onto an appropriate vessel in a rotary evaporator.

2. Disperse the film into the aqueous buffer by gentle shaking. Stock concentrations in the range of 10 mM total lipid are generally useful.

3. Freeze-thaw the aqueous phospholipid dispersion ten times.

4. Extrude the dispersion ten times through 0.1 μm pore diameter polycarbonate membranes in a stainless steel high pressure extrusion device (75).

5. Determine the phospholipid concentration, using a phosphate assay as described in Protocol 4, or as in ref. 76.

In another study, the pyrene label was part of the *sn*-2 acyl chain of anionic phosphatidylglycerol (PG) molecules (77). When incorporated into a membrane with PC, a significant increase in excimer-to-monomer ratio was observed upon binding of annexin IV, indicating that the annexin binding laterally segregates the anionic PG molecules, probably into fluid patches under the protein. By contrast, annexin binding to pure PG membranes containing the PG probe led to a decrease in excimer-to-monomer ratio, as seen with the PC probe in highly anionic membranes. Neither the pyrene-PC nor the pyrene-PG probe would be expected to concentrate in association with bound annexin molecules in essentially pure anionic lipid membranes. Therefore, it is likely that the decrease in excimer-to-monomer ratio results from a restriction in lateral mobility of the probes by the annexin-associated patches in both cases. These data illustrate the richness of information that can be obtained, as well as the importance of multiple approaches to avoid the potential ambiguity in interpreting the response of such probes.

Similar results can be obtained with fluorescence energy transfer pairs of lipid probes or self-quenched probes. Any change in segregation of species or lateral mobility due to protein binding can be potentially observed. In preliminary studies, we have observed changes in the donor-to-acceptor fluorescence ratio of NBD/rhodamine RET pair of lipid probes, or self-quenched NBD probes that apparently follow the same pattern as the excimer-to-monomer ratio.

3.2 Detection with intrinsic protein-associated fluorophores

One of the most common methods for monitoring protein binding to membranes is via the intrinsic protein fluorescence, particularly due to tryptophans. For proteins with one or a low number of tryptophan residues, the fluorescence changes can be interpreted readily.

3.2.1 Emission wavelength shift

Tryptophan fluorescence is sensitive to the polarity of the surrounding solvent. In a polar solvent, the solvent molecules can reorient dipoles around the excited state of the fluorophore such that the energy of the excited state is minimized (78). Therefore the emission wavelength is shifted more to the red than it may be in a solvent or environment lacking such dipoles. The polar solvent molecules also provide a relaxation mechanism for the excited state, such that the quantum yield tends to be lower in such an environment. Thus when a tryptophan group moves from an aqueous solvent into a non-polar environment, there is a shift to a more blue emission wavelength and a generally higher quantum yield.

Binding of human recombinant annexin V to phospholipid membranes exhibits a behaviour that can be monitored by a change in emission intensity and an emission wavelength shift (79). The single tryptophan of annexin V exhibits a relatively blue-shifted emission wavelength and is relatively inaccessible to quenchers (see below), consistent with a location within a hydrophobic pocket in the interior of the protein. Upon addition of sufficient Ca^{2+}, a pronounced red shift is observed, concomitant with accessibility to aqueous quenchers. This can be explained by the exposure of tryptophan to the aqueous solvent. These data presented the unusual situation where a fluorescent method gave information with regard to the crystal structure of the protein. The first Ca^{2+}-bound crystal form of annexin V showed a buried tryptophan residue (80, 81). Subsequent studies with rat annexin V demonstrated the Ca^{2+}-induced movement of this tryptophan from a buried to an exposed position (82), consistent with the fluorescence studies in solution (79, 83).

In the presence of liposomes containing anionic lipids, the Ca^{2+}-induced red shift of the tryptophan fluorescence is maintained, but is accompanied by a large increase in emission intensity. While this behaviour correlates with binding to the membrane as determined by other techniques, the actual origin of this effect is not clear. There may be a relatively immobile population of tryptophans at the interfacial region of the membrane where slow reorientation of polar solvent dipoles still occurs in response to the excited state. There may also be specific hydrogen bonding effects in operation in the interfacial region that shift and enhance tryptophan fluorescence.

3.2.2 Fluorescence quenching

Another method of detection of protein binding to liposomes is via the quenching of intrinsic protein fluorescence, by membrane-bound or aqueous quenchers. The classic aqueous quenchers, acrylamide and iodide, are generally excluded from the hydrophobic interior of phospholipid bilayers. Therefore the localization of a tryptophan in the aqueous or hydrophobic membrane environment can be distinguished by the degree of quenching by such reagents. In general, quenching can be described by the Stern–Volmer plot if it is primarily collisional in nature (78). The Stern–Volmer plot relates the ratio of the fluorescence in the presence or absence of the quencher to the quencher concentration. A plot of these quantities from experimental data leads ideally to a line that has a slope of K_D, the quenching constant (Protocol 10).

Data from the emission wavelength suggested that the annexin V tryptophan localizes in a hydrophobic pocket of the protein, unless Ca^{2+} ions are bound to the protein. Indeed, annexin V displays an acrylamide K_D of 5.2 M^{-1} in the absence of Ca^{2+} and 36 M^{-1} in its presence, consistent with the expected solvent exposure revealed by the emission wavelength. When bound to membranes containing anionic lipids via Ca^{2+}, the constant is only 6.7 M^{-1} (79). Therefore, the membrane-bound state of this protein shields the fluorophore from acrylamide, although it does not seem to involve a primarily hydrophobic environment.

Protocol 10

Tryptophan quenching experiments

Equipment and reagents

- Fluorometer with stirred cuvette
- Acrylamide
- Liposomes

Method

1 Perform fluorescence measurements using a fluorometer with sufficient stray light rejection. Set the excitation monochromator at 295 nm and monitor the emission spectra from 300 to 400 nm.

2 Maintain samples at constant temperature in a stirred cuvette and add small aliquots of concentrated stocks of acrylamide or other quencher to obtain the appropriate data. Make corrections to the fluorescence values for volume dilution.

3 Generate a plot of F_0/F against Q, where F_0 is the initial fluorescence, F is the quenched fluorescence, and Q is the quencher concentration. The slope of this curve is the Stern–Volmer quenching constant, K_D, calculated from a least squares fit to the data.

Membrane-localized quenchers have also been used to monitor protein binding to membranes. This method can give an indication of the depth of the fluorophore within the membrane if the quencher is localized well with respect to the depth of the membrane. Two main types of quenchers have been utilized, nitroxide spin labels and bromine groups (84, 85). These groups are covalently attached to acyl chains or head groups of phospholipids such that they localize at various average depths within the bilayer. In the parallax analysis, a hard sphere approximation of the distance dependence of quenching is utilized. Knowing the average depth of two different quenchers, the two-dimensional concentration of quenchers, and the observed fluorescence intensity of the fluorophore in the presence of the quenchers, the average depth of the fluorophore can be calculated by this method (84). While the parallax method gives the most physically reasonable results with the available spin-labelled quenchers, other methods of analysis may be advantageous in specific situations (86). A qualitative version of this method has also been applied to annexin. Upon membrane binding, its tryptophan 187 is strongly quenched by phospholipid nitroxide spin labels localized near the surface of the membrane, but not by those localized in the interior of the membrane (83), indicating that it is available for contact with phospholipid membranes when exposed following Ca^{2+} binding.

Similar experiments can be performed by energy transfer between tryptophan and membrane-associated acceptor fluorophores. For instance, the depth of membrane penetration of a single tryptophan within cytochrome $b5$ was estimated via energy transfer between the tryptophan and membrane-bound dansyl or trinitrophenyl acceptor groups (87). Binding of annexin IV was measured using RET between tryptophans and dansyl labelled lipids in the membrane (88). In an extension of this methodology, membranes symmetrically and asymmetrically labelled with acceptor probe were compared to determine the location of the tryptophan residue of peptides partitioned into liposomal membranes (89).

While fortuitous localization of tryptophans or reactive groups for labelling has been used in the past, site-directed mutagenesis has allowed selection of desired target sites within a protein for investigation. Thus, a more detailed picture of the orientation of the protein on the membrane can potentially be obtained. One of the most common approaches is to insert tryptophan residues in desired locations, usually as a conservative replacement of another hydrophobic amino acid. Another approach is to insert reactive cysteine residues, allowing labelling with a variety of fluorophores, often more easily detectable than tryptophan. Tryptophan residues have been placed strategically in the diphtheria toxin A and B chains (90) and in a Ca^{2+} binding loop of synaptotagmin (91) to assess interactions with spin-labelled lipid quenchers in the liposome membrane.

Fluorescence methods offer a unique, rapid means of assessing the extent of binding of a protein to a membrane. Interpretation of the data is greatly assisted, however, by the existence other structural information and by the use of complementary methods. The clearest picture of annexin binding to liposomes emerged only after several fluorescence techniques had been utilized to measure binding. Careful application of fluorescent techniques to other membrane-binding or membrane-associated proteins should continue to be a foundation on which to build a better understanding of protein–lipid interactions.

4 Liposomes as pH sensors in the study of cellular interactions

Liposomes fill dual roles in research, both as model membranes used in the study of physical and biological processes, and as delivery vehicles to convey drugs and macromolecules to cells and tissues. In both roles, there has been considerable interest in the preparation of liposomes containing pH-sensing reporter molecules. In studies ranging from measurement of rates for transmembrane proton transport to the investigation of cellular and tissue interactions of liposomes, a variety of pH-sensing fluorescence methods have been used. Here we will focus on the use of pH-sensing liposomes for the study of liposome–cell interactions. The nature of such interactions is a critical step in the delivery of molecules to the cell interior, an objective that has both experimental and therapeutic utility. Liposomes of the appropriate composition interact with the cell surface, and undergo either charge-mediated binding to unspecified surface components or (in the case of 'active targeting' approaches) ligand-directed binding to specific surface receptors. The result, depending on the cellular dynamics of the binding site, may include internalization of the liposome into the endocytotic apparatus of the cell.

Details are not fully available on the various intracellular fates of liposomes. It is anticipated that most of the sequelae observed for various macromolecules that are internalized by cells—endocytosis, transcytosis, recycling to the cell surface following internalization, routing to degradative or biosynthetic intracellular compartments—are possible fates for internalized liposomes. Liposomes which are internalized into cells are exposed rapidly to a compartment of somewhat acidic pH, the depth of acidification depending on a wide range of factors. For this reason, assays that seek to discriminate surface-bound from cell-internalized liposomes frequently use the acidification of the liposome environment as a means for determining internalization.

4.1 The pyranine (HPTS) assay

Pyranine (hydroxy-pyrene-[1,3,6]-trisulfonate) (Figure 5) was originally used as a proton-sensitive probe of the liposome interior and aqueous interfacial region (92, 93). More recently, we and others have employed pyranine-containing liposomes to evaluate the extent and rate of liposome internalization, or to compare the internalization of liposomes among different cell types (94–98) (Protocol 11). The main difference between studies of membrane permeability to protons and the application of detecting cellular internalization lies in the concentration of dye: cell studies are performed with high concentrations of dye in the liposome to provide adequate signal intensity, whereas in proton permeability studies, these concentrations of dye would dampen the fluorescence response through buffering action. The basic method for observing endocytosis employs fluorescent dyes having both pH-sensitive and pH-insensitive ('reference') regions of their spectra. Ratio methods employing fluorescein or derivatives such as

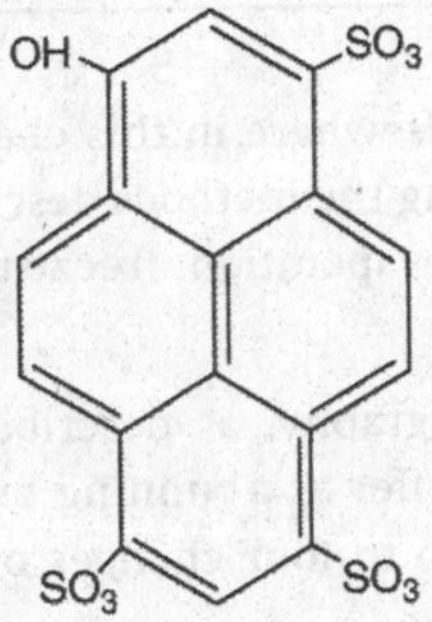

Pyranine
(hydroxy-pyrene-[1,3,6]-trisulfonate)

Figure 5 Structure of pyranine, a pH-sensitive fluorophore with physical properties appropriate for encapsulation in liposomes.

carboxyfluorescein have been used previously to measure pH in the endocytotic pathway (99–101). A pH calibration curve is obtained by computing a ratio of fluorescence obtained at pH-sensitive and pH-insensitive wavelengths, with the dye held at various known pH. The advantage of ratio methods is that the pH-invariant reference signal obviates the requirement that the probe concentration be known or constant in each cellular compartment.

Protocol 11

Encapsulation of pyranine in liposomes for use as a probe of cellular uptake

Equipment and reagents

- Spectrophotometer (for determining the concentration of pyranine)
- Gel filtration medium (Sephadex G-75, Pharmacia) or dialysis membranes for removal of unentrapped dye (see Protocol 1)
- Purified phospholipids and equipment for preparing liposomes (see protocols on liposome preparation)

- Pyranine (hydroxy-pyrene-[1,3,6]-trisulfonate) (Molecular Probes, or other supplier of high quality fluorescent probes)
- Aqueous calcium/magnesium-free buffer that is isotonic with cell growth medium: e.g. 150 mM NaCl, 10 mM HEPES pH 7.4
- Detergent such as Triton X-100 for lysing liposomes (see Section 2.1)

Method

1   Prepare a solution containing 35 mM pyranine in 10 mM HEPES buffer pH 7.4, containing sufficient NaCl (approx. 100 mM) to maintain isotonicity with the buffer to be used with cells. Adjust the pH to 7.2–7.4.

Protocol 11 continued

2 Encapsulate pyranine in liposomes using the protocols elsewhere in this chapter. Liposomes may be made by a variety of protocols, including the methods described here for multilamellar, small unilamellar, reverse-phase evaporation, freeze-thaw, or extruded liposomes.

3 Remove unencapsulated pyranine by column chromatography, as described in Protocol 1, using the isotonic calcium/magnesium-free buffer as a running buffer. Alternatively, place liposomes in a dialysis bag, with two to four changes of the external buffer, in the cold.

4 Determine the liposome phospholipid concentration (Protocol 4) for studies in which a defined concentration of liposomes or liposome:cell ratio is of interest.

5 Determine the concentration of pyranine encapsulated using spectrophotometry: dilute a sample of liposomes serially in buffer containing detergent such as 0.1% Triton X-100. Dilute similarly a pyranine stock of known concentration in the same buffer to provide a standard curve. Determine the concentration of pyranine from the absorbance at 413 nm, the isosbestic point.

Although the excitation spectrum of fluorescein has both pH-sensitive and -insensitive regions (99), fluorescence emission at the pH-insensitive wavelengths is weak, and fluorescein lacks a consistent isosbestic wavelength. In addition, the pH-sensitive and reference wavelengths are relatively closely-spaced, posing difficulties for use in fluorescence microscopy; filters or laser sources may not provide the optimal wavelengths for the determination of pH. In contrast, pyranine has a strong intensity at both pH-sensitive and -insensitive regions of its excitation spectrum, a well-defined isosbestic point (Figure 6), and a pH-invariant emission wavelength. Furthermore, not only are the excitation and emission spectra within ranges achievable with common optical elements on fluorescence microscopes, but also the pH-sensitive and -insensitive spectral regions are widely spaced and easily discriminated, thus providing a high signal-to-noise ratio.

An example of the use of pyranine as an intracellular pH sensor, employing both spectrofluorometer and fluorescence microscopy, is provided in ref. 96 (Protocols 12 and 13). Spectrofluorometry has the advantage of providing a population average of the pH at which liposomes reside in cells, while fluorescence microscopy provides greater detail on the fraction of liposomes internalized, the heterogeneity of liposome fate, and the correlation of liposome deposition with specific cellular structures. An example of data analysis to estimate the fraction of liposomes internalized by cells is provided in ref. 95. A detailed example of image processing methods to determine the pH of individual fluorescent accretions within cells is given in ref. 102.

Protocol 12

Cellular uptake of liposomes by spectrofluorometry

Equipment and reagents

- Spectrofluorometer: temperature control, scanning, and a stirring cell are useful features
- Small magnetic stir-bars for cuvette (if suspension cells are used)
- Aqueous isotonic buffer (e.g. PBS pH 7.4) for cell incubation, additionally containing 0.5 mM each Ca^{2+} and Mg^{2+} for incubations in which the cells are grown in monolayer culture

- Liposomes containing pyranine (see Protocol 11)
- Methylamine calibration solutions: concentrated (0.5–1 M) if suspension cells are used, or 50 mM methylamine in PBS, adjusted to various pH
- Cells for study; grown on sterile glass coverslips if monolayer cells

Method

1. If cells growing in monolayer culture are to be used, analyse them at the appropriate time by removing them from the culture dish and placing them in suspension in the spectrofluorometer. Alternatively, subculture cells onto sterile rectangular glass coverslips of such dimension as to fit diagonally into a cuvette, and analyse them *in situ*. Use a diamond-tipped pen to score and break larger coverslips into the appropriate dimensions. Sterilize coverslips by soaking in 95% ethanol, and then briefly flaming over an alcohol lamp to remove the ethanol. Place the coverslips in the bottom of a cell culture dish and add suspended cells in tissue culture medium. In some cases, experimentation is necessary to determine whether coverslips must be coated or treated to enhance cell adhesion. Proceed with the experiments when the desired confluency is achieved.

2. Remove the tissue culture growth medium by washing twice in buffered saline. If monolayer cells are used, include sufficient concentrations of Ca^{2+} and Mg^{2+} (typically 0.5 mM each) to maintain cell adhesion. In this and following steps, if suspension cells are used, wash the cells twice with buffer by centrifugation at low force g (typically 300 g), and suspended in buffer at 10^6 cells/ml.

3. Add liposomes in buffer to cells. For many cell types, 500 mM of liposome phospholipid per 10^6 cells may saturate cellular uptake mechanisms. The concentration of liposomes is often an experimental variable. The volume of fluid should be sufficient to cover the cell monolayer. Incubation proceeds at 37 °C.

4. The time of liposome–cell interaction is frequently an experimental variable. Typically, the majority of binding is complete in 15–30 min. However, much shorter incubation times permit the observation of early events and more synchronous observation.

Protocol 12 continued

5 To terminate the interaction, remove unbound liposomes by washing cells twice with buffer. In some cases, culture medium may be added to cells for continued incubation and cellular processing. If so, remove culture medium by washing twice with buffer prior to fluorescence determinations.

6 If monolayer cells are to be analysed, remove them from the culture dish by a combination of trypsin/EDTA treatment and/or scraping.

7 Place the cells in a quartz cuvette and transfer to a spectrofluorometer; to reduce light scattering, analyse cells in suspension at the lowest density that permits adequate detection of a fluorescent signal. Typically, 10^5 cells/ml are detected easily. Stir suspension cells gently with a stir-bar. Maintain temperature at 37 °C if possible. For monolayer cells to be analysed *in situ*, place coverslips diagonally in a quartz cuvette, and place the cuvette in a spectrofluorometer. Some experimentation with the position of the coverslip in the cuvette and the orientation of the cells (toward/ away from the excitation beam) is necessary to reduce scattering and refraction by the glass coverslip.

8 Perform fluorescence excitation scans over a range of 400–490 nm, with the emission fixed at 510 nm. The characteristic spectrum of pyranine (Figure 6A) should be observed. For monolayer cells *in situ* on a coverslip, the position in the cuvette may require adjustment, as scattering and refraction are manifested as distortions of the pyranine spectrum. Scans may be repeated over time as an experimental variable. For long-term observation, cells may require glucose for maintaining metabolic activity.

9 Calculate the ratio of fluorescence at pH-sensitive and pH-insensitive wavelengths. Typically, use 450 versus 413 nm excitation (λ_{EX} 450/413 nm). However, other wavelength pairs, including 403 versus 413 nm excitation (λ_{EX} 403/413 nm), are useful.

10 Perform fluorescence calibrations to determine the pH reported. For pyranine, two methods of calibration can be compared. First, dilute (5–10 mM) solutions of pyranine can be prepared in buffers pH-adjusted to the range of interest, typically pH 4.5–7.4, and each one scanned (Figure 6A). Alternatively, the more appropriate calibration is an *in situ* calibration, in which a lipophilic amine (e.g. methylamine) and/or a proton ionophore (e.g. monensin) are used to clamp intracellular pH to values approaching the extracellular pH. Typically, add methylamine from a concentrated stock to a final concentration of 50 mM in the cell-containing buffer. Then acquire fluorescence scans with the buffer at pH 7.4 and at several other (acidic) pH. The pH is verified using a pH meter, permitting the corroboration of the *in situ* calibration curve with that of dilute pyranine in buffers of known pH. Typically, the results of both methods agree well.

Protocol 13

Cellular uptake of liposomes by fluorescence microscopy

Equipment and reagents

- Fluorescence microscope equipped with image capture device, and excitation and emission filters suitable for pyranine fluorescence. Filters are needed that provide excitation in the pH-insensitive band of the spectrum (413 nm) and in the pH-sensitive band (440–490 nm; peak is 450 nm). Emission is detected at ≥510 nm. The image capture device must be capable of low-light image acquisition, and it must be possible to capture images under fixed gain and photomultiplier voltage.

- Image processing software that allows pixel-by-pixel division of two images, and the elimination of non-regions of interest (ROI) by masking (e.g. NIH Image for Macintosh, National Institutes of Health, Bethesda, MD, *http://rsb.info.nih.gov/nih-image/*)

- Liposomes containing pyranine (see Protocol 11)

- Cells for study; grown on sterile glass coverslips if monolayer cells (see Protocol 12)

- Aqueous isotonic buffer (e.g. PBS pH 7.4) for cell incubation, additionally containing 0.5 mM each Ca^{2+} and Mg^{2+} for incubations in which the cells are grown in monolayer culture

- Methylamine calibration solutions: 50 mM methylamine in PBS, adjusted to various pH

Method

1 Prepare cells, optionally on coverslips, as described in Protocol 12, except that standard 22 × 22 mm glass coverslips may be used in place of rectangular coverslips. Wash cells free of culture medium, incubate with pyranine liposomes, and wash free of unbound liposomes, as described in Protocol 12.

2 For analysis by fluorescence microscopy, mount the coverslip on a standard glass slide, and seal on only two parallel edges. This permits solutions to be changed underneath the coverslip by wicking them away from one side with a tissue while adding fresh solution to the other side.

3 Place the coverslip on a fluorescent microscope having excitation and emission filters appropriate for pyranine, and bring the cells into focus. Typically, a ×60 objective is necessary for sufficient excitation intensity.

4 Acquire images of each cell field, with the sample irradiated using the two different excitation bands appropriate for pyranine. Care must be taken to avoid any movement of the cells. The image capture device must be operated in a non-automatic fixed-gain mode. Automatic adjustment of detector gain, black level, and phototube voltage (if a video device) will compensate for the differing levels of intensity in the sample, thus obscuring the pH-dependent changes in fluorescence that one seeks to observe.

Protocol 13 continued

5 Perform the calibration of the sample in two ways, as described in Protocol 12, with modifications.

(a) Wick standard solutions of dilute pyranine at known pH under a coverslip that is mounted on a slide in the same position and focal plane as a cell sample. Several images of each field are acquired, as in step 4.

(b) Treat the cell sample with methylamine solutions of known pH, again by wicking each solution under the coverslip, while the cell sample remains in place. After cells are equilibrated in each solution, acquire images at each excitation wavelength, as in step 4.

6 Process the data using an image processing program. Calculate a ratio image using pixel-by-pixel division of images acquired at one excitation wavelength by the corresponding image acquired at the other wavelength. Division algorithms must re-scale the data to display fractional data resulting from division to the intensity range used for displaying images (i.e. a scale of 0–256 for 8-bit images). The background region beyond the border of a cell typically has very low intensity, but nonetheless may yield a valid ratio upon division. Therefore, apply a binary 'mask' to each ratio image, usually based on a threshold that eliminates low-intensity background regions. Details of ratioing and masking are illustrated in ref. 102. Often a pseudocolour palette is used to display the ratio image, with each colour calibrated to display a different pH range.

7 Analyse the data for the two calibration methods: from (a) images of dilute dye at known pH and (b) images of cells clamped to known pH using methylamine, as described in step 6. Prepare a standard curve by plotting the known pH against the ratios calculated: either the average ratio of whole fields in method (a) or the average ratio determined for numerous objects in method (b). The resulting ratios for each method typically agree, and comprise the standard curve by which pH values can be determined for each location containing fluorescence in the ratio images of cells.

4.2 The dual-fluorophore assay

One problem noted with pyranine-based measurements of pH reported by intracellular liposomes is a blunting of the pH responsiveness of the dye, especially at early time points or when using highly stable liposomes (103) (Y.-K. Oh and R. M. Straubinger, submitted). The effect can be manifested spectrally as an apparent acidification of the liposome lumen when liposomes are known to be at neutral pH. The source of this artefact appears to lie partly in the interaction of pyranine with the membrane interfacial region, and partly with dye–dye interactions at the high concentrations used. Although the pyranine method is simple and provides accurate measurements of intracellular pH, alternative methods are preferable at longer incubation times (when liposomes have begun to leak) or when using less stable liposomes. The method is based on fluorescence ratios, as with pyranine, but utilizes dual fluorophores and locates the fluorophores on the liposome exterior, covalently attached through a hydrophilic spacer arm (Y.-K. Oh and R. M. Straubinger, submitted).

Ratio methods involving fluorescein as the pH-sensitive fluorophore (99) in combination with a pH-insensitive reference fluorophore such as rhodamine have been used to observe cellular internalization of diverse materials such as

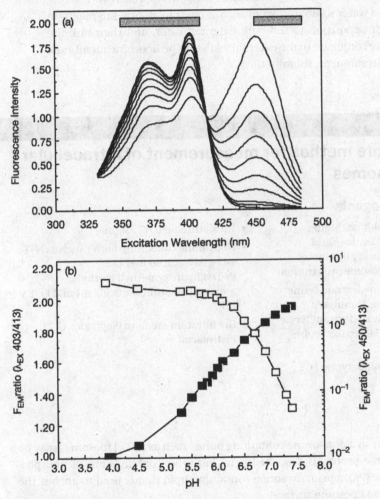

Figure 6 Spectral properties of pyranine, and construction of a calibration curve. (A) Excitation spectra of 7 mM pyranine at various pH over the range of 7.4–4.5. The emission wavelength was 510 nm. The pH 7.5 curve can be identified as the one with the highest intensity at 450 nm and the lowest intensity at 350–400 nm. The pH-insensitive isosbestic wavelength is 413 nm. Stippled bars over the spectra indicate the excitation wavelength ranges for typical filter sets used in fluorescence microscopy. (B) Ratios were calculated for fluorescence emission intensity (F_{EM}) of 510 nm as a function of pH. Two excitation wavelength ratios were calibrated, given the two spectral domains (403 nm and 450 nm) which are pH-sensitive. Open symbols: λ_{EX} 450/413 nm; filled symbols: λ_{EX} 403/413 nm (redrawn from ref. 96, with permission).

peptides, ligand–polymer complexes, yeast, and bacteria (100, 102, 104, 105). The use of a second, spectrally-distinct reference fluorophore provides wide separation of the pH-sensitive and reference signals into regions of the spectrum that are achieved easily with conventional lasers. Furthermore, the ability to vary the ratio of the probes allows matching of the dynamic range of the assay to that of the video or photomultiplier detectors, thereby providing greater accuracy in the pH measurement (Protocol 14). A key modification of our approach was to link the fluorophores to a water soluble polymer such as dextran, in order to maintain the probes in closer apposition to the bulk external water, and then link the polymer/fluorophore conjugate to the external leaflet of the liposome membrane (Y.-K. Oh and R. M. Straubinger, submitted).

Protocol 14

Dual-fluorophore method for measurement of intracellular pH using liposomes

Equipment and reagents

- Purified phospholipids (including phosphatidylethanolamine), and equipment for preparing liposomes (see protocols on liposome preparation)
- Aminated fluorescein–dextran 'lysine fixable' (MW 3000) and aminated tetramethylrhodamine–dextran 'lysine fixable' (MW 3000) (Molecular Probes)
- Sulfosuccinimidyl 4-(*p*-maleimidophenyl)butyrate (Sulfo-SMPB; Pierce)

- Dithiothreitol (DTT; Sigma)
- Non-amine containing buffer such as NTE: 145 mM NaCl, 10 mM TES (*N*-Tris[hydroxymethyl]-methyl-2-aminoethane sulfonic acid), 0.1 mM EDTA pH 7
- Gel filtration medium (Sephadex G-75, Pharmacia)

Method

1 Prepare liposomes in a non-amine containing buffer such as NTE. Liposomes may be made by any of the protocols described here, but must contain 3 mole% phosphatidylethanolamine (PE), a primary amine containing lipid that is used to anchor the fluorophores to the liposome surface.

2 Thiolate liposomes by incubating for 4 h in a mixture of sulfo-SMPB and DTT, using a molar ratio of liposomal PE/sulfo-SMPB/DTT of 1:10:100.

3 Separate liposomes from unreacted materials by gel filtration on Sephadex G-75.

4 Conjugate fluorescent dyes via the amino dextran spacer arm by incubating overnight with a mixture of aminated fluorescein–dextran, rhodamine–dextran, and sulfo-SMPB in a molar ratio of 1:1:2.

5   Separate liposomes from reactants by gel filtration on Sephadex G-75.

6   Utilize liposomes for pH measurements as described in Protocols 12 and 13, taking into account the optimal wavelengths for excitation and emission of fluorescein and rhodamine. Typically, 490/520 nm are used for the fluorescein excitation/emission wavelengths, respectively, and 540/580 nm are used for the excitation/emission wavelengths of tetramethylrhodamine, respectively. Prepare calibration curves by incubating liposomes in buffers of known pH, and calculating the ratio of fluorescein:rhodamine fluorescence as a function of pH. Perform *in situ* calibrations of pH within cells using methylamine-containing buffers, as described in Protocols 12 and 13.

5 Two-photon excitation fluorescence microscopy to detect lipid phases in giant liposomes

The effect of temperature on phase equilibria in lipid mixtures has been studied for many years using different experimental techniques and phase diagrams have been constructed, providing important thermodynamic information for several lipid mixtures (106–111). One interesting temperature region in a lipid mixture's phase diagram is that corresponding to the formation of a stable lipid domain structure. The coexistence of ordered (tightly packed) and disordered (loosely packed) lipid phases plays a central role in the stabilization of multi-component vesicles and in the fission of small vesicles after budding (112). Fluorescence recovery after photobleaching (FRAP) has also been used to study lipid domain structure and phase coexistence (113, 114). The information extracted from these different experimental techniques is useful to understand the possible occurrence of phase separation phenomena in cell membranes. It is important to note that the presence of phase coexistence in cell membranes is still a matter of controversy. However, experimental evidence is being accumulated favouring the presence of lateral organized domains in biological membranes (115–117).

5.1 Direct visualization of lipid domain coexistence in bilayers

Although coexistence of lipid phases is well accepted in model systems (monolayers and bilayers), the *direct visualization* of lipid domains was successfully accomplished only in lipid films at the air water interface, using fluorescence microscopy (118, 119). Changes in lateral pressure induce the formation of coexisting lipid phases in lipid monolayers composed of pure lipids or lipid mixtures. The direct observation of this phenomenon generally involves the use of different fluorescent probes with preferential partitioning to one of the coexisting lipid phases (see below). The direct visualization of lipid domains in bilayers at the phase coexistence region was achieved by electron microscopy

(120). However, no direct and detailed knowledge of the shape and formation of domains in bilayers was available. Here we introduce an experimental approach that allows visualization of temperature-dependent lipid phase equilibria at the level of single, unilamellar 'giant' liposomes, using two-photon fluorescence microscopy and particular fluorescent probes.

5.2 Giant unilamellar liposomes

To mimic the lipid lateral organization of the cell plasma membrane it would be ideal to use cell-sized liposomes as a model membrane system. Giant unilamellar vesicles (GUV) have a mean diameter of approx. 20 μm, and constitute an attract-ive experimental system to study phase equilibria of pure lipid systems and lipid mixtures by fluorescence microscopy, mainly because single liposomes can be observed under the microscope (121). The first lipid domains to be observed with GUV were those induced by Ca^{2+} in liposomes composed of mixtures of PC and acidic phospholipids, or erythrocyte lipids (122).

Two important conditions are required to prepare GUV:

(a) The temperature during the vesicle preparation must be higher than the phase transition temperature of the lipids (this is also valid in the formation of multilamellar, and small or large unilamellar liposomes).

(b) The samples should not be agitated during vesicle formation.

Experimental conditions, including ionic strength, pH, lipid composition, the substrate on which the lipid film is dried, and the presence of some sugars, appear to be critical parameters to obtain giant liposomes (123–128). Low ionic strength (<10 mM) is usually required to prepare giant vesicles (124, 127). Physiological conditions can be used by including a percentage of charged lipids in the lipid sample (126). A technique based on organic solvent evaporation in aqueous solution can produce liposomes up to 50 μm in diameter (123). The drawbacks of these techniques are that the yield of GUV is no more than 20%, and that the vesicle size distribution is broad (128).

5.2.1 The electroformation method

A useful technique to generate giant liposomes consists of hydration of the dried lipid films above the phase transition temperature in the presence of electric fields, yielding about 95% GUV with a relatively narrow size distribution (5–60 μm) in a reasonable period of time (60–90 min) (127, 129) (Protocol 15). This method requires a special chamber and a simple function generator. The total cost of the equipment is relatively low. Figure 7 shows a Teflon chamber, with the same dimensions as a microscope slide on the bottom, designed to be used in an inverted microscope (130–132). Air objectives with long working distances are recommended to avoid a temperature gradient through the objective. Such gradients can easily damage the microscope objectives when working at high temperatures.

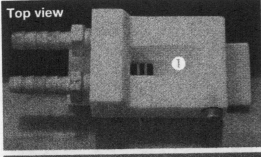

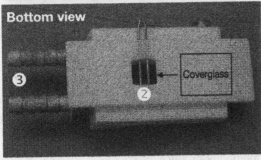

① water container
② Pt wires
③ water bath circulation

Figure 7 Chamber for GUV formation. The chamber contains two main parts, the liposome formation chamber that contains Pt wires and the water circulation part that allows temperature control (from 5–80 °C) by circulating water inside the body of the unit. A coverglass is attached to seal the part that contains the Pt wires, using vacuum grease or epoxy glue, making it possible to visualize the liposomes (lower panel). The Pt wires have a diameter of 1 mm, the centre-to-centre separation between the wires is 3 mm, and the distance from the bottom of the chamber to the centre of the Pt wires is minimal.

Protocol 15

Preparation of giant unilamellar liposomes (GUV)

Equipment and reagents

- Liposome formation chamber
- Inverted phase contrast microscope, preferably with a CCD colour video camera (CCD-Iris, Sony)
- Lyophilizer or vacuum oven
- A phospholipid stock solution of 0.2 mg/ml in chloroform[a]

Method

1 Spread approx. 2 μl of the lipid stock solution, drop to drop, on each Pt wire with a Hamilton syringe under a nitrogen stream. Excess of lipid can cause high incidence of multilamellar vesicles.

2 Introduce the chamber into a lyophilizer or vacuum oven under high vacuum for 30 min to remove traces of organic solvent.

3 Attach the coverglass to the bottom of the chamber.

4 Put the chamber on the microscope and connect the water-bath to the chamber. Attach a thermocouple close to the Pt wires. Wait a few minutes until the chamber warms up.

5 Place water (Millipore water 17.5 MΩ/cm), previously heated to the desired temperature, into the chamber (the water temperature must be above the lipid mixture phase transition). Immediately connect the Pt wires to a low frequency AC field function (sinusoidal wave function with a frequency of 10 Hz and an amplitude of 3 V) for 90 min.

6 Monitor liposome formation via the microscope (preferably phase contrast). A CCD video camera may be used to follow liposome growth and to select one liposome for further observation.

7 Once vesicle formation is achieved, turn off the AC field. Note that the liposomes remain adsorbed to the Pt wires, allowing long-term observation of a single GUV.

[a] Since mainly lipid-like fluorescent probes are used in the experiments, the desired amount of fluorescent molecule is pre-mixed with the lipid stocks (0.25 mol%). However, the alternative approach of addition of the fluorescent molecules in very small volumes of organic solvents (such as DMSO or DMF) after vesicle formation do not produce differences in the final results (130–132).

The 'sectioning effect' of the two-photon excitation microscope allows one to easily distinguish the unilamellar from the multilamellar liposomes. To check lamellarity, up to 20 fluorescently-labelled vesicles in different regions of the Pt wires are imaged at the equatorial region using the two-photon excitation microscope. The fluorescent intensity obtained in pixels that contain the membrane is proportional to the number of bilayers in the giant vesicles. The existence of multilamellar liposomes would give rise to different intensity values due to the presence of different numbers of labelled lipid bilayers (131, 132).

5.3 Two-photon excitation microscopy

Two-photon excitation is a non-linear process in which a fluorophore absorbs two photons simultaneously. Each photon provides half the energy required for excitation. The high photon densities required for two-photon absorption are achieved by focusing a high peak power laser light source on a diffraction-limited spot through a high numerical aperture objective (133). Therefore, in the areas above and below the focal plane, two-photon absorption does not occur, because of insufficient photon flux. This phenomenon allows a sectioning effect that allows observation of the liposome surface, without background contributions (which is essential to observe the formation of lipid domains), and without using emission pin-holes as in conventional one-photon confocal microscopy. An important advantage of two-photon excitation is the low extent of photobleaching and photodamage above and below the focal plane. One-photon excitation has dramatic photobleaching effects on 6-lauroyl-2-(*N*,*N*-dimethylamino) naphthalene (LAURDAN) fluorescence (T. Parasassi, L. Bagatolli, and E. Gratton, unpublished). Using two-photon excitation, however, a LAURDAN-labelled giant vesicle can be imaged for hours. Another advantage is that one wavelength can be used to excite many different fluorescent molecules simultaneously, without changing the excitation wavelength.

5.3.1 Experimental apparatus for two-photon excitation fluorescence microscopy measurements

A scanning two-photon fluorescence microscope is employed for these measurements (134). An LD-Achroplan 20X long working distance air objective (Zeiss, Holmdale, NJ) with a numerical aperature (N.A.) of 0.4 is used to observe the giant liposomes. Although the N.A. of this objective is not so high (the higher the N.A. of the objective the higher the efficiency of two-photon excitation), it circumvents the problem of high temperature in the chamber. The excitation wavelength is set to 780 nm. The laser power is attenuated to 50 mW before the light enters the microscope through a polarizer. The fluorescence emission is observed through a broad bandpass filter from 350 nm to 600 nm (BG39 filter; Chroma Technology, Inc., Brattleboro, VT). Miniature photomultipliers (R5600-P, Hamamatsu, Brigdewater, NJ) are used for light detection in the photon counting mode. The scanning rate is controlled by the input signal of a home-built computer card and a frame rate of 5 s^{-1} is used to acquire the images (256 × 256 pixels). The pixel size corresponds to 0.52 μm.

5.3.2 Fluorescent probes

Lipid domain coexistence has been observed with fluorescent molecules that partition differently between the ordered and disordered phases (118, 119, 131, 132, 135). LAURDAN (Figure 8) is a polarity-sensitive molecule that displays homogeneous partition between the ordered and disordered lipid domains, providing information on the local physical characteristics of the lipid domain together with the lipid domain morphology (136, 137). This family of probes also includes 6-propionyl-2-(*N*,*N*-dimethylamino) naphthalene (PRODAN) and 2'-(*N*,*N*-dimethylamino)-6-naphthoyl-4-*trans*-cyclohexanoic acid (DANCA). These probes all possess large excited state dipoles. In polar solvents, and when the molecular dynamics of solvent dipoles occur on a time scale of the probe's fluorescence lifetime, a reorientation of solvent dipoles around the probe excited state dipole may occur. The energy required for this reorientation results in a red shift of the fluorescence emission spectrum (138). LAURDAN's emission and excitation spectra are sensitive to the packing of lipid molecules and thus to their phase state. At the lipid phase transition LAURDAN's emission spectrum shows a continuous red shift with no isoemissive point, and its excitation maximum changes (111, 138, 139). During the phospholipid phase transition (gel → fluid) a continuous red shift of LAURDAN's emission spectrum is observed, and is attributed to the reorientation of water molecules at the lipid interface near LAURDAN's fluorescent

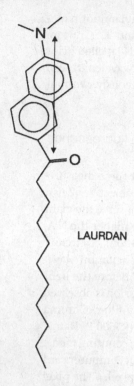

Figure 8 The structure of 6-lauroyl-2-(N,N-dimethylamino) naphthalene LAURDAN.

LAURDAN

moiety (140). Water molecules penetrate into the phospholipid interface during the main phase transition. To reorient with respect to LAURDAN's excited state dipole, the rotational dynamics of these water molecules must occur in the same time scale as LAURDAN's fluorescence lifetime (3–4 ns). Part of LAURDAN's excited state energy is utilized for the reorientation of the water dipoles causing an emission red shift (138).

The 50 nm emission shift of LAURDAN from the gel to the fluid phase together with the homogeneous partition between the coexisting lipid phases allows one to distinguish between the ordered (blue fluorescence) and disordered (green fluorescence) lipid phases from the fluorescent intensity images (130–132, 141). Another way to quantify the extent of water dipolar relaxation in lipid interfaces is based on the relationship between the emission intensities obtained in the blue and red side of the emission spectrum. This relationship, called Generalized Polarization (GP), was defined analogous to the fluorescence polarization function as:

$$GP = (I_B - I_R) / (I_B + I_R)$$

where the intensities at the blue and red edges of the emission spectrum are designated I_B and I_R, respectively (138, 140). GP images can be obtained from the intensity images obtained with blue and green bandpass filters on the microscope, allowing characterization of the coexisting lipid phases, for domains equal to or bigger than the resolution of the microscope, approx 0.3 μm (130–132, 141, 142). The images must be obtained at the equatorial region of the GUVs to avoid artefacts arising from the photoselection effect because of the particular locations of the LAURDAN probe in the lipid bilayer.

5.3.3 The photoselection effect

The parallel orientation of LAURDAN excited state dipole to the lipid molecules in the bilayer offers an extra advantage to ascertain lipid phase coexistence from the fluorescent images using the photoselection effect (130–132, 142). In the

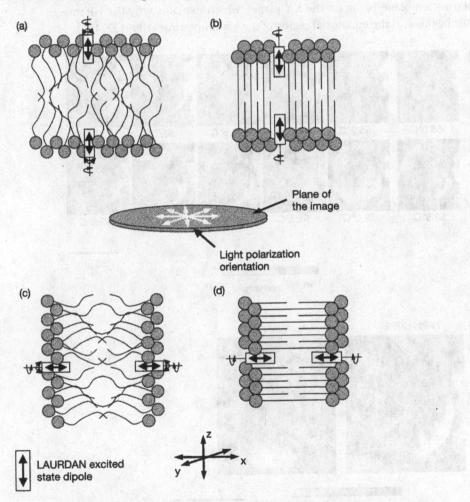

Figure 9 Sketch of LAURDAN's orientation on the lipid bilayer with respect to the polarization plane of the excitation light. (A) Fluid phase (loose packed) bilayer observed at the polar region, and (C) in the equatorial region of GUV. Green emission is observed in both cases; the emission intensity is lower in (A) relative to (C) because of the photoselection effect. (B) Gel phase bilayer observed at the polar region, and (D) in the equatorial region. In this case only blue emission is observed in D (being zero in B) because of the photoselection effect. To obtain the GP images the total emission intensity from both phases is necessary (C and D).

photoselection effect only those fluorophores that are aligned parallel or nearly so, to the plane of polarization of the excitation light become excited. Using circularly polarized light, only fluorescence coming from the fluid part at the polar region of the GUV is observed (Figure 9). In this last case, a component of LAURDAN's transition dipole is always parallel to the excitation polarization because of the relatively low lipid order, i.e. the wobbling movement of the LAURDAN molecule increases relative to the gel phase where no fluorescent intensity is observed. This effect is only evident at the polar region of the vesicle where the LAURDAN molecules are located along the Z axis (the excitation light polarization plane being on the X-Y plane), which explains why the GP images must be taken at the equatorial region of the giant liposome (130–132, 143).

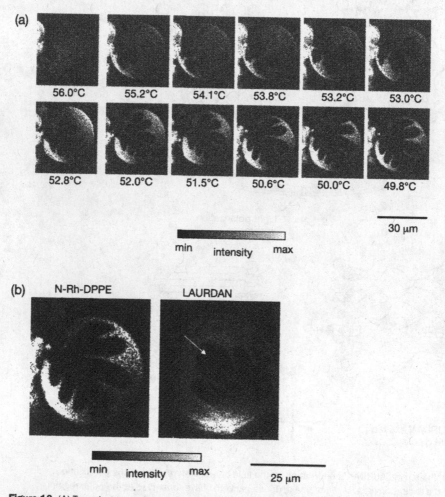

Figure 10 (A) Two-photon excitation fluorescence intensity images of N-Rh-DPPE-labelled GUV composed of DPPE/DPPC 7:3 mol/mol as a function of temperature. (B) Comparison between N-Rh-DPPE- and LAURDAN-labelled GUV composed of DPPE/DPPC 7:3 mol/mol at the phase coexistence temperature region. The images have been taken at the top part of the GUV. The probe concentration was below 0.25 mol% (adapted from ref. 131).

5.4 Visualization of gel/fluid phase coexistence in binary phospholipid mixtures

Temperature-dependent lipid domain formation at the phase coexistence temperature regime of a dipalmitoylphosphatidylcholine (DPPC)/dipalmitoylphosphatidylethanolamine (DPPE) mixture, labelled with lissamine-rhodamine B-1,2-dihexadecanoyl-sn-glycero-3-phosphoethanolamine (N-Rh-DPPE) is shown in Figure 10A. The dark domains correspond to the gel phase (131). The phase state of the lipid domains is ascertained by using the photoselection effect on LAURDAN fluorescence (Figure 10B). LAURDAN is distributed homogeneously in the lipid bilayer but in images obtained at the polar region of the GUV only LAURDAN in the fluid phase is excited. N-Rh-DPPE in this particular binary mixture is segregated from the gel phase and only provides information related to the shape of the lipid domains.

The technique outlined above provides important novel information on the correlation of domain shape with lipid mixture composition, and the lipid domain compositional and energetic differences among different phospholipid mixtures can be extracted directly from fluorescent images. The reader is encouraged to explore refs 141–145 that confirm the advantages of using this experimental approach on different lipid systems, including cholesterol-containing membranes, lipid bilayers composed of natural lipid extracts, and lipid–protein interaction studies.

Acknowledgements

L. A. B.'s research was supported by Fundacion Antorchas (Argentina) and NIH Grant RR03155 (that supports the Laboratory for Fluorescence Dynamics). He would like to thank Dr E. Gratton for his stimulating opinions about the experimental results and his support during L. A. B.'s stay in his laboratory, and Dr D. M. Jameson for critical reading of Section 5. MEMPHY-Center for Biomembrane Physics is supported by the Danish National Research Foundation.

References

1. Nir, S., Bentz, J., Wilschut, J., and Düzgüneş, N. (1983). *Prog. Surf. Sci.*, **13**, 1.
2. Düzgüneş, N. (1985). In *Subcellular biochemistry* (ed. D. B. Roodyn), Vol. 11, p. 195. Plenum Press, New York.
3. Düzgüneş, N. and Nir, S. (1995). In *Liposomes as tools in basic research and industry* (ed. J. R. Philippot and F. Schuber), p. 103. CRC Press, Boca Raton.
4. Düzgüneş, N. (1995). In *Trafficking of intracellular membranes: from molecular sorting to membrane fusion* (ed. M. C. Pedroso de Lima, N. Düzgünes, and D. Hoekstra), p. 97. Springer–Verlag, Berlin.
5. Wilschut, J., Düzgüneş, N., Fraley, R., and Papahadjopoulos, D. (1980). *Biochemistry*, **19**, 6011.
6. Düzgüneş, N. and Wilschut, J. (1993). In *Methods in enzymology* (ed. N. Düzgünes), Vol. 220, p. 3. Academic Press, San Diego.

7. Düzgüneş, N., Wilschut, J., Fraley, R., and Papahadjopoulos, D. (1981). *Biochim. Biophys. Acta*, **642**, 182.

8. Bentz, J., Düzgüneş, N., and Nir, S. (1983). *Biochemistry*, **22**, 3320.

9. Nir, S., Düzgüneş, N., and Bentz, J. (1983). *Biochim. Biophys. Acta*, **735**, 160.

10. Düzgüneş, N., Paiement, J., Freeman, K. B., Lopez, N. G., Wilschut, J., and Papahadjopoulos, D. (1984). *Biochemistry*, **23**, 3486.

11. Bentz, J., Alford, D., Cohen, J., and Düzgüneş, N. (1988). *Biophys. J.*, **53**, 593.

12. Bentz, J. and Düzgüneş, N. (1985). *Biochemistry*, **24**, 5436.

13. Ohki, S. (1984). *J. Membr. Biol.*, **77**, 265.

14. Wilschut, J., Düzgüneş, N., Hoekstra, D., and Papahadjopoulos, D. (1985). *Biochemistry*, **24**, 8.

15. Bentz, J., Düzgüneş, N., and Nir, S. (1985). *Biochemistry*, **24**, 1064.

16. Sundler, R., Düzgüneş, N., and Papahadjopoulos, D. (1981). *Biochim. Biophys. Acta*, **649**, 751.

17. Düzgüneş, N., Hong, K., and Papahadjopoulos, D. (1980). In *Calcium binding proteins: structure and function* (ed. F. L. Siegel, E. Carafoli, R. H. Kretsinger, D. H. MacLennan, and R. H. Wasserman), p. 17. Elsevier/North Holland, New York.

18. Aranda, F. J., Sanchez-Migallon, M. P., and Gomez-Fernandez, J. C. (1996). *Arch. Biochem. Biophys.*, **333**, 394.

19. Shavnin, S. A., Pedroso de Lima, M. C., Fedor, J., Wood, P., Bentz, J., and Düzgüneş, N. (1988). *Biochim. Biophys. Acta*, **946**, 405.

20. Schuber, F., Hong, K., Düzgüneş, N., and Papahadjopoulos, D. (1983). *Biochemistry*, **22**, 6134.

21. Düzgüneş, N., Hoekstra, D., Hong, K., and Papahadjopoulos, D. (1984). *FEBS Lett.*, **173**, 80.

22. Hoekstra, D. and Düzgüneş, N. (1986). *Biochemistry*, **25**, 1321.

23. Hong, K., Düzgüneş, N., and Papahadjopoulos, D. (1981). *J. Biol. Chem.*, **256**, 3641.

24. Hong, K., Düzgüneş, N., Ekerdt, R., and Papahadjopoulos, D. (1982). *Proc. Natl. Acad. Sci. USA*, **79**, 4642.

25. Meers, P., Ernst, J. D., Düzgüneş, N., Hong, K., Fedor, J., Goldstein, I. M., *et al.* (1987). *J. Biol. Chem.*, **262**, 7850.

26. Bartlett, G. R. (1959). *J. Biol. Chem.*, **234**, 466.

27. Ellens, H., Bentz, J., and Szoka, F. C. (1985). *Biochemistry*, **24**, 3099.

28. Düzgüneş, N., Straubinger, R. M., Baldwin, P. A., Friend, D. S., and Papahadjopoulos, D. (1985). *Biochemistry*, **24**, 3091.

29. Parente, R. A. and Lentz, B. R (1986). *Biochemistry*, **25**, 6678.

30. Nieva, J. L., Goni, F. M., and Alonso, A. (1989). *Biochemistry*, **28**, 7364.

31. Luk, A. S., Kaler, E. W., and Lee, S. P. (1993). *Biochemistry*, **32**, 6965.

32. Boesze-Battaglia, K., Lamba, O. P., Napoli, A. A. Jr, Sinha, S., and Guo, Y. (1998). *Biochemistry*, **37**, 9477.

33. Hoekstra, D. and Düzgüneş, N. (1993). In *Methods in enzymology* (ed. N. Düzgüneş), Vol. 220, p. 15. Academic Press, San Diego.

34. Struck, D. K., Hoekstra, D., and Pagano, R. E. (1981). *Biochemistry*, **20**, 4093.

35. Düzgüneş, N., Allen, T. M., Fedor, J., and Papahadjopoulos, D. (1987). *Biochemistry*, **26**, 8435.

36. Rosenberg, J., Düzgüneş, N., and Kayalar, C. (1983). *Biochim. Biophys. Acta*, **735**, 173.

37. van Meer, G., Davoust, J., and Simons, K. (1985). *Biochemistry*, **24**, 3593.

38. Maezawa, S., Yoshimura, T., Hong, K., Düzgüneş, N., and Papahadjopoulos, D. (1989). *Biochemistry*, **28**, 1422.

39. Düzgüneş, N., Goldstein, J. A., Friend, D. S., and Felgner, P. L. (1989). *Biochemistry*, **28**, 9179.

40. Cajal, Y., Boggs, J. M., and Jain, M. K. (1997). *Biochemistry*, **36**, 2566.

144

41. El Baraka, M., Pecheur, E. I., Wallach, D. F., and Philippot, J. R. (1996). *Biochim. Biophys. Acta*, **1280**, 107.

42. Wilschut, J., Scholma, J., Bental, M., Hoekstra, D., and Nir, S. (1985). *Biochim. Biophys. Acta*, **821**, 45.

43. Walter, A. and Siegel, D. P. (1993). *Biochemistry*, **32**, 3271.

44. Driessen, A. J., Hoekstra, D., Scherphof, G., Kalicharan, R. D., and Wilschut, J. (1985). *J. Biol. Chem.*, **260**, 10880.

45. Oshry, L., Meers, P., Mealy, T., and Tauber, A. I. (1991). *Biochim. Biophys. Acta*, **1066**, 239.

46. Meers, P., Ali, S., Erukulla, R., and Janoff, A. S. (2000). *Biochim. Biophys. Acta*, **1467**, 227.

47. Weinstein, J. N., Yoshikami, S., Henkart, P., Blumenthal, R., and Hagins, W. A. (1977). *Science*, **195**, 489.

48. Szoka, F. C. Jr., Jacobson, K., and Papahadjopoulos, D. (1979). *Biochim. Biophys. Acta* **551**, 295.

49. Allen, T. M. and Cleland, L. G. (1980). *Biochim. Biophys. Acta*, **597**, 418.

50. Ralston, E., Hjelmeland, L. M., Klausner, R. D., Weinstein, J. N., and Blumenthal, R. (1981). *Biochim. Biophys. Acta*, **649**, 133.

51. Straubinger, R. M., Hong, K., Friend, D. S., and Papahadjopoulos, D. (1983). *Cell*, **32**, 1069.

52. Straubinger, R. M., Düzgüneş, N., and Papahadjopoulos, D. (1985). *FEBS Lett.*, **179**, 148.

53. Kayalar, C. and Düzgüneş, N. (1986). *Biochim. Biophys. Acta*, **860**, 51.

54. Rapaport, D., Peled, R., Nir, S., and Shai, Y. (1996). *Biophys. J.*, **70**, 2502.

55. Liu, X. Y., Nakamura, C., Yang, Q., and Miyake, J. (2001). *Anal. Biochem.*, **293**, 251.

56. Tian, P., Ball, J. M., Zeng, C. Q., and Estes, M. K. (1996). *J. Virol.*, **70**, 6973.

57. Fan, Q., Relini, A., Cassinadri, D., Gambacorta, A., and Gliozzi, A. (1995). *Biochim. Biophys. Acta*, **1240**, 83.

58. Kono, K., Zenitani, K., and Takagishi, T. (1994). *Biochim. Biophys. Acta*, **1193**, 1.

59. Babbitt, B., Burtis, L., Dentinger, P., Constantinides, P., Hillis, L., McGirl, B., *et al.* (1993). *Bioconjug. Chem.*, **4**, 199.

60. Ellens, H., Bentz, J., and Szoka, F. C. (1984). *Biochemistry*, **23**, 1532.

61. Shiffer, K., Hawgood, S., Düzgüneş, N., and Goerke, J. (1988). *Biochemistry*, **27**, 2689.

62. Chang, R., Nir, S., and Poulain, F. R. (1998). *Biochim. Biophys. Acta*, **1371**, 254.

63. Shiffer, K., Goerke, J., Düzgüneş, N., Fedor, J., and Shohet, S. B. (1988). *Biochim. Biophys. Acta*, **937**, 269.

64. Düzgüneş, N. and Gambale, F. (1988). *FEBS Lett.*, **227**, 110.

65. Düzgüneş, N. and Shavnin, S. A. (1992). *J. Membr. Biol.*, **128**, 71.

66. Nicol, F., Nir, S., and Szoka, F. C. Jr. (2000). *Biophys. J.*, **78**, 818.

67. Hristova, K., Selsted, M. E., and White, S. H. (1997). *J. Biol. Chem.*, **272**, 24224.

68. Alford, D., Renugopalakrishnan, V., and Düzgüneş, N. (1996). *Int. J. Peptide Protein Res.*, **47**, 84.

69. Swairjo, M. A. and Seaton, B. A. (1994). *Annu. Rev. Biophys. Biomol. Struct.*, **23**, 193.

70. Galla, H.-J. and Sackmann, E. (1974). *Biochim. Biophys. Acta*, **339**, 103.

71. Hartmann, W. and Galla, H.-J. (1978). *Biochim. Biophys. Acta*, **509**, 474.

72. Freire, E., Markello, T., Rigell, C., and Holloway, P. (1983). *Biochemistry*, **22**, 1675.

73. Jones, M. E. and Lentz, B. R. (1986). *Biochemistry*, **25**, 567.

74. Meers, P., Daleke, D., Hong, K., and Papahadjopoulos, D. (1991). *Biochemistry*, **30**, 2903.

75. Mayer, L. D., Hope, M. J., and Cullis, P. R. (1986). *Biochim. Biophys. Acta*, **858**, 161.

76. Kingsley, P. B. and Feigenson, G. W. (1979). *Chem. Phys. Lipids*, **24**, 135.

77. Junker, M. and Creutz, C. E. (1993). *Biochemistry*, **32**, 9968.

78. Lakowicz, J. R. (1999). *Principles of fluorescence spectroscopy* (2nd edn). Plenum Press, New York.

79. Meers, P. and Mealy. T. R. (1993). *Biochemistry*, **32**, 5411.

80. Huber, R., Schneider, M., Mayr, I., Romisch, J., and Paques, E.-P. (1990). *FEBS Lett.*, **275**, 15.

81. Huber, R., Berendes, R., Burger, A., Schneider, M., Karshikov, A., Luecke, H., *et al.* (1992). *J. Mol. Biol.*, **223**, 683.

82. Concha, N. O., Head, J. F., Kaetzel, M. A., Dedman, J. R., and Seaton, B. A. (1993). *Science*, **261**, 1321.

83. Meers, P. (1990). *Biochemistry*, **29**, 3325.

84. Chattopadhyay, A. and London, E. (1987). *Biochemistry*, **26**, 39.

85. Markello, T., Zlotnick, A., Everett, J., Tennyson, J., and Holloway, P. W. (1985). *Biochemistry*, **24**, 2895.

86. Kaiser, R. D. and London, E. (1998). *Biochemistry*, **37**, 8180.

87. Fleming, P. J., Koppel, D. E., Lau, A. L. Y., and Strittmatter, P. (1979). *Biochemistry*, **18**, 5458.

88. Junker, M. and Creutz, C. E. (1994). *Biochemistry*, **33**, 8930.

89. Wimley, W. C. and White, S. H. (2000). *Biochemistry*, **39**, 161.

90. Wang, Y., Kachel, K., Pablo, L., and London, E. (1997). *Biochemistry*, **36**, 16300.

91. Chapman, E. R. and Davis, A. F. (1998). *J. Biol. Chem.*, **273**, 13995.

92. Kano, K. and Fendler, J. H. (1978). *Biochim. Biophys. Acta*, **509**, 289.

93. Biegel, C. M. and Gould, J. M. (1981). *Biochemistry*, **20**, 3474.

94. Straubinger, R. M., Lopez, N. G., Debs, R., Hong, K., and Papahadjopoulos, D. (1988). *Cancer Res.*, **48**, 5237.

95. Daleke, D. L., Hong, K., and Papahadjopoulos, D. (1990). *Biochim. Biophys. Acta*, **1024**, 352.

96. Straubinger, R. M., Papahadjopoulos, D., and Hong, K. (1990). *Biochemistry*, **29**, 4929.

97. Lee, K.-D., Hong, K., Nir, S., and Papahadjopoulos, D. (1993). *Biochemistry*, **32**, 889.

98. Miller, C. R., Bondurant, B., McLean, S. D., McGovern, K. A., and O'Brien, D. F. (1998). *Biochemistry*, **37**, 12875.

99. Ohkuma, S. and Poole, B. (1978). *Proc. Natl. Acad. Sci. USA*, **75**, 3327.

100. Murphy, R. F., Powers, S., and Cantor, C. R. (1984). *J. Cell Biol.*, **98**, 1757.

101. Maxfield, F. R. (1989). In *Methods in enzymology* (ed. S. Fleisher and B. Fleisher), Vol. 173, p. 745. Academic Press, San Diego.

102. Oh, Y.-K. and Straubinger, R. M. (1996). *Infect. Immun.*, **64**, 319.

103. Oh, Y.-K. and Straubinger, R. M. (1993). *Pharm. Res.*, **10**, S191.

104. Lee, R. J., Wang, S., and Low, P. S. (1996). *Biochim. Biophys. Acta*, **1312**, 237.

105. Downey, G. P., Botelho, R. J., Butler, J. R., Moltyaner, Y., Chien, P., Schreiber, A. D., *et al.* (1999). *J. Biol. Chem.*, **274**, 28436.

106. Lentz, B. R., Barenholz, Y., and Thompson, T. E. (1976). *Biochemistry*, **15**, 4529.

107. Mabrey, S. and Sturtevant, J. M. (1976). *Proc. Natl. Acad. Sci. USA*, **73**, 3862.

108. Van Dijck, P. W. M., Kaper, A. J., Oonk, H. A. J., and De Gier, J. (1977). *Biochim. Biophys. Acta*, **470**, 58.

109. Shimshick, E. J. and McConnell, H. M. (1973). *Biochemistry*, **12**, 2351.

110. Maggio, B., Fidelio, G. D., Cumar, F. A., and Yu, R. K. (1986). *Chem. Phys. Lipids*, **42**, 49.

111. Bagatolli, L., Maggio, B., Aguilar, F., Sotomayor, C. P., and Fidelio, G. D. (1997). *Biochim. Biophys. Acta*, **1325**, 80.

112. Sackmann, E. and Feder, T. (1995). *Mol. Membr. Biol.*, **12**, 21.

113. Vaz, W. L. C., Melo, E. C. C., and Thompson, T. E. (1989). *Biophys. J.*, **56**, 869.

114. Schram, V., Lin, H. N., and Thompson, T. E. (1996). *Biophys. J.*, **71**, 1811.

115. Simons, K. and Ikonen, E. (1997). *Nature*, **387**, 569.

116. Jacobson, K. and Dietrich, C. (1999). *Curr. Opin. Cell Biol.*, **9**, 84.

117. Brown, D. A. and London, E. (1998). *Annu. Rev. Cell Dev. Biol.*, **14**, 111.

118. Weis, R. M. and McConnell, H. M. (1984). *Nature*, **310**, 47.

119. Möhwald, H., Dietrich, A., Böhm, C., Brezesindki, G., and Thoma, M. (1995). *Mol. Membr. Biol.*, **12**, 29.

120. Sackmann, E. (1978). *Ber. Bunsenges. Phys. Chem.*, **82**, 891.

121. Menger, F. M. and Keiper, J. S. (1998). *Curr. Opin. Chem. Biol.*, **2**, 726.

122. Haverstick, D. M. and Glaser, M. (1987). *Proc. Natl. Acad. Sci. USA*, **84**, 4475.

123. Moscho, A., Orwar, O., Chiu, D. T., Modi, B. P., and Zare, R. N. (1996). *Proc. Natl. Acad. Sci. USA*, **93**, 11443.

124. Reeves, J. P. and Dowben, R. M. (1969). *J. Cell. Physiol.*, **73**, 49.

125. Käs, J. and Sackmann, E. (1991). *Biophys. J.*, **60**, 825.

126. Akashi, K., Miyata, H., Itoh, H., and Kinosita, K. Jr. (1996). *Biophys. J.*, **71**, 3242.

127. Angelova, M. I. and Dimitrov, D. S. (1988). *Progr. Colloid Polym. Sci.*, **76**, 59.

128. Bagatolli, L. A., Parasassi, T., and Gratton, E. (2000). *Chem. Phys. Lipids*, **105**, 135.

129. Mathivet, L., Cribier, S., and Devaux, P. F. (1996). *Biophys. J.*, **70**, 1112.

130. Bagatolli, L. A. and Gratton, E. (1999). *Biophys. J.*, **77**, 2090.

131. Bagatolli, L. A. and Gratton, E. (2000). *Biophys. J.*, **78**, 290.

132. Bagatolli, L. A. and Gratton, E. (2000). *Biophys. J.*, **79**, 434.

133. Denk, W., Strickler, J. H., and Webb, W. W. (1990). *Science*, **248**, 73.

134. So, P. T. C., French, T., Yu, W. M., Berland, K. M., Dong, C. Y., and Gratton, E. (1996). In *Chemical analysis series*, Vol. 137 (ed. X. F. Wang and B. Herman), p. 351. John Wiley and Sons, New York.

135. Korlach, J., Schwille, P., Webb, W. W., and Feigenson, G. W. (1999). *Proc. Natl. Acad. Sci. USA*, **96**, 8461.

136. Weber, G. and Farris, F. J. (1979). *Biochemistry*, **18**, 3075.

137. Parasassi, T., Conti, F., and Gratton, E. (1986). *Cell. Mol. Biol.*, **32**, 103.

138. Parasassi, T., Krasnowska, E., Bagatolli, L. A., and Gratton, E. (1998). *J. Fluoresc.*, **8**, 365.

139. Bagatolli, L. A., Gratton, E., and Fidelio, G. D. (1998). *Biophys. J.*, **75**, 331.

140. Parasassi, T., De Stasio, G., Ravagnan, G., Rusch, R. M., and Gratton, E. (1991). *Biophys. J.*, **60**, 179.

141. Dietrich, C., Bagatolli, L. A., Volovyk, Z., Thompson, N. L., Levi, M., Jacobson, K., *et al.* (2001). *Biophys. J.*, **80**, 1417.

142. Parasassi, T., Gratton, E., Yu, W., Wilson, P., and Levi, M. (1997). *Biophys. J.*, **72**, 2413.

143. Nag, K., Pao, J. S., Harbottle, R. R., Possmayer, F., Petersen, N. O., and Bagatolli, L. A. (2002). *Biophys. J.*, **82**, 2041.

144. Sanchez, S., Bagatolli, L. A., Gratton, E., and Hazlett, T. (2002). *Biophys. J.* **82**, 2232.

145. Bagatolli, L. A., and Gratton, E. (2001). *J. Fluoresc.*, **11**, 141.

Chapter 5
Stability, storage, and sterilization of liposomes[1]

Nicolaas Jan Zuidam
Present address: Unilever Research & Development, Vlaardingen, The Netherlands.

Ewoud van Winden
Regulon, Athens, Greece.

Remco de Vrueh
OctoPlus Technologies, Leiden, The Netherlands.

Daan J. A. Crommelin
OctoPlus Technologies, Leiden, The Netherlands; and Department of Pharmaceutics, Utrecht Institute for Pharmaceutical Sciences, Utrecht University, The Netherlands.

1 Introduction

During the preparation process or upon storage liposomes may undergo chemical degradation or physical changes. In this chapter, the types of degradation, the consequences, and measures of prevention or minimization are discussed. Methods to establish the degree of degradation are presented in Chapter 2. Most of the relevant data on liposome stability published in the public domain was collected with bilayers based on phosphatidylcholine, phosphatidylglycerol, and phosphatidylethanolamine often in combination with cholesterol. Therefore, our conclusions are particularly relevant for liposomes composed of those lipids. A number of review articles/chapters dealing with liposome stability issues have been published by our group (1–5).

2 Prevention of chemical degradation

2.1 Phospholipid oxidation

Even in the absence of specific oxidants, the fatty acid chains of phospholipids can be oxidized. It occurs via a free radical chain mechanism. The initiation step is the

---

[1] Major parts of the text and figures of this chapter were taken from the first edition of 'Liposomes: a practical approach', edited by R. R. C. New.

abstraction of a hydrogen atom from the lipid chain, which can be catalysed by trace amounts of transition metal ions, radiation, or sonication. Although any lipid can form radicals by this mechanism, the most susceptible to oxidation are lipids containing double bonds. The higher the level of unsaturation, the more susceptible they are. In the presence of oxygen, the process can develop further, e.g. by formation of aldehydes, chain scissions, and formation of lipid hydro-peroxides (see Figure 1). In natural phospholipids, which contain multiple unsaturations, rearrangements of non-conjugated double bonds into conjugated ones might occur upon oxidation (see Figure 2). In the absence of oxygen, this rearrangement can take place without the appearance of any peroxides. Most oxidation products are subject to further degradation. To monitor oxidative lipid degradation, one might consider measuring one or more stages in the oxidation process, i.e. conjugation of isolated double bonds, formation of peroxides and aldehydes, and chain scission. In Chapter 2 analytical methodology for these stages in the oxidation process are presented.

The head group of phospholipids may be subject to oxidation as well. TLC analysis based on separation of phospholipids according to differences in head group shows the appearance of several spots upon gamma irradiation of aqueous liposome dispersions. Some of the structures of these degradation products have been elucidated by TLC/fast atom bombardment mass spectrometry (6).

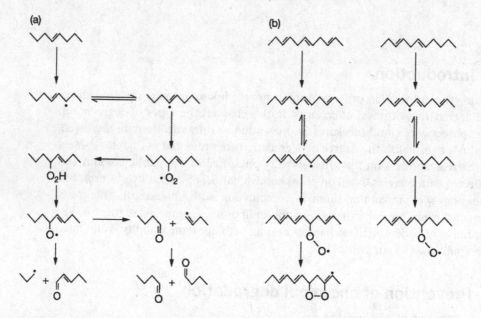

Figure 1 Lipid oxidation. (a) Radical abstraction in fatty acids with an isolated double bond, showing some of the chain-breaking reactions which can occur upon exposure to oxygen. (b) Formation of peroxides in polyunsaturated fatty acid chains. Di-unsaturated acids are less likely to form cyclic peroxides than tri-unsaturates, since rearrangements giving the di-oxygen radical adjacent to a $-CH_2-CH=CH-$ group in di-unsaturates can only take place if the opportunity to form conjugated dienes by abstraction is sacrificed.

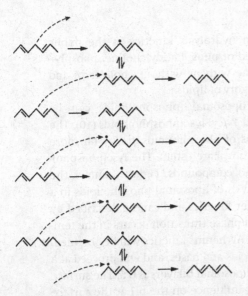

Figure 2 Rearrangement of double bonds by radical abstraction. After a hydrogen atom has been removed from a methylene group in between two double bonds, the radical species thus formed is stabilized by delocalization of the free electron over the five carbons encompassing those two unsaturations. This species can itself abstract a hydrogen atom from adjacent lipid molecules, to continue the chain reaction, but the hydrogen will return to a different carbon in the chain from the one that left, so that the double bonds can end up adjacent to each other (that is, conjugated—a configuration energetically more favourable than being isolated from each other by a methylene group). Note that this process can take place without the participation of oxygen.

One of the consequences of lipid oxidation is an increase in the permeability of bilayers (7, 8). Not much is known about the impact of oxidation on liposome behaviour and safety *in vivo* (9).

Oxidation of liposomal lipids can be minimized by taking the following precautions:

(a) Use high quality lipids purified from hydroperoxides and transition metals.

(b) Use (partially) hydrogenated, natural phospholipids or entirely synthetic saturated ones such as DMPC, DPPC, or DSPC.

(c) Use freshly distilled and deoxygenated solvents.

(d) Avoid procedures which involve high temperatures or sonication.

(e) Carry out the liposomal preparation process in the absence of oxygen.

(f) Use an antioxidant (such as α-tocopherol, butyl hydroxytoluene, or vitamin C) and/or a transition metal ion chelator (such as EDTA or desferal).

(g) Store liposomes at low temperatures, at low oxygen pressure, and protected from light.

151

2.2 Hydrolysis of phospholipids

Here again, most detailed information on hydrolysis kinetics in the public domain is available for liposomes composed of phosphatidylcholine, phosphatidylglycerol, and phosphatidylethanolamine with or without cholesterol and our comments specifically apply to that category of lipids.

In an aqueous liposome dispersion, liposomal (phospho)lipids can be hydrolysed to free fatty acids and 2-acyl- and 1-acyl-lyso(phospho)lipids (10). The carboxy esters at the *sn*-1 and *sn*-2 positions of phospholipids are by far more sensitive to chemical hydrolysis than the phosphate esters. The lyso(phospho)-lipids hydrolyse further to glycero phospho compounds. Figure 3 shows the hydrolysis scheme of phospholipids. Hydrolysis of liposomal phospholipids in a buffered dispersion follows pseudo-first order kinetics and can be described by Arrhenius kinetics. However, if a major lipid phase transition occurs in the temperature range under investigation, biphasic Arrhenius kinetics will be obtained. Hydrolysis of phospholipids is catalysed by acids and bases, and will proceed at a minimal rate when the pH at the surface of liposomal bilayers is 6.5. The surface potential of charged bilayers has a dramatic influence on the pH at the surface

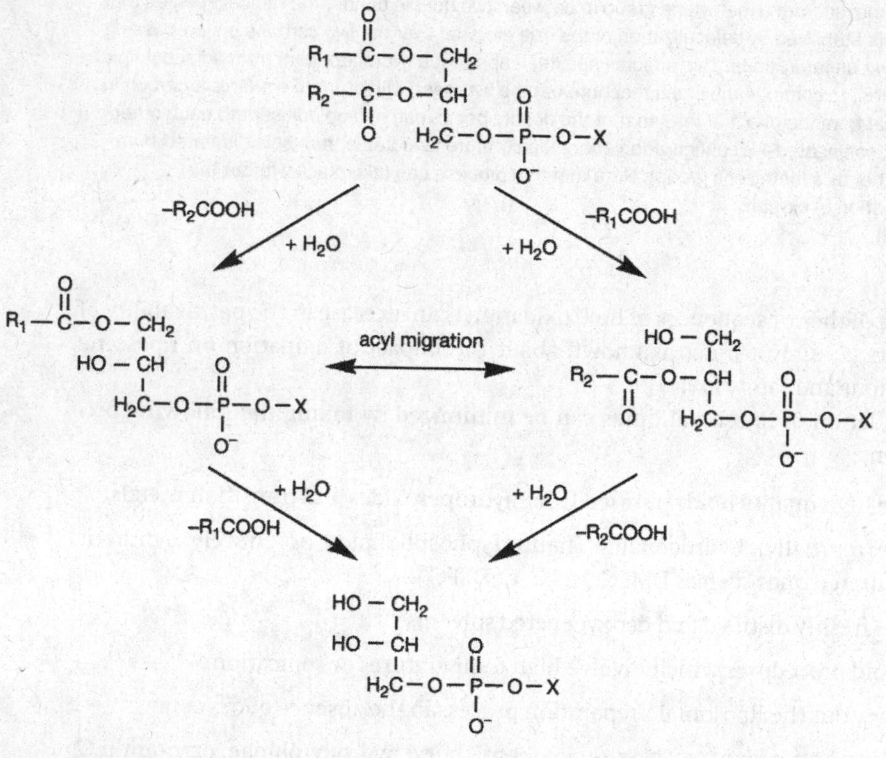

Figure 3 Hydrolysis reactions of a phospholipid in an aqueous environment results in both isomers of its lysophospholipid form. These compounds are intermediates, and hydrolyse further to water soluble glycero phospho compounds. X is the head group (e.g. choline, glycerol, or a proton), and R_1 and R_2 are hydrocarbon moieties of fatty acids.

(pH$_{surface} \neq$ pH$_{bulk}$), and therefore on the hydrolysis kinetics of phospholipids (11, 12). The influence of the physical state of the bilayers is less dramatic, although at low temperatures it may become significant. The hydrolysis rates of bilayers at 4 °C and at pH 4.0 increase in the order DSPC < DPPC < EPC $\cong$ DMPC $\cong$ DPPC/Chol 10/4. However, no such differences could be found at 20 °C or 30 °C (12). Charged buffer species may induce a slight increase in hydrolysis rate (10). The presence of α-tocopherol, cryoprotectants, or salts does not influence the hydrolysis of phospholipids in neutral liposomes at pH 4.0 and 30 °C (12).

Upon chemical hydrolysis of phospholipids in bilayers in aqueous dispersions several physical changes may occur:

(a) Liposomal bilayers become less permeable for water soluble, non-bilayer interacting marker molecules such as carboxyfluorescein up to 10% hydrolysis of bilayer phospholipids, and more permeable above that degree of hydrolysis (13).

(b) The phospholipid configuration converts from a bilayer into a micellar one, if the liposomes pass through the gel-to-liquid phase transition, and if the degree of chemical hydrolysis exceeds a critical value which depends on the type of phospholipid(s) (14).

(c) Liposome size increases and the size distribution curve widens up above about 40% hydrolysis (14).

(d) Melting characteristics of bilayers are affected in a pH-dependent manner (15, 16).

Hydrolysis of phosphatidylcholine-based liposomes can be minimized by taking the following precautions:

(a) Design the liposomal formulation in such a way that the pH at the surface of the bilayers is about 6.5.

(b) Limit the (charged) buffer concentration.

(c) If possible, compose the liposomal bilayers of 100% pure phospholipids with long, saturated, acyl chain phospholipids, such as DSPC or hydrogenated, natural phospholipids.

(d) Avoid manufacture procedures which involve high temperatures.

(e) Store liposomes at a low temperature (4 °C) or in a freeze-dried form (see Section 4).

Another method to avoid acyl chain hydrolysis altogether might be the use of bilayer forming non-ionic surfactants containing ether links between the polar head group and acyl chain(s) (e.g. niosomes). Vesicles containing these ether lipid amphiphiles may offer advantages when used for non-parenteral purposes, e.g. for dermatological applications. However, for parenteral use much less safety data are available than for phosphatidylcholine-based liposomes.

3 Prevention of physical changes

Liposomal aggregation, bilayer fusion, and drug leakage affect the shelf-life of liposomes. Aggregation is the formation of larger units composed of individual liposomes. This process is reversible by for example, applying mild shear forces, changing the temperature, or by binding metal ions that initially induced aggregation. Fusion of bilayers, however, is irreversible and consequently new liposomal structures are formed. In contrast to aggregation, fusion of liposomes may induce drug leakage, in particular when the encapsulated drug is water soluble and does not interact with the bilayer. In general, properly made, large liposomes do not fuse with time (14). However, bilayer defects may enhance fusion. These irregularities may disappear by a process termed 'annealing': incubating the liposomes at a temperature above the phase transition to allow differences in packing density between opposite sides of the bilayer leaflets to equalize by transmembrane 'flip-flop'. Bilayer defects can also be induced during a phase transition, so it is recommended to handle and store aqueous liposome dispersions at a temperature well above or below the phase transition temperature range. Alternatively, one could include a sufficient amount of cholesterol in the membrane (up to about an equimolar content to the phospholipids) to reduce or completely annihilate the bilayer phase transition process. Bilayer defects may also be induced by freezing (see Section 4 of this chapter). Size effects play a role in the tendency to aggregate as well. Very small (<<100 nm) liposomes are more prone to fusion than larger liposomes due to stress coming from the high curvature of their membrane.

Drug leakage depends both on the liposome composition and on the drug characteristics. Large polar or ionic, water soluble drugs will be retained much more effectively than low molecular weight, amphiphilic compounds. In general, membranes composed of saturated phospholipids (with acyl chains of $C \geq 16$) and/or membranes which contain a sufficient fraction of cholesterol are the least permeable ones. However, these rigid bilayers may be undesirable for use *in vivo*, because release of encapsulated drug *in vivo* may be too slow. Drug leakage of water soluble drugs is also enhanced by bilayer defects (see above).

Charged drug compounds may interact with oppositely charged bilayers (e.g. positively charged basic drugs interacting with phosphatidylglycerol containing bilayers). This interaction increases liposome encapsulation efficiency compared to compounds that show no bilayer interaction and slows down drug release. Drug leakage may also be minimized by forming a complex of the (charged) drug inside the liposomes (e.g. complex of doxorubicin with sulfate) (17).

Lipophilic compounds may phase separate in or from the liposomal bilayers with time or upon storage at a low temperature, and phase separated material can be found within the dispersion (this material can be observed for example, with a light microscope). Incorporation of larger amounts of lipophilic compounds into liposomal bilayers during liposome preparation (supersaturation) may lead to low entrapment efficiencies in the final product, which can be explained by a higher chance of the occurrence of phase separation.

Physical changes in liposome dispersions can be minimized by taking the following precautions:

(a) Design the manufacture procedure of the liposomes in such a way that the bilayers are free of local defects (if necessary through 'annealing').

(b) Avoid compositions of liposomes which have a phase transition at manufacturing and/or storage conditions such as 100% DMPC.

(c) Use a transition metal ion chelator (such as EDTA or desferal).

(d) If leakage of a water soluble drug is a problem, select phospholipid(s) with saturated acyl chains (e.g. DPPC or hydrogenated soybean PC) and/or cholesterol to compose the liposomes.

(e) Alternatively, drug leakage can be minimized by increasing the affinity between the drug and the bilayer through electrostatic interaction or through derivatization of the drug.

(f) Stabilize the liposomes against aggregation or fusion by including a small fraction of negatively charged lipids in the bilayer, e.g. 10% PG or cholesterol hemisuccinate (CHEMS), or attach to the bilayers synthetic hydrophilic polymers such as poly(ethylene glycol) (PEG).

(g) Avoid freezing of liposomes in the absence of cryoprotectants (see Section 4).

(h) Store liposomes at low temperatures or in a (by cryoprotectants) stabilized freeze-dried form (see Section 4).

4 Freeze-drying of liposomes

4.1 Introduction

Application of the freeze-drying (or lyophilization) technique to improve the storage stability of liposomes is mainly based on two considerations:

(a) Removal of water prevents hydrolysis of phospholipids.

(b) Other chemical and physical degradation processes are retarded by a low molecular mobility in the solid phase.

Unfortunately, liposomes may also be damaged by the freeze-drying process itself. Freeze-drying and rehydration of liposomes without protective agents (called lyoprotectants) results in fusion and aggregation of liposomes, and extensive leakage of an entrapped water soluble compound upon rehydration. However, if MLVs are the liposome type aimed for, and if the drug interacts with the bilayers, freeze-drying of just the lipids and the drug from, e.g. a butanol solution, may be an attractive option. However, in most other cases, the protection of liposomes during the freeze-drying process is necessary. Both the design of the liposome formulation and the freeze-drying process determine whether the freeze-dried liposomes can be easily rehydrated with preservation of their properties (size, % encapsulated compound). For more extensive literature the reader is referred to refs 3, 18, and 19, and references therein.

4.2 Important factors for freeze-drying of liposomes

4.2.1 Addition of a lyoprotectant

A schematic presentation of the processes that occur during freeze-drying is given in Figure 4. Lyoprotectants (e.g. disaccharides) exert their effect via one or more of the following mechanisms:

(a) Glass formation. This provides an amorphous matrix between the vesicles which prevents fusion or bilayer damage by crystal formation.

(b) Interaction with the phospholipids. The hydroxyl groups of the sugar molecules form hydrogen bonds with the phosphate moiety of the phospholipid head groups in the dry state, and thus replace water ('water substitution theory').

Although substantial evidence has appeared in the literature for both mechanisms, the factors involved in lyoprotection are still subject of ongoing research, and for details the reader is referred elsewhere (e.g. 3, 18, 20). In order to be optimally effective, the lyoprotectant should be present both in- and outside the liposomes. Moreover, the concentration of lyoprotectant and encapsulated compound should be chosen such that the intra- and extra-liposomal media have the same osmolarity. The sugar/phospholipid ratio that is required for the full protective action depends on the lyoprotectant involved. Generally, optimal protection can be achieved when amorphous sugar is present at ratios above, e.g. 2 g sugar/g phospholipid. The total solute concentration should be at least about 2.5% (w/v) in order to obtain a proper cake after freeze-drying.

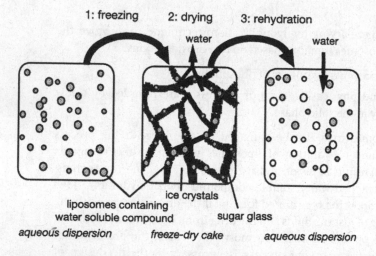

Figure 4 Freeze-drying/rehydration cycle of liposomes. During freezing ice crystals are formed with a concentrate of the remaining solutes (lyoprotectant (sugar), buffer components) and the liposomes. In the drying stage, the ice is sublimated and the water content in the remaining amorphous, porous structure is reduced. The sugar glass protects the liposomes against damage by crystal formation and fusion processes (see text).

4.2.2 Selection of a lyoprotectant

Disaccharides, such as sucrose, lactose, and trehalose, are currently the most preferred lyoprotectants. A monosaccharide, such as glucose or sorbitol, or high concentrations of other excipients with a low MW, such as amino acids and inorganic salts, should be avoided, because of their low glass transition and collapse temperature in the frozen state (see below). The use of the high MW polyol dextran was reported to provide sufficient protection for dipalmitoyl-phosphatidylcholine (DPPC) liposomes, but not for egg phosphatidylcholine (EPC) liposomes (21). This effect was ascribed to a poor interaction between dextran and the phospholipids. This interaction is especially required to protect EPC liposomes during the freeze-drying and rehydration process. The use of excipients that crystallize during the freezing process and form porous cakes, such as mannitol, has not been described in the literature on freeze-dried liposome formulations

4.2.3 Selection of vesicle size

Until now, high retention of a water soluble, non-bilayer interacting encapsulated compound (>80%) has only been reported for SUVs of c. 0.1 μm. Both smaller and larger liposomes show a more pronounced leakage upon rehydration, even if freeze-dried in the presence of a lyoprotectant. The reason for this is not fully clear, and this subject is discussed elsewhere (3, 19).

4.2.4 Avoid quick cooling

Slow cooling (0.5 °C/min) of lyoprotected, 0.1 μm liposomes resulted in a higher retention of the encapsulated water soluble marker carboxyfluorescein after freeze-drying and rehydration than after quick cooling by submerging the samples in boiling nitrogen (22). This effect of cooling protocol depended on the rigidity of the liposomes. The damage caused by quick cooling was most pronounced for rigid liposomes (e.g. liposomes consisting of DPPC, without cholesterol), but was not observed for EPC containing liposomes. The damaging effect of the high cooling rate only developed during the drying and/or rehydration step of the freeze-drying process and was not observed after a freezing-thawing cycle. The exact mechanism behind the effects of the cooling rate is unclear, but is probably related to differences in crystallization patterns of ice. Slow cooling results in undercooling of the dispersion below 0 °C, until the whole sample freezes nearly instantaneously. Quick cooling induces formation of dendritic ice crystals that grow upwards from the bottom of the vial. As a result, solutes are pushed upwards during freezing, leading to the formation of a nearly closed layer of amorphous material at the top of the freeze-dried cake. This layer may inhibit the drying process, and can be recognized by a shiny appearance of the dried cake.

4.2.5 Use of charged liposomal bilayers

Addition of phosphatidylserine (PS) to EPC liposomes (0.1 μm) in a molar ratio of EPC/PS of 10:1 increased the CF retention after freeze-drying/rehydration (19).

The inclusion of charged phospholipid species may be important to reduce fusion processes. However, for the addition of another negatively charged phospholipid (phosphatidylglycerol) no, or even a negative effect on the CF retention after freeze-drying/rehydration has been reported (23).

4.2.6 Avoid collapse of the cake during freeze-drying

Generally, an optimized freeze-drying process should fulfil two major requirements:

(a) The resulting product should have a large specific surface area (high porosity), which allows a quick, nearly instantaneous reconstitution of the liposomes after the addition of water. Therefore, the porous structure of the amorphous matrix that is formed during freezing should be preserved throughout the process.

(b) The freeze-drying time should be minimal.

For design of a proper freeze-drying process, a basic understanding of the drying process is required (see also refs 24–27). Two phases can be distinguished in the drying process:

(a) The 'primary' drying phase, in which the ice crystals are sublimated.

(b) The 'secondary' drying phase in which the residual water content of the remaining solid matrix is further reduced.

An overview of factors that play a role in the freeze-drying process is given in Figure 5.

i. Freeze-dry *c.* 4 °C below the collapse temperature during primary drying

Freeze-drying results in a freeze-dried cake with a large surface area if the porous structure of the amorphous matrix that is formed during freezing is preserved throughout the process. This can be achieved by maintaining the temperature at which the ice is sublimated (T_{front}, see Figure 5) below the so-called 'collapse temperature' (T_c) of the glassy matrix. The nature of the process(es) occurring at the T_c (also denoted in literature as glass transition ($T_{g'}$) or softening (T_s) temperature) of a freeze-concentrate is still subject of investigation (see e.g. ref. 28), but it is clear that the viscosity of the freeze-concentrate is strongly reduced by heating the sample to temperatures above T_c. The T_c of the freeze-concentrate is mainly dependent on:

(a) The molecular weight.

(b) Molecular structure.

(c) The mass fraction of its components.

The T_c can be measured by means of (modulated temperature) differential scanning calorimetry ((MT)DSC) (see e.g. refs 29 and 30) or electrical resistance analysis (31). The T_c values of some carbohydrates are listed in Table 1.

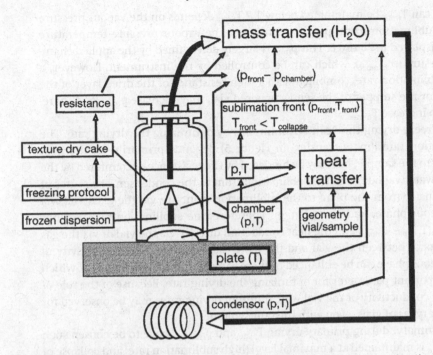

Figure 5 Overview of the main factors that influence the freeze-drying process. At any location, the relation between the temperature (T) and the pressure (p) is given by the curve in Figure 6. The figure is based on data from refs 22, 23, and 25. For more details, see text.

Table 1 Collapse temperatures (T_c) of freeze-concentrated solution of different carbohydrates[a]

Carbohydrate	Collapse temperature (°C)	References
Glucose	−40 or −43 to −46	30, 34, 38, 39
Sorbitol	−42 to −46	31, 34, 38, 39
Sucrose	−32 to −33.5	31, 34, 37−40
Maltose	−30 to −31	34, 38−40
Trehalose	−30 to −31	30, 31, 34, 38, 40
Lactose	−28 to −30	31, 34, 38, 40
Cellobiose	−29	34, 38
Raffinose	−26.5	34, 39
Maltotriose	−23.5	34
Dextran (MW: c. 9 k)	−13.5	31, 34

[a] In order to preserve the porous texture of the freeze-dried cake, primary drying should be performed at c. 4 °C below T_c (see text). The values of T_c were determined by means of electrical thermal analysis (31), DSC (31, 34, 37–39), or MTDSC (30, 40). Apart from variability caused by different techniques and analysis protocols, differences in T_c may also originate from differences in the freezing protocol (28, 41).

How can T_{front} be maintained below T_c? T_{front} depends on the vapour pressure at the sublimation front (p_{front}), according to the vapour pressure temperature curve displayed in Figure 6. This p_{front} is largely determined by the applied chamber pressure ($p_{chamber}$), which can be controlled by the instrument. However, a high sublimation rate, combined with a high resistance of the dried layer of the sample or the stopper of the semi-stoppered vial, may increase p_{front}, and therefore also increase T_{front}.

The freeze-drying time can be minimized by optimizing the drying rate. The sublimation rate ('mass transfer' in Figure 5) depends primarily on the heat transfer to the sample, but may be hindered by the resistance encountered by the flow of water vapour from the sublimation front to the condenser. The routes of heat transfer from the plate to the sublimation front are via the glass vial, via the gaseous phase, and via radiation. Therefore, the sublimation rate depends both on ($T_{plate} - T_{front}$), and the heat conduction directly via the vial or via the gas in the space between the vial and the plate (see Figure 5). The conductivity of this gaseous phase can be enhanced by increasing the gas density ($p_{chamber}$), which is an important parameter for optimizing the drying rate. Because of the role of the heat conductivity of the vial wall, different drying rates may be observed for different types of vials, even with the same volume.

In summary, during primary drying T_{plate} and $p_{chamber}$ have to be chosen such that T_{front} is maintained at a maximal level (high sublimation rate) and collapse of the sample is prevented ($T_{front} < T_c$, with a safety margin of $c.$ 4 °C).

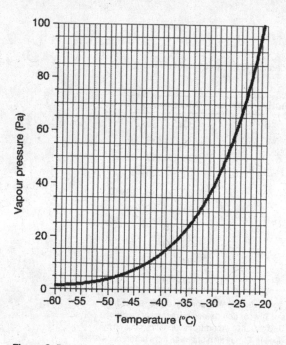

Figure 6 Relation between temperature and vapour pressure.

ii. Keep the sample temperature below the T_g during secondary drying

After the completion of ice sublimation, the temperature of the sample approaches T_{plate}. In this secondary drying phase, the residual water content of the porous matrix is further decreased and quickly (in few hours) approaches a level which depends on T_{plate} (24). An important characteristic of the dry cake is its glass transition temperature (T_g). Exposure of the cake to temperatures above its T_g strongly decreases its viscosity and results in reduction of its surface area by collapse of the porous matrix. The T_g depends, as T_c, on the molecular weight and structure and weight fraction of its components. Importantly, T_g increases with decreasing residual water content. A sudden, strong increase in T_{plate} during secondary drying may result in passage of T_g and (partial) collapse of the sample before the residual water content has been sufficiently reduced. Obviously, the plate temperature should never exceed the T_g of the anhydrous cake. The T_g of a freeze-dried cake can be determined by (MT)DSC as an increase in the heat capacity of the sample, or by thermomechanical analysis as an expansion of the material (e.g. refs 30 and 32).

During secondary drying, $p_{chamber}$ is often further reduced, since the relatively small amount of water that needs to be removed from the sample only requires a small heat transfer rate. However, at this stage the drying rate is hardly affected by the chamber pressure (0–27 Pa), but mainly depends on the specific surface area of the sample (24).

4.3 Stability in the freeze-dried state

Until now, only a limited number of studies on the stability of lyoprotected liposomes in the dried state have appeared (see for a review ref. 3). Therefore, insufficient data are available to predict the storage stability of freeze-dried liposomes. In literature on the stability of dry, amorphous products, the role of the T_g is generally strongly emphasized. At temperatures above T_g the high molecular mobility allows pronounced chemical and physical degradation (33, 34). However, instability of freeze-dried liposomes has also been observed for samples stored at temperatures below T_g (40, 42). The stability of the freeze-dried product may depend on its specific characteristics, such as the physicochemical nature and concentration of the encapsulated compound, residual water, choice of phospholipids, and (freeze-)drying protocol. Water molecules can increase the molecular mobility of the amorphous matrix, and decrease T_g. The effect of the water content on the stability of freeze-dried liposomes is exemplified by Figure 7, which shows the degradation of doxorubicin in freeze-dried liposomes. In these samples degradation occurred below the T_g as measured with MTDSC, which was explained by the non-homogeneous nature of freeze-dried, lyoprotected liposomes. For example, the solid state characteristics of the drug containing matrix encapsulated by the liposomes may differ from the characteristics of the extra-liposomal matrix (40).

Despite all uncertainties, it can be recommended to avoid the use of lyo-protectants with a low molecular weight, such as glucose or sorbitol, which have

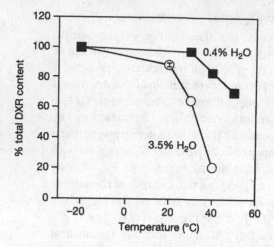

Figure 7 Doxorubicin content in freeze-dried liposomes after six months of storage. The liposomes were freeze-dried to different residual water contents, with sucrose as a lyoprotectant. The values for the glass transition temperature (T_g) of the freeze-dried samples were about 38 °C (3.5% H_2O) and 70 °C (0.4% H_2O). Lipid composition: DPPC/DPPG/Chol = 10:1:4. Data from ref. 42.

a low T_g in the anhydrous state. For doxorubicin liposomes, no differences in storage stability were observed when using lactose, trehalose, and maltose as a lyoprotectant, whereas the same liposomes freeze-dried with sucrose showed a slightly less stable behaviour (40). Further, for optimal stability the residual water content should be as low as possible (e.g. <0.5%). In this respect, packaging materials play an important role. Different types of rubber closures may exhibit differences in water release and permeability to water (35). In order to minimize such problems, the water content of the closures can be reduced by drying (e.g. at 110 °C for 5 h) prior to usage. Alternatively, glass ampoules can be employed.

4.4 Example of a freeze-drying protocol

Although in the literature many examples of successful lyoprotection of liposomes were described with manifold freeze-dryers, the use of tray dryers with a controllable plate temperature (e.g. –40 to 40 °C) and chamber pressure is preferred, since these process parameters affect the characteristics of the final product (see above). The protocol below has been designed for a plate freeze-dryer and is aimed to:

(a) Prevent high temperature gradients in the sample during primary drying.

(b) Result in samples of different residual water contents.

However, the T_{plate} during primary drying may be increased in order to accelerate the drying process, taking into account the considerations described above.

Protocol 1

Freeze-drying of liposomes

Equipment

- Vials: 10 ml glass freeze-dry vial
  (e.g. from Dura B.V., Uithoorn,
  The Netherlands)
- Plate freeze-dryer[a]

- Rubber closures: (e.g. type V1972 DZ,
  FM 257/5 C from Helvoet Pharma, Alken,
  Belgium) dried at 110 °C for 5 h prior to
  usage

A. Liposome preparation

1 Prepare >1 ml of 0.1 μm DPPC/DPPG (10:1) liposomes at a total lipid concentration
   of about 25 mM according to standard procedures. The extra-liposomal medium is
   10% lactose and 30 mM sodium citrate pH 6.5, and the intra-liposomal medium is
   5 mM CF, 10% lactose, and 30 mM sodium citrate pH 6.5.

2 Put 0.4 ml of the liposomes in a freeze-dry vial.

B. Freeze-drying procedure

1 Prepare the freeze-dryer (switch on condenser cooling). The condenser temperature
   in this example is assumed to be about –55 °C.

2 Place the semi-stoppered vials containing the samples on the plate and cool to
   –40 °C or lower with 0.5 °C/min.

3 Keep the temperature of the plate temperature (T_{plate}) constant for 0.5 h.

4 Decrease the $p_{chamber}$ to a value between 11–13 Pa.

5 Set T_{plate} to –37 °C, for 30 h.

6 Increase T_{plate} to –30 °C, for 2 h. Vials closed after completion of this stage will
   contain c. 3% residual water (A).[b]

7 Increase T_{plate} to –16 °C, for 2 h (B).[b]

8 Increase T_{plate} to +20 °C, for 2 h (C).[b]

9 Close the vials preferably without opening the freeze-dryer.

10 Use dry nitrogen for releasing the pressure to prevent an increase in the residual
   water content of the samples.[c]

[a] Plate freeze-dryers manufacturers are, e.g. FTS/kinetics (www.ftssystems.com), Martin Christ
GmbH (www.martinchrist.de), Virtis (www.virtis.com), Hull Company (www.hullcompany.com),
Labcongo Corp. (www.labconco.com), and Serail (www.serail.com).

[b] The residual water contents of the cakes are approx. (when closing at point A) 3%, 1.5% (B), or
0.5% (C). However, different residual water contents may be obtained with different condenser
and plate temperatures, vial and sample volumes, etc.

[c] If the pressure is released after closing the vials, a vacuum will be present inside the vials,
which facilitates tight closing of the vial by the rubber caps before the vial is sealed. If the vials
are closed after opening the freeze-dryer, minimize the exposure time of the hygroscopic
samples to the atmosphere.

Methods often used for the determination of the residual water content are Karl-Fisher titration or thermogravical analysis (36). Since freeze-dried lipid/sugar samples are very hygroscopic, sampling should be performed under dry nitrogen conditions in order to prevent changes in the residual water content. Samples with, for example 0.3% water quickly attract water from an ambient environment, whereas freeze-dried carbohydrate samples containing, for example 4% water will further dry when stored in a dry nitrogen atmosphere over P_2O_5. Finally, the rehydration can be performed by adding water (example: 0.36 ml) up to the original volume or sample weight, followed by shaking for a few seconds.

5 Preparation of sterile liposome formulations

Liposomes to be used for parenteral administration, for pulmonary administration, or to be administered to open wounds, have to be sterile. Liposomes can be produced under aseptic conditions (43), but this procedure is complex and expensive. Sterilization of aqueous liposome dispersions by autoclaving (15 min at 121 °C) is possible (15, 44), but may not be acceptable when using a non-neutral pH (because of hydrolysis), when using insufficient quality of unsaturated phospholipids (because of oxidation), or when using a water soluble (because of drug leakage) or a heat-labile drug. Filtration through a 0.22 μm filter is non-destructive to small liposomes, but is limited to liposomes smaller than 0.2 μm and has the drawbacks that removal of the bacterial contaminants does not take place in the final container (which increases the chance of contamination) and that it does not remove virions and small spores. The present state of technology excludes the use of gamma irradiation (using a regularly recommended dose of 25 kGy) as a sterilization technique, because it is too destructive to liposome dispersions (5).

References

1. Barenholz, Y. and Crommelin, D. J. A. (1994). In *Encyclopedia of pharmaceutical technology*, Vol. 9 (ed. J. Swarbrick and J. C. Boylan), p. 1. Marcel Dekker, Inc., NY.
2. Crommelin, D. J. A., Talsma, H., Grit, M., and Zuidam, N. J. (1993). In *Handbook of phospholipids* (ed. G. Cevc), p. 335. Marcel Dekker, Inc., NY.
3. Van Winden, E. C. A., Zuidam, N. J., and Crommelin, D. J. A. (1998). In *Medical applications of liposomes* (ed. D. D. Lasic and D. Papahadjopoulos), p. 567. Elsevier Sciences, B.V., Amsterdam.
4. Grit, M., Zuidam, N. J., and Crommelin, D. J. A. (1993). In *Liposome technology*, 2nd edn (ed. G. Gregoriadis), Vol. I, p. 455. CRC Press, Boca Raton, FL.
5. Zuidam, N. J., Talsma, H., and Crommelin, D. J. A. (1996). In *Handbook of nonmedical applications of liposomes. From design to microreactors* (ed. Y. Barenholz and D. D. Lasic), Vol. III, p. 71. CRC Press, Boca Raton.
6. Zuidam, N. J., Versluis, C., Vernooy, E. A. A. M., and Crommelin, D. J. A. (1996). *Biochim. Biophys. Acta*, **1280**, 135.
7. Asayama, K., Aramak, Y., Yoshida, T., and Tsuchiya, S. (1992). *J. Liposome Res.*, **2**, 275.
8. Zhang, D., Yasuda, T., and Okada, S. (1993). *J. Clin. Biochem. Nutr.*, **14**, 83.

9. Storm, G., Oussoren, C., Peeters, P. A. M., and Barenholz, Y. (1993). In *Liposome technology* (ed. G. Gregoriadis), Vol. III, p. 345. CRC Press, Boca Raton, FL.

10. Grit, M. and Crommelin, D. J. A. (1993). *Chem. Phys. Lipids*, **64**, 3.

11. Grit, M. and Crommelin, D. J. A. (1993). *Biochim. Biophys. Acta*, **1167**, 49.

12. Zuidam, N. J. and Crommelin, D. J. A. (1995). *J. Pharm. Sci.*, **84**, 1113.

13. Grit, M. and Crommelin, D. J. A. (1992). *Chem. Phys. Lipids*, **62**, 113.

14. Zuidam, N. J., Gouw, H. K., Barenholz, Y., and Crommelin, D. J. A. (1995). *Biochim. Biophys. Acta*, **1240**, 101.

15. Zuidam, N. J., Lee, S. S. L., and Crommelin, D. J. A. (1993). *Pharm. Res.*, **10**, 1591.

16. Zuidam, N. J. and Crommelin, D. J. A. (1995). *Int. J. Pharm.*, **126**, 209.

17. Barenholz, Y. (2001). *Curr. Opin. Colloid Interface Sci.*, **6**, 66.

18. Crowe, J. H., Hoekstra, F. A., Nguyen, K. H. N., and Crowe, L. M. (1996). *Biochim. Biophys. Acta*, **1280**, 187.

19. Crowe, J. H. and Crowe, L. M. (1993). In *Liposome technology* (ed. G. Gregoriadis), Vol. I. CRC Press, Boca Raton, FL.

20. Koster, K. L., Webb, M. S., Bryant, G., and Lynch, D. V. (1994). *Biochim. Biophys. Acta*, **1193**, 143.

21. Crowe, J. H., Leslie, S. B., and Crowe, L. M. (1994). *Cryobiology*, **31**, 355.

22. Van Winden, E. C. A., Zhang, W., and Crommelin, D. J. A. (1997). *Pharm. Res.*, **14**, 1151.

23. Harrigan, P. R., Madden, T. D., and Cullis, P. R. (1990). *Chem. Phys. Lipids*, **52**, 139.

24. Pikal, M. J., Shah, S., Roy, M. L., and Putman, R. (1990). *Int. J. Pharm. Sci.*, **60**, 203.

25. Pikal, M. J. (1990). *BioPharm*, **10**, 18.

26. Essig, D., Oschmann, R., and Schwabe, W. (1993). In *Lyophilisation, Paperback APV*. Wissenschaftliche Verlagsgesellschaft mbH, Stuttgart.

27. Ybema, H., Kolkman-Roodbeen, L., Te Booy, M. P., and Vromans, H. (1995). *Pharm. Res.*, **12**, 1260.

28. Sahagian, M. E. and Goff, H. D. (1994). *Thermochim. Acta*, **246**, 271.

29. Her, L. M. and Nail, S. L. (1994). *Pharm. Res.*, **11**, 54.

30. Van Winden, E. C. A., Talsma, H., and Crommelin, D. J. A. (1998). *J. Pharm. Sci.*, **87**, 231.

31. Her, L. M., Jefferis, R. P., Gatlin, L. A., Braxton, B., and Nail, S. L. (1994). *Pharm. Res.*, **11**, 1023.

32. Brown, M. E. (1988). In *Introduction to thermal analysis. Techniques and applications.* Chapman and Hall, London.

33. Sun, W. Q., Leopold, A. C., Crowe, L. M., and Crowe, J. H. (1996). *Biophys. J.*, **70**, 1769.

34. Levine, H. and Slade, L. (1988). *J. Chem. Soc. Faraday Trans. 1*, **84**, 2619.

35. Vromans, H. and Van Laarhoven, J. A. H. (1992). *Int. J. Pharm.*, **79**, 301.

36. Ford, J. L. and Timmins, P. (1989). In *Pharmaceutical thermal analysis*, p. 279. Ellis Horwood Ltd., Chisester.

37. Shalaev, E. Y. and Franks, F. (1995). *J. Chem. Soc. Faraday Trans.*, **91**, 1511.

38. Taylor, L. S. (1996). Thesis from the University of Bradford, Bradford, UK.

39. Franks, F. (1982). In *Water a comprehensive treatise*, Vol. 7: *Water and aqueous solutions at subzero temperatures*, p. 313. Plenum Press, New York.

40. Van Winden, E. C. A. and Crommelin, D. J. A. (1997). *Eur. J. Pharm. Biopharm.*, **43**, 295.

41. Roos, Y. and Karel, M. (1991). *Int. J. Food Sci. Technol.*, **26**, 553.

42. Van Winden, E. C. A. and Crommelin, D. J. A. (1999). *J. Control. Rel.*, **58**, 69.

43. Amselem, S., Gabizon, A., and Barenholz, Y. (1993). In *Liposome technology* (ed. G. Gregoriadis), Vol. I, p. 501. CRC Press, Boca Raton, FL.

44. Cherian, M., Lenk, R. P., and Jedrusiak, J. A. (1990). PCT Int. Appl. Patent, No. WO 90/03808.

Chapter 6
Encapsulation of weakly-basic drugs, antisense oligonucleotides, and plasmid DNA within large unilamellar vesicles for drug delivery applications

David B. Fenske and Norbert Maurer
Department of Biochemistry and Molecular Biology, University of British Columbia, 2146 Health Sciences Mall, Vancouver, BC V6T 1Z3, Canada.

Pieter R. Cullis
Department of Biochemistry and Molecular Biology, University of British Columbia, 2146 Health Sciences Mall, Vancouver, BC V6T 1Z3, Canada; and
Inex Pharmaceuticals Corporation, 100–8900 Glenlyon Parkway, Burnaby, BC V5J 5L8, Canada.

1 Introduction

Liposomes are microscopic spheres consisting of one or more lipid bilayers arranged concentrically about a central aqueous core. Liposomes were first described over thirty-five years ago (1), and it was not long after that their usefulness as models of biological membranes and their potential as systems for the systemic delivery of drugs was recognized (2). Development of this potential required techniques for the generation of unilamellar vesicles and encapsulation of drugs and macromolecules within them. Although a wide variety of methods were developed for the formation of liposomes (3, 4), many of them were technically demanding, time-consuming, and did not generate liposomes of optimal size and polydispersity. Likewise, early attempts at encapsulating drugs within liposomes relied on passive entrapment methods, which resulted in low encapsulation levels (<30%) and poor retention of drugs (5). Nevertheless, early *in vivo* experiments on liposomal drug systems were encouraging enough to fuel further development (see ref. 5 and references therein).

A major step forward came with the development of extrusion methodology for the rapid generation of monodisperse populations of unilamellar vesicles (6, 7). This led to the characterization of a wide variety of liposomal systems, both in terms of their physical properties and their behaviour in the circulation. From this information it became clear that ideal drug delivery systems would possess a small size (on the order of 100 nm) and long circulation lifetimes (half-life > 5 h in mice). Large unilamellar vesicles (LUVs) with a diameter of 100 nm were found to be large and stable enough to carry adequate quantities of encapsulated material, but were small enough to circulate for a time adequate to reach sites of disease, such as tumours or sites of inflammation. Vesicles much larger or smaller were quickly cleared from the circulation. Furthermore, circulation lifetimes and drug retention were found to be greatly enhanced in systems made from phosphatidylcholine (or sphingomyelin) and cholesterol (8–11). Further improvements in circulation longevity was achieved by the inclusion of ganglio-side G_{M1} in the vesicle formulation (12–14), or by grafting water soluble polymers such as poly(ethylene glycol) (PEG) onto the vesicle surface, thereby generating what have come to be known as 'stealth' liposomes (13, 15–17).

A second major advance in the development of liposomal delivery systems came with the recognition that many chemotherapeutic drugs could be accumulated within vesicles in response to transmembrane pH gradients (ΔpH) (18–20). The ability of ΔpH to influence the equilibrium transmembrane distributions of certain weak bases and weak acids had long been recognized (see ref. 20 and references therein), and had stimulated studies in our laboratory to investigate the transport of these substances into liposomes in response to ΔpH. This work has demonstrated the transbilayer movement of a wide variety of drugs, biogenic amines, amino acids, peptides, lipids, and ions in LUVs exhibiting a ΔpH (for a review, see ref. 20).

The observation that many of the important chemotherapeutic drugs were weak bases led to the development of several liposomal anticancer systems which exhibit improved therapeutic properties over free drug. Initial efforts were directed at doxorubicin, the most commonly employed chemotherapeutic agent, which is active against a variety of ascitic and solid tumours, yet exhibits a variety of toxic side-effects. Early studies (see ref. 5 and references therein) had shown that reduced side-effects with equal or enhanced efficacy could be obtained in liposomal systems, despite low encapsulation levels and poor drug retention. The pH gradient approach (5, 8, 9, 21, 22) was expected to provide significant improvements in overall efficacy due to high drug-to-lipid ratios and excellent retention observed both in vitro and in vivo. This has been realized in liposomal doxorubicin preparations which are currently either in advanced clinical trials (23, 24), or have been approved by the US FDA for clinical use (25). Other liposomal doxorubicin formulations (26–35) are in various Phase I or II clinical trials, often with promising results. A variety of other liposomal drugs are currently in preclinical or clinical development; these include vincristine (11, 36–39), daunorubicin (25, 40, 41), ciprofloxacin (42, 43), and topotecan (44), to name a few. Of these, our group has been prominent in devising methods for

168

the encapsulation of doxorubicin, vincristine, and ciprofloxacin, and thus the examples for encapsulation of conventional drugs discussed in this review will focus on these three drugs.

Liposomal delivery systems are finally reaching a stage of development where significant advances can reasonably be expected in the short-term. The first of the conventional drug carriers are reaching the market while new liposomal drugs are being developed and entered into clinical trials. These advances stem from the fact that the design features required of drug delivery systems that have systemic utility are becoming better defined. Based on the studies indicated above, we now know that liposomal systems that are small (diameter ≤ 100 nm) and that exhibit long circulation lifetimes (half-life ≥ 5 h in mice) following i.v. injection exhibit a remarkable property termed 'disease site targeting' or 'passive targeting' that results in large improvements in the amounts of drug arriving at the disease site. For example, liposomal vincristine formulations can deliver 50- to 100-fold higher amounts of drug to a tumour site relative to the free drug (8, 10–12, 39, 45). This can result in large increases in efficacy (12). These improvements stem from the increased permeability of the vasculature at tumour sites (46, 47) or sites of inflammation which results in preferential extravasation of small, long-circulating carriers in these regions.

The insights gleaned from conventional drug carriers have implications for the design of liposomal systems for the delivery of larger macromolecules. There is currently much interest in developing systemic vectors for the delivery of therapeutic genetic drugs such as antisense oligonucleotides or plasmid DNA. In order to get appreciable amounts of a vector containing the antisense oligonucleotides or therapeutic gene to the site of disease, the vector must be stable, small, and long-circulating. Of course, the vector must also be accumulated by target cells, escape the endocytotic pathway, and be delivered to the nucleus, but these are ultimately secondary, albeit crucially important, requirements.

Over the past twenty years, our laboratory has played a major role in the development of liposomal systems optimized for the delivery of both conventional drugs and, more recently, genetic drugs. Our early studies on the production of LUVs by extrusion led to the characterization of several liposomal drug delivery systems (12, 18–20, 23, 48–52), the development of new approaches for the loading of drugs via generation of ΔpH (51–53), and finally new methods for the encapsulation of antisense oligonucleotides (54–56) and plasmid DNA (56–60) within liposomes. In this paper, we will provide a brief overview of these methods, along with detailed protocols for the encapsulation of both conventional and genetic drugs within liposomes.

2 Measurement of phospholipid concentration

An important assay used in all aspects of liposome research (despite dating back to 1925) is that of Fiske and Subbarow for the quantitative determination of inorganic phosphate (61). The combination of simplicity, accuracy, and high reproducibility makes this essential for determining the concentration of phospholipid stock solutions or of LUV preparations. The assay is based on the ability of perchloric acid to liberate and oxidize phosphorus, forming phosphate ions which form a coloured complex that is quantified by absorbance spectrophotometry. The entire assay takes about two hours, including preparation of standard curve and clean up.

Protocol 1

Determination of lipid concentrations using a phosphate assay

Equipment and reagents

- Pyrex test-tubes (16 × 150 mm, or 18 × 150 mm)
- Glass marbles (20–30 mm diameter)
- Aluminium test-tube blocks (on hot plates)
- Thermometer (0–350 °C)
- Boiling water-bath (or frying pan)
- UV/visible spectrophotometer
- Plastic cuvettes (disposable, 1 cm path length)
- Fume hood suitable for perchloric acid digestion
- Reagent dispenser bottles for perchloric acid, Fiske–Subbarow, and ammonium molybdate solutions
- Ammonium molybdate solution: dissolve 4.4 g of ammonium molybdate in 1.5 litres distilled water. Slowly add 40 ml sulfuric acid (conc.), and make up to a final volume of 2 litres with distilled water.

- Fiske–Subbarow solution: dissolve 150 g $NaHSO_3$ (sodium bisulfite) and 5 g Na_2SO_3 (sodium sulfite) in 1 litre distilled water. Add 2.5 g 1-amino-2-naphthol-4-sulfonic acid (ANS), and stir at 40 °C in the dark for 1–2 h until dissolved (keep covered due to fumes). Store overnight in the dark at room temperature, then filter off any insoluble material with a Buchner funnel and Whatman (No. 1) filter paper. The solution is stored in an amber glass bottle.
- 70% perchloric acid
- 1 mM Na_2HPO_4 in water (anhydrous disodium hydrogen orthophosphate standard)

Method

1   Preparation of standard curve: pipette 0, 50, 100, 150, and 200 nmoles of phosphate (from 1 mM standard) into a series of Pyrex tubes (in duplicate).

2   Preparation of samples: pipette aliquots of samples (dilute if necessary) containing 100–200 nmoles phosphate into Pyrex tubes (in duplicate). Samples can be aqueous or organic (for volumes in the μl range). For larger volumes of organic samples, remove solvent under a stream of nitrogen gas. Samples containing sucrose should be dialysed prior to analysis. Sample volume should not exceed 200 μl.

3   Carefully add 0.7 ml perchloric acid into assay tubes, cover tube with a marble, and vortex. Place tubes in heating block in fume hood for 1–2 h, ensuring the temperature remains between 180–210 °C.

Protocol 1 continued

4   Remove tubes from heating block and let cool to room temperature. Add 0.75 ml Fiske–Subbarow solution followed by 7 ml ammonium molybdate solution, and vortex.

5   Place tubes (with marbles on top) in boiling water-bath in fume hood for 15 min, then place tubes in cold water-bath to cool to room temperature.

6   Read the absorbance of all standards and samples at 815 nm. If possible, use the spectrophotometer to generate a standard curve so that samples can be quantified as nmol PO_4/tube.

7   To determine the phosphate concentration of the original samples (mM), divide nmol PO_4/tube by the volume of sample (in μl) added to the assay tube, accounting for any dilutions.

8   After reading absorbance values, contents of tubes are diluted down the sink with a large quantity of cold water. The Pyrex tubes are immediately rinsed several times with tap-water followed by distilled water, and allowed to dry. Phosphate assay tubes should never be cleaned using any detergent.

3 The formation of large unilamellar vesicles by extrusion through polycarbonate filters with defined pore size

The development of the extrusion method was largely driven by investigations on the effect of ion and pH gradients on lipid asymmetry (20, 62). It soon became clear that model membranes such as multilamellar vesicles were not appropriate for such topics, and that methods for producing unilamellar vesicles would be required. The methods available for the generation of LUVs, which included dispersion of lipids from organic solvents (63), sonication (64), detergent dialysis (65), and reversed-phase evaporation (66), had serious drawbacks (62). However, Papahadjopolous and co-workers (67) had observed that sequential extrusion of MLVs through a series of filters of reducing pore size under low pressure gave rise to LUV systems. This led to the approach developed in our laboratory, in which MLVs are directly extruded, at relatively high pressures (200–400 psi), through polycarbonate filters with a pore size ranging from 30–400 nm, giving rise to narrow, monodisperse vesicle populations with diameters close to the chosen pore size (Figure 1) (6, 7). The method is rapid and simple, and can be performed for a wide variety of lipid compositions and temperatures. As it is necessary to extrude the lipid emulsions at temperatures 5–10 °C above the gel to liquid-crystalline phase transition temperature, the system is manufactured so that it may be attached to a circulating water-bath.

Protocol 2 details the generation of 100 nm LUVs composed of DSPC/cholesterol, with a lipid concentration of 30 mM, and a total volume of 2 ml. This highly ordered lipid mixture is frequently chosen for drug delivery applications as it has a good circulation lifetime and drug retention properties.

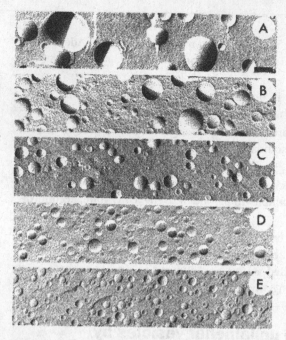

Figure 1 Freeze-fracture electron micrographs of egg phosphatidylcholine LUVs prepared by extrusion through polycarbonate filters with pore sizes of (A) 400 nm, (B) 200 nm, (C) 100 nm, (D) 50 nm, and (E) 30 nm. The bar in panel (A) represents 150 nm. Reproduced from ref. 3, with permission.

Protocol 2

Preparation of LUVs (DSPC/Chol, 55:45) by extrusion

Equipment and reagents

- Extruder (Northern Lipids)
- Nuclepore polycarbonate membranes (0.1 μm pore size; 25 mm diameter) (Whatman)
- Cryovials and holders
- Circulating water-bath
- Liquid nitrogen
- DSPC (Avanti Polar Lipids; Northern Lipids) and cholesterol (Sigma-Aldrich; Northern Lipids)
- Cholesteryl hexadecyl ether ([³H] or [¹⁴C]) (Perkin Elmer Life Sciences Canada)

Method

1   Prepare stock solutions of DSPC and Chol in $CHCl_3$ with concentrations in the range of 100–200 mM. Verify DSPC concentration using the phosphate assay (see Protocol 1).

Protocol 2 continued

2   Add 33 μmol DSPC and 27 μmol Chol to a 13 × 100 mm test-tube. If desired, add a trace of a radioactive tracer such as [^{3}H]cholesteryl hexadecyl ether ([^{3}H]CHE) to give a specific activity of 10–30 dpm/nmol lipid. Remove CHCl$_3$ under a gentle stream of nitrogen gas while immersing tube in hot water (50–60 °C).

3   Place lipid film under high vacuum for a minimum of 1 h.

4   Hydrate lipid film with 2 ml of appropriate buffer (internal buffer), such as 300 mM citrate pH 4.0 (pH gradient loading), 300 mM ammonium sulfate (for amine loading), or 300 mM MgSO$_4$ pH 6.5 (for ionophore loading). Vortex at 65 °C until lipid emulsion is obtained and lipid film can no longer be seen on glass tube. This step must always be performed at a temperature approx. 10 °C higher than the gel to liquid-crystalline phase transition temperature (T$_m$) of the phospholipid being used.

5   Transfer to cryovial tubes. Immerse cryovials in liquid nitrogen for 3–5 min, then transfer to lukewarm water (for 1 min) and then to water-bath at 65 °C. Let thaw completely, and then vortex vigorously. Repeat freeze-thaw cycle four more times.

6   Assemble extruder with two polycarbonate filters with pore size of 0.1 μm, and connect to a circulating water-bath equilibrated at 65 °C. Extrude ten times through filters under pressure of approx. 400 psi. For larger LUVs (200–400 nm), lower pressures will be adequate (100–200 psi). After each pass the sample is cycled back to the extruder. Start at low pressure and gradually increase until each pass takes less than 1 min.

7   Determine lipid concentration of LUVs by a phosphate assay (see Protocol 1) or by liquid scintillation counting.

4 Accumulation of weakly-basic drugs within LUVs in response to transmembrane pH gradients

The recognition that a variety of chemotherapeutic drugs could be accumulated within LUVs exhibiting transmembrane pH gradients followed earlier studies on membrane potentials and the uptake of weak bases used for measurement of ΔpH (62). The technique is based on the membrane permeability of the neutral form of weakly basic drugs such as doxorubicin. When doxorubicin (pK$_a$ = 8.6) is incubated in the presence of LUVs exhibiting a ΔpH (interior acidic), the neutral form of the drug will diffuse down its concentration gradient into the LUV interior, where it will be subsequently protonated and trapped (the charged form is membrane impermeable). As long as the internal buffer (300 mM citrate pH 4) is able to maintain the ΔpH, diffusion of neutral drug will continue until either all the drug has been taken up, or the buffering capacity of the interior has been overwhelmed. This process is illustrated in Figure 2 for the uptake of doxorubicin into EPC/Chol and EPC LUVs, where it is seen that uptake is dependent on time, temperature, and lipid composition (68). Under appropriate conditions high drug-to-lipid ratios can be achieved with high trapping efficiencies

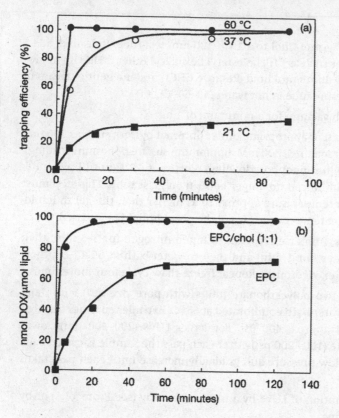

Figure 2 (A) Effect of incubation temperature on uptake of doxorubicin into 200 nm EPC/cholesterol (55:45 mol/mol) LUVs exhibiting a transmembrane pH gradient (pH 4 inside, 7.8 outside). Doxorubicin was added to LUVs (D/L = 0.3 wt:wt) equilibrated at 21 °C (■), 37 °C (○), and 60 °C (●). Reproduced from ref. 9, with permission. (B) Effect of cholesterol on the uptake of doxorubicin at 20 °C into 100 nm LUVs exhibiting a transmembrane pH gradient (pH 4.6 inside, 7.5 outside). Lipid compositions were EPC (■) and EPC/cholesterol (1:1 mol/mol) (●). The initial D/L ratio was 100 nmol/μmol. Reproduced from ref. 18, with permission.

(98% and higher) and excellent drug retention. A diagrammatic illustration of this process is given in Figure 3 (left column). Interestingly, much higher levels of doxorubicin can be loaded than would be predicted on the basis of the magnitude of ΔpH (20, 69). It would now appear that this is due to the formation of doxorubicin precipitates within the LUV interior, which provides an additional driving force for accumulation (70, 71). These precipitates can be visualized by cryo-electron microscopy, where they are seen to give the LUVs a 'coffee bean' appearance (Figure 4). We have recently observed that very high levels of uptake can be achieved in the absence of a pH gradient by the formation of doxorubicin-Mn^{2+} complexes (72).

In Protocol 3, the lipids are hydrated in 300 mM citrate pH 4.0 prior to extrusion. A pH gradient with ΔpH ~ 3 is then formed by buffer exchange on a column of Sephadex G-50 hydrated in HEPES-buffered saline pH 7.5. This basic

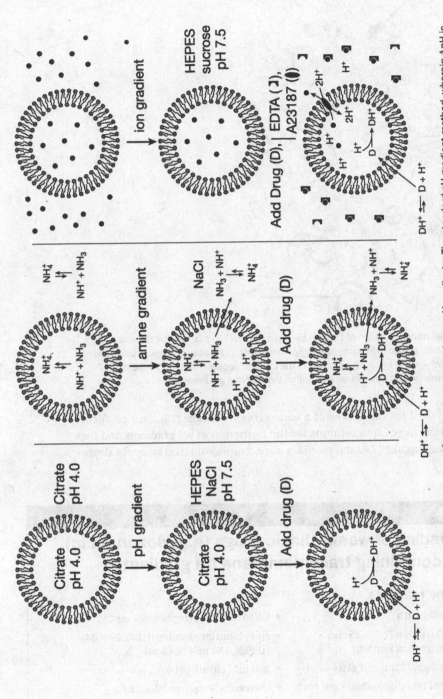

Figure 3 Diagrammatic representations of drug uptake in response to transmembrane pH gradients. The standard pH gradient method, wherein ΔpH is established by buffer exchange on a gel exclusion column, is summarized in the *left column*. A second method for generating ΔpH involves the initial formation of a transmembrane gradient of ammonium sulfate, which leads to an acidified vesicle interior as neutral ammonia leaks from the vesicles (*centre column*). Transmembrane pH gradients can also be established by ionophores (such as A23187) in response to transmembrane ion gradients (e.g. Mn^{2+}, represented as solid circles) (*right column*). A23187 couples the external transport of one Mn^{2+} ion (down its concentration gradient) to the internal transport of two protons, resulting in acidification of the vesicle interior. An external chelator such as EDTA is required to bind Mn^{2+} ions as they are transported out of the vesicle. See text for more details.

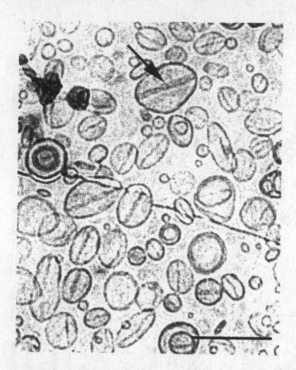

Figure 4 Cryo-electron micrograph of 100 nm EPC/cholesterol LUVs containing doxorubicin (D/L = 0.3 mol/mol) loaded in response to a transmembrane pH gradient (inside acidic). The additional internal structure (arrow), which gives the LUV the appearance of a 'coffee bean', represents doxorubicin that has precipitated within the LUV in a gel-like state.

system can be used for the uptake of a wide variety of drugs (19). This protocol also describes the use of spin columns for the formation of pH gradients and for monitoring drug uptake (73), and provides a spectrophotometric assay for doxorubicin.

Protocol 3

Remote loading of weakly basic drugs (e.g. doxorubicin) into LUVs containing transmembrane pH gradients

Equipment and reagents

- Circulating water-bath
- Sephadex G-50 column (1.5 × 15 cm) (Amersham Pharmacia Biotech)
- Disposable syringes (1 ml) and glass wool
- Plastic cuvettes (1 ml disposable, 1 cm path length)
- UV/visible spectrophotometer
- HEPES-buffered saline (HBS): 20 mM HEPES, 150 mM NaCl pH 7.5
- 300 mM citrate pH 4.0
- Doxorubicin (Sigma-Aldrich)

Method

1 Prepare DSPC/Chol (55:45) LUVs (diameter = 100 nm) as described in Protocol 2 ([lipid] = 30 mM, volume = 2 ml). Use 300 mM citrate pH 4.0 as the hydration buffer.

2 Prepare spin columns for monitoring drug uptake with time. On the day prior to drug loading, prepare a slurry of Sephadex G-50 in HBS. Add a small volume (2–3 ml) of dry G-50 to 200–300 ml HBS, and swirl. Add as necessary until settled G-50 occupies about half the aqueous volume. Let sit overnight. To prepare spin columns, pack a tiny plug of glass wool into the end of a 1 ml disposable syringe, which is then placed in a 13 × 100 mm glass test-tube. Swirl the G-50 slurry, and fill syringes using a Pasteur pipette. Place syringes (in test-tubes) in a desktop centrifuge, and pack gel by bringing speed to 2000 r.p.m. (670 g) momentarily. Add more G-50 and repeat centrifugation. When finished, the moist G-50 bed should be 0.9–1.0 ml. Cover spin columns with Parafilm to prevent drying, and use within the day.

3 Form pH gradient by running an aliquot (200 μl) of the LUVs down a column (1.5 × 15 cm) of Sephadex G-50 eluted in HBS. Collect LUV fraction, which will elute at the void volume and can be seen by eye. The final volume will be ~2 ml and the lipid concentration will be around 15 mM. Alternatively, form gradient using spin columns prepared in HBS (spin 4 × 100 μl), and pool the fractions.

4 Doxorubicin is often loaded at a drug-to-lipid (D/L) ratio of 0.2 mol:mol. Prepare a doxorubicin standard solution by dissolving 1.0 mg of drug in 0.5 ml of saline (150 mM NaCl). Verify concentration on the spectrophotometer using doxorubicin extinction coefficient $\varepsilon = 1.06 \times 10^4$ M^{-1} cm^{-1} (74). Pipette 5 μmol of lipid and 1 μmol of doxorubicin (approx. 0.5 mg) into a glass test-tube (or plastic Eppendorf tube) with HBS to give a final volume of 1 ml (5 mM lipid concentration). Incubate at 65 °C for 30 min. At appropriate time points (0, 5, 15, 30 min) apply an aliquot (50–100 μl) to a spin column and centrifuge at 2000 r.p.m. for 2 min. LUVs containing entrapped drug will elute off the column, while free doxorubicin will be trapped in the gel. Save an aliquot (50 μl) of the initial lipid–drug mixture for determination of initial D/L.

5 Assay the initial mixture and each time point for doxorubicin and lipid. Lipid can be quantified by the phosphate assay (Protocol 1), by liquid scintillation counting of an appropriate radiolabel, or by measuring the fluorescence of LUVs containing 0.5–1 mol% of rhodamine-PE (see Protocol 6). Doxorubicin is quantified by an absorbance assay (see step 6). The per cent uptake at any time point (e.g. t = 30 min) is determined by:

$$\% \text{ uptake} = [(D/L)_{t = 30 \text{ min}}] \times 100 / [(D/L)_{\text{initial}}].$$

6 Doxorubicin assay. Prepare a standard curve consisting of four or five cuvettes containing 0–150 nmol doxorubicin in a volume of 0.1 ml. Add 0.9 ml of 1% (v/v) Triton X-100 (in water). Prepare assay samples in the same manner, and read absorbance at 480 nm.

The pH gradient approach described above has been applied successfully to many different drugs (19). However, not all drugs can be easily loaded using this approach. A case in point is the antibiotic ciprofloxacin, a commercially successful, quinolone antibiotic widely used in the treatment of respiratory and urinary tract infections (50). Ciprofloxacin is a zwitterionic compound that is charged and soluble under acidic and alkaline conditions, but is neutral and poorly soluble in the physiological pH range. Less than 20% uptake is achieved when the drug is loaded using the standard technique (Protocol 3). However, high levels of encapsulation can be achieved using an alternate ΔpH loading method that is based on transmembrane gradients of ammonium sulfate (50, 70, 75). In brief, the drug of interest is incubated in the presence of LUVs containing internal ammonium sulfate and external saline. A small amount of neutral ammonia will diffuse out of the vesicle, creating an unbuffered acidic interior with a pH ~ 2.7 (50). The neutral form of externally added drug can diffuse into the vesicle interior, where it will consume a proton and become charged and therefore trapped. As the incoming drug uses up the supply of protons, more neutral ammonia will diffuse out, creating more protons to drive drug uptake. This continues until all the drug has been loaded, or until the internal proton supply is depleted. Over the course of drug loading the internal pH rises to about 5.1 (50). The technique is ideal for ciprofloxacin as the drug is supplied as an HCl salt, and thus is acidic and soluble when dissolved in water. A diagrammatic scheme of the uptake is given in Figure 3 (*centre column*).

This technique has been applied to a variety of drugs including doxorubicin (51, 70, 71, 75), epirubicin (51), ciprofloxacin (50, 51, 70, 76), and vincristine (51). A variety of alkylammonium salts (e.g. methylammonium sulfate, propyl-ammonium sulfate, amylammonium sulfate) can be used in place of ammonium sulfate (51). Some drugs, such as doxorubicin, precipitate and form a gel in the vesicle interior (70, 71), while others, such as ciprofloxacin, do not (70, 76). The physical state of encapsulated drug will clearly affect retention and therefore may impact efficacy.

Protocol 4 describes the uptake of ciprofloxacin into SPM/Chol LUVs. Prior to assaying for ciprofloxacin, a Bligh–Dyer extraction (77) into 200 mM NaOH is performed to remove lipid, which interferes at the wavelength used for measuring drug.

Protocol 4

Remote loading of weakly basic drugs (e.g. ciprofloxacin) into LUVs containing transmembrane amine gradients

Equipment and reagents

- See Protocols 2 and 3
- Egg sphingomyelin (Avanti Polar Lipids; Northern Lipids; Sigma-Aldrich)
- Ciprofloxacin (Bayer Corporation)
- Saline: 150 mM NaCl
- 300 mM $(NH_4)_2SO_4$ (ammonium sulfate)

Method

1 Co-dissolve 275 μmol egg sphingomyelin (193 mg) and 225 μmol Chol (87 mg) in 7 ml t-butanol. If desired, add 12 μCi of [^{3}H]cholesteryl hexadecyl ether (CHE) or [^{14}C]CHE. To obtain specific activity of lipid mixture, determine the activity of an aliquot by liquid scintillation counting, and measure SPM concentration via the phosphate assay (Protocol 1), removing t-BuOH by lyophilization prior to assay (freeze tubes in liquid nitrogen and place under high vacuum for 30 min). Express specific activity as dpm/μmol lipid. Divide lipid into ten glass Pyrex tubes (50 μmol lipid per tube), freeze in liquid nitrogen, and lyophilize. Prepare SPM/Chol (55:45) LUVs (diameter = 100 nm) using 50 μmol lipid as described in Protocol 2 ([lipid] = 25 mM, volume = 2 ml). Use 300 mM ammonium sulfate as the hydration buffer.

2 Prepare spin columns (using saline rather than HBS) for monitoring drug uptake with time, as described in Protocol 3, step 2.

3 Form amine gradient by running an aliquot (200 μl) of the LUVs down a column (1.5 × 15 cm) of Sephadex G-50 eluted in saline, as described in Protocol 3, step 3. Alternatively, form gradient using spin columns (spin 2 × 100 μl), and pool the fractions (see Protocol 3, step 2).

4 Ciprofloxacin is often loaded at a drug-to-lipid (D/L) ratio of 0.3 mol:mol. Prepare a ciprofloxacin standard solution (4 mM) in water. Pipette 5 μmol of lipid and 1.5 μmol of ciprofloxacin into a glass test-tube (or plastic Eppendorf tube), adding saline to give a final volume of 1 ml (5 mM lipid concentration). Incubate at 65 °C for 30 min. At appropriate time points (0, 5, 15, 30 min) apply an aliquot (50–100 μl) to a spin column and centrifuge at 2000 r.p.m. (670 g) for 2 min. Save an aliquot (50 μl) of the initial lipid–drug mixture for determination of initial D/L.

5 Assay the initial mixture and each time point for ciprofloxacin and lipid. Lipid can be quantified as described in Protocol 3, step 5. Ciprofloxacin is quantified by an absorbance assay following removal of drug from lipid by a Bligh–Dyer extraction procedure (77) (see step 6). The per cent uptake is determined as described in Protocol 3, step 5.

6 Ciprofloxacin assay:

(a) Prepare a standard curve of six glass test-tubes containing 0, 50, 100, 150, 200, and 250 nmol ciprofloxacin (in water). Make up to 1 ml volume with 200 mM NaOH. For the blank, use 1 ml of 200 mM NaOH. Each LUV sample to be assayed should contain <250 nmol ciprofloxacin in a volume of 1 ml.

(b) To each standard and assay sample, add 2.1 ml methanol and 1 ml chloroform. Vortex gently. Only one phase should be present (if two phases form, add 0.1 ml methanol and vortex again).

(c) Add 1 ml of 200 mM NaOH and 1 ml chloroform to each tube, and vortex on high. Two phases should form, an aqueous phase containing the ciprofloxacin with a volume of 4.1 ml (top), and an organic phase containing the lipid with a volume of 2 ml (bottom). If a clean separation is not obtained, centrifuge at 2000 r.p.m. for 2 min in a desktop centrifuge.

Protocol 4 continued

(d) Carefully remove the aqueous phase, and read the absorbance at 273.5 nm. Divide nmol cipro (obtained from the standard curve) by the original sample volume (in μl), multiplying by any dilution factor, to obtain the sample drug concentration (mM).

Recently, we have developed a new method for remote loading of weakly basic drugs that is based on the ionophore-mediated generation of a secondary pH gradient in response to transmembrane gradients of monovalent and divalent cations (52). The process is diagrammed in Figure 3 (*right column*). Initially, an ion gradient is established: LUVs are hydrated in a 300 mM solution of K_2SO_4, $MnSO_4$, or $MgSO_4$, after which they are passed down a column containing 300 mM sucrose. The choice of sulfate salts is important, as chloride ion can dissipate pH gradients by forming neutral HCl which can diffuse out of the vesicle. Likewise, sucrose is chosen as the external solution rather than saline, as chloride ion can interfere with some ionophores (78). After establishing the primary ion gradient, the drug (this protocol has been utilized for doxorubicin, ciprofloxacin, and vincristine, and should be generally applicable to other drugs that are weak bases) is added. The ionophore nigericin is added to LUVs containing a potassium salt, whereas A23187 and the chelator EDTA are added to LUVs containing either Mn^{2+} or Mg^{2+}. In both cases, the ionophore transports the cations out of the LUV, down their concentration gradients, and at the same time transports protons in, acidifying the interior. This creates a pH gradient which drives drug uptake (as in Protocols 3 and 4). The EDTA appears to chelate calcium and magnesium as they are transported out of the vesicles, and is required to drive drug uptake when using divalent cations. The method gives high levels of encapsulation for the drugs ciprofloxacin and vincristine (80–90%), and excellent *in vitro* retention (52). The A23187-loaded systems exhibit *in vivo* circulation and drug retention properties that are comparable to systems loaded by the citrate or amine methods (Protocols 3 and 4, respectively).

Protocol 5

Ionophore-mediated loading of weakly basic drugs (e.g. vincristine) into LUVs containing transmembrane ion gradients

Equipment and reagents

- See Protocols 2 and 3
- Egg sphingomyelin (Avanti Polar Lipids; Northern Lipids; Sigma-Aldrich)
- HEPES-buffered sucrose: 20 mM HEPES, 300 mM sucrose pH 7.5
- Vincristine sulfate (Eli Lilly Canada)
- 300 mM $MnSO_4$
- 300 mM sucrose
- Ionophore A23187 (2.0 mg/ml in ethanol) (Sigma-Aldrich)

Method

1 Prepare SPM/Chol (55:45) LUVs (diameter = 100 nm) using 50 μmol lipid as described in Protocols 2 and 4 ([lipid] = 25 mM, volume = 2 ml). Use 300 mM $MnSO_4$ (in water) as the hydration solution.

2 Prepare spin columns (hydrated in 300 mM sucrose) for monitoring drug uptake with time, as described in Protocol 3, step 2.

3 Form manganese gradient by running an aliquot (200 μl) of the LUVs down a column (1.5 × 15 cm) of Sephadex G-50 eluted in HEPES-buffered sucrose pH 7.5 containing 3 mM Na_2EDTA. Alternatively, form gradient using spin columns prepared in the same buffer (spin 2 × 100 μl), and pool the fractions (see Protocol 3, step 2).

4 Vincristine sulfate (commercially available at 1 mg/ml) is added to give a drug-to-lipid (D/L) ratio of 0.03 mol:mol. Pipette 5 μmol of lipid and 0.15 μmol of vincristine into a glass test-tube, adding HEPES-buffered sucrose containing 3 mM Na_2EDTA to give a final volume of 1 ml (5 mM lipid concentration). Incubate at 60 °C for 10 min. Save an aliquot (50 μl) for determination of initial D/L ratio. Apply an aliquot (50–100 μl) to a spin column to assess any drug uptake prior to addition of ionophore.

5 At time t = 0, the A23187 (dilute original stock to 0.1 μg/μl) is added in a volume of approx. 5 μl to give a concentration of 0.1 μg/μmol lipid. At appropriate time points (0, 5, 15, 30 min) apply an aliquot (100 μl) to a spin column and centrifuge at 2000 r.p.m. for 2 min.

6 Assay the initial mixture and each time point for vincristine and lipid. Lipid can be quantified as described in Protocol 3, step 5. Vincristine is quantified by an absorbance assay (see step 7), with the per cent uptake determined as described in Protocol 3, step 5.

7 Vincristine assay. Prepare a standard curve consisting of four or five tubes containing 0–150 nmol vincristine in a volume of 0.2 ml. Add 0.8 ml of 95% ethanol. Prepare assay samples in the same manner, and read absorbance at 295 nm.

5 Liposomal systems for the encapsulation of genetic drugs: long-circulating vectors for the systemic delivery of genes and antisense oligonucleotides

A current focus in the field of gene therapy is on the development of genetic drugs, such as antisense oligonucleotides or plasmid DNA carrying a therapeutic gene, capable of treating acquired diseases such as cancer and inflammation. The systemic nature of these diseases requires the development of gene delivery vehicles capable of accessing distal disease sites following systemic (intravenous) administration. Unfortunately, while numerous methods exist for effective *in vitro* gene delivery, many current systems, such as viral vectors, lipoplexes, and lipopolyplexes, have limited utility for systemic applications (79). Viral vectors cannot carry plasmids that exceed a certain size, and often elicit strong immune responses. Lipoplexes and lipopolyplexes tend to be cleared rapidly from the circulation due to their large size and positive charge characteristics, and suffer from toxicity issues (see ref. 79 and references therein). Liposomal carriers of genetic drugs that possess the characteristics of the conventional drug carriers discussed above, i.e. small size, serum stability, and long circulation lifetimes, have been difficult to achieve (80), as large, highly charged molecules are not easily encapsulated within relatively small vesicles. Recently, though, we have developed two very different methods for the generation of liposomes capable of carrying either antisense oligonucleotides or plasmid DNA. The first of these employs a detergent dialysis approach for the formation of liposomal DNA carriers known as stabilized plasmid–lipid particles (SPLP) (57, 58, 60), which are described in Protocol 6. The second method, to be described in Protocol 7, involves entrapping polynucleotides, via electrostatic interactions, within pre-formed ethanol destabilized cationic liposomes (54–56).

SPLP are small (~70 nm), monodisperse particles that consist of a single plasmid encapsulated in a unilamellar lipid vesicle composed of DOPE, a cationic lipid (usually DODAC), and PEG-ceramide (PEGCer) (57, 58). The plasmid DNA can be visualized within the particles by cryo-EM (Figure 5). SPLP are formed from mixtures of plasmid and lipid by a detergent dialysis procedure involving octyl-glucopyranoside (OGP). SPLP protect plasmid DNA from DNase I and serum nucleases (57), possess extended circulation half-lives (6–7 h) (58), and have been

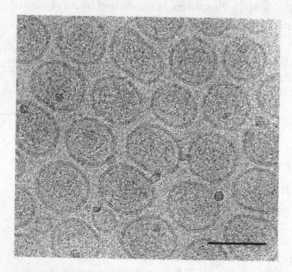

Figure 5 Cryo-electron micrographs of purified SPLP, prepared from DOPE/ DODAC/ PEGCerC$_{20}$ (83: 7: 10; mol:mol:mol) and pCMVluc as described in the text. The bar indicates 100 nm. Reprinted from ref. 58, with permission.

shown to accumulate in distal tumour sites with subsequent gene expression in mouse tumour models following i.v. injection (79). These vectors are clearly capable of disease site targeting, making them promising vectors for *in vivo* gene transfer.

Protocol 6 outlines the production of SPLP for smaller scale *in vitro* or *in vivo* studies. A detailed protocol for the production of a large scale SPLP batch, suitable for animal studies, has been published elsewhere (60).

Protocol 6

Encapsulation of plasmid DNA within stabilized plasmid–lipid particles (SPLP) via a detergent dialysis procedure

Equipment and reagents

- Glass test-tubes (13 × 100 mm)
- Spectrum Spectra/Por® Molecular porous 10 mm membrane tubing 12 000–14 000 MWCO (Spectrum Laboratories)
- Beckman SW41 ultracentrifuge rotor with polycarbonate tubes (Beckman Ultra-clear centrifuge tubes, 14 × 89 mm, No. 344059)
- Nicomp Model 370 Submicron Particle Sizer (or equivalent QELS unit)
- Assorted sterile syringes and 18G1/2 needles
- Millipore 0.22 μm syringe filtration unit
- Pasteur pipettes
- Plasmid DNA (1 mg/ml)

- DOPE (Avanti Polar Lipids; Northern Lipids)
- PEGCerC$_{20}$ (Northern Lipids; Inex Pharmaceuticals)
- DODAC (Inex Pharmaceuticals)
- Rhodamine-DOPE [1,2-dioleoyl-*sn*-glycero-3-phosphoethanolamine-N-(lissamine rhodamine B sulfonyl)] (Avanti Polar Lipids)
- 1 M octyl-glucopyranoside (OGP) in water (Sigma-Aldrich)
- 10% (v/v) Triton X-100 in water (Sigma-Aldrich)
- Picogreen DNA quantitation reagent (Molecular Probes)

Method

This protocol describes the preparation of SPLP beginning with 200 μg of plasmid DNA in a total volume of 1 ml. The basic procedure involves solubilizing lipid and plasmid in a detergent solution of appropriate ionic strength, and removing the detergent by dialysis to form SPLP and empty vesicles. Unencapsulated DNA is removed by ion exchange chromatography, and empty vesicles by sucrose density gradient centrifugation.

1 Prepare 2 litres of 10 × HBS (1 × = 20 mM HEPES, 150 mM NaCl pH 7.4).

2 Prepare lipid stock solutions (dissolve lipids in chloroform or in methanol). Examples of convenient lipid concentrations would be 100 mM for DOPE, 25.8 mM (15 mg/ml) for DODAC, 9.3 mM (25 mg/ml) for PEGCerC$_{20}$, and 0.78 mM (1 mg/ml) for rhodamine-PE. Combine required amounts of solutions for a preparation consisting of 10 μmol total lipid and composition DOPE/ DODAC/ PEGCerC$_{20}$/ Rho-PE (81.5: 8: 10: 0.5). Remove chloroform under a stream of nitrogen gas and then remove residual traces of solvent under high vacuum for 1 h.

3 To 10 μmol dry lipid, add 200 μl of 1 M OGP. Heat and vortex until lipid is mostly dissolved, and no longer sticking to glass. Then add 600 μl HBS and vortex with heating until clear. Add 200 μg plasmid DNA and vortex gently. This will give a 1 ml solution with 200 μg plasmid DNA, [lipid] = 10 mM, and [OGP] = 200 mM.

4 Encapsulation of plasmid and formation of SPLP is highly sensitive to the cationic lipid content and the salt concentration of the dialysis buffer. In general, a salt concentration is selected that gives high levels of encapsulation (50–70%), a small diameter (80–100 nm), and a monodisperse particle distribution (a χ^2 value of three or less, obtained from QELS). In practice, it is often necessary to test a range of salt concentrations to achieve optimal encapsulation. This is particularly critical when preparing SPLP with high DODAC content (14–24 mol%), which requires inclusion of a polyanionic salt such as citrate or phosphate in addition to NaCl (81, 82). For SPLP containing 8 mol% DODAC, particle formation should occur for 20 mM HEPES pH 7.5 containing 140–150 mM NaCl. As it may be necessary to test several salt concentrations for a given lipid formulation, the sample size may need to be increased. Thus, a 4 ml sample could be prepared using 40 μmol lipid, 800 μg plasmid DNA, with [lipid] = 10 mM, and [OGP] = 200 mM.

5 To determine optimal encapsulation conditions, dialyse 250 μl aliquots of the above preparation in 1 cm diameter dialysis tubing overnight against 1 litre of 20 mM HEPES pH 7.5 containing 140, 145, and 150 mM NaCl.

6 The next day, perform QELS analysis (not described; see manufacturers manual) and a picogreen assay. The picogreen assay is as follows:

(a) Pipette 5 μl aliquots of each formulation into disposable 1 cm fluorescence cuvettes.

(b) Add 1.8 ml of picogreen buffer (containing 1 μl of picogreen per 2 ml HBS) to cuvette. Read fluorescence in the absence and presence of Triton X-100. The excitation and emission wavelengths of picogreen are 480 and 520 nm, respectively (set slit width to 5 nm). After reading fluorescence in the absence of detergent (– Triton value), add 30 μl of 10% Triton X-100 to the cuvette, mix thoroughly, and then read fluorescence again (+ Triton value). The % encapsulation = {([+ Triton] – [– Triton]) × 100} / [+ Triton].

7 The optimal NaCl concentration is determined by the per cent of plasmid encapsulation and particle size. The optimal NaCl provides for 50–80% encapsulation and a single population with a particle size of ≤100 nm. Particle sizes greater than 120 nm indicate a 'crashed' preparation where the vesicles have aggregated. Determine the optimal NaCl concentration and prepare 4 × 2 litres of dialysis buffer for a 48 h dialysis.

8 Dialyse the initial lipid solution for 48 h using the optimal buffer conditions. Transfer the dialysis bags to fresh dialysis buffer every 12 h.

9 Perform a picogreen assay and QELS on the resulting material. Expect a per cent encapsulation of approx. 50–80%. If this is not achieved, perform another salt curve

Protocol 6 continued

before proceeding to the next step (the lipid–DNA mixture can be re-solubilized in OGP, and re-dialysed with a different buffer).

10 Following formation of SPLP, unencapsulated DNA is removed by DEAE-Sepharose chromatography. Up to 0.64 mg of DNA can be loaded per 1 ml stationary volume of the DEAE-Sepharose CL-6B (Sigma) column. Pour the column in a small plastic holder (such as a 3 ml disposable syringe stopped with a small plug of glass wool) and wash with ten column volumes of $1 \times$ HBS.

11 Once the column has settled, slowly load the formulation suspension to the resin, and elute with HBS. Collect a final volume equal to 1.5 times the sample volume to completely elute all of the formulation from the column.

12 The final step in the purification of SPLP is removal of empty vesicles from those containing plasmid DNA. This is accomplished by sucrose density gradient ultra-centrifugation in a Beckman ultracentrifuge using an SW41 rotor. Prepare desired volumes of 1.0%, 2.5%, and 10.0% (w/v) sucrose in $1 \times$ HBS and filter sterilize into a sterile container. Store at 4 °C.

13 Pull a long glass pipette to a small point using forceps and a Bunsen burner. Place the elongated pipette into the ultracentrifuge tube and pour 3.6 ml of 1.0% sucrose solution into the pipette using a second pipette. Avoid air bubbles in the narrow part of the pipette.

14 Pour the sucrose layers in order of increasing density; 3.6 ml of 1.0%, 3.6 ml of 2.5%, and 3.6 ml of 10.0%. Load 1 ml of SPLP on top of the gradients.

15 Balance all the tubes with $1 \times$ HBS to within 0.01 g and place the tubes in the SW41 buckets. Spin for 2 h at 36 000 r.p.m. at 20 °C. Make sure the brake is off when the run is complete.

16 The SPLP will be visible as a pink (rhodamine) band layered at the interface of the 2.5% and 10% sucrose solutions (lower band). The empty vesicles will either be banded at the 1–2.5% interface, or spread throughout the 1% and 2.5% solutions. Puncture the tube 2 mm below the SPLP band using an 18G needle with a 3 ml syringe, and slowly aspirate the SPLP band. Pool all of the SPLP bands and place the formulation into a dialysis bag overnight in $1 \times$ HBS to remove the sucrose.

17 Perform a picogreen assay to determine the per cent encapsulation and DNA concentration, and measure the size by QELS.

18 Ideally, the SPLP concentration should be in the range of 0.1 mg DNA/ml. If necessary, the sample can be concentrated using an Amicon filtration device, or by using Aquacide.

19 Filter sterilize the final volume through a sterile Millipore 0.22 μm filter unit in a Biological Safety Cabinet and adjust the final volume so that the DNA concentration is exactly 0.1 mg/ml. Store SPLP in sterile vials at 4 °C for up to two years. If desired, the lipid concentration can be determined from a phosphate assay, and agarose gel electrophoresis can be used to verify the integrity of the plasmid.

Antisense oligonucleotides are another class of genetic drugs that may benefit . from encapsulation within a liposomal carrier (54). Recently, we have described a novel formulation process that utilizes an ionizable aminolipid (DODAP) and an ethanol-containing buffer for encapsulating large quantities of polyanionic antisense oligonucleotide in lipid vesicles (54–56). The resulting particle is known as a 'stabilized antisense–lipid particle,' or SALP. Initially, an ethanolic liposome solution is formed by addition of ethanol to preformed vesicles consisting of DSPC/Chol/PEGCerC$_{14}$/DODAP, or by addition of lipids dissolved in ethanol to an aqueous buffer with subsequent extrusion. A citrate buffer is used to acidify the ethanol-containing buffer (pH 4) to ensure that the cationic lipid is protonated. The addition of oligonucleotide to the ethanolic liposome solution leads to the formation of multilamellar liposomes (as well as some unilamellar and bilamellar vesicles), which trap oligonucleotides between the bilayers. Upon dialysis against acidic and then neutral buffers, the ethanol is removed and any externally bound oligonucleotide is released from the uncharged liposome surface. Unencapsulated ODN is then removed by anion exchange chromatography. The end result is a multilamellar vesicle with a small diameter (70–120 nm), and a maximum entrapment of 0.16 mg ODN/mg lipid, which corresponds to ~2200 oligonucleotide molecules per 100 nm liposome (56) (Figure 6). The SALP exhibit

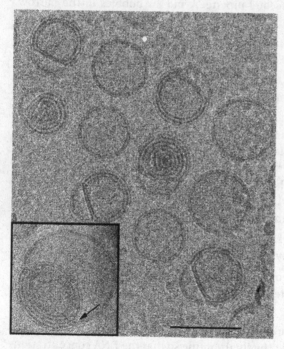

Figure 6 Cryo-electron micrographs of DSPC/ Chol/ PEGCerC$_{14}$/ DODAP (20: 45: 10: 25 mol%) liposomes entrapping oligonucleotides (SALP). The inset is an expanded view of a multilamellar liposome showing two initially separated membranes forced into close apposition by bound oligonucleotides (*arrow*). The entrapped antisense-to-lipid weight ratio was 0.125 mg/mg. The bar represents 100 nm. Reprinted from ref. 56, with permission.

extended circulation half-lives, ranging from 5–6 h for particles formed with PEGCerC$_{14}$ to 10–12 h for particles formed with PEGCerC$_{20}$ (54). The combination of high entrapment efficiencies, small size, and extended circulation lifetimes suggests that the SALP system should prove of utility for the liposomal delivery of antisense drugs.

Protocol 7

Encapsulation of antisense oligonucleotides within stabilized antisense–lipid particles (SALP) via ethanol-dependent uptake of polynucleotides into preformed vesicles

Equipment and reagents

- Extruder
- Spectra/Por dialysis tubing (12–14 000 MWCO) (Spectrum Laboratories)
- Absolute ethanol (≥ 99%)
- Stock solutions of 1,2-dioleoyl-3-dimethylammoniumpropane (DODAP) (Inex Pharmaceuticals), DSPC, Chol, and PEGCerC$_{14}$ (Northern Lipids; Inex Pharmaceuticals) in chloroform or ethanol

- Oligonucleotide (ODN) stock solution: e.g. human c-myc (16-mer), 5'-TAACGTTGAGGGGCAT-3' at 20 mg/ml in distilled water or buffer (Inex Pharmaceuticals)
- Buffer solutions: 300 mM citrate pH 4, HBS (20 mM HEPES, 145 mM NaCl pH 7.5)
- DEAE-Sepharose CL-6B (Sigma-Aldrich)

Method

1. Prepare a lipid mixture containing 25 mg total lipid, with a molar ratio of DSPC/Chol/ PEGCerC$_{14}$/ DODAP of 20: 45: 10: 25. Remove solvent under a stream of N$_2$ followed by high vacuum for 1 h. Hydrate the lipid film in 1 ml of citrate buffer pH 4, and subject to five freeze-thaw cycles (Protocol 2, steps 4 and 5).

2. Form LUVs by extrusion at 60 °C as described in Protocol 2, step 6.

3. Slowly add ethanol to the LUVs with rapid vortexing up to a concentration of 40% (to avoid high local concentrations). The total lipid concentration should be 10 mg/ml. Slow addition of ethanol and rapid mixing are important as liposomes become unstable and coalesce into large lipid structures as soon as the ethanol concentration exceeds a certain upper limit, which depends on the lipid composition. The final liposomes should be around 100 nm in diameter. If necessary, the ethanolic liposome dispersions can be additionally extruded (2 ×).

4. LUVs can also be prepared by slow addition of the lipids dissolved in ethanol (total volume of 0.4 ml) to citrate buffer at pH 4 (0.6 ml) followed by extrusion through two stacked 100 nm filters (two passes) at room temperature. Typical liposome diameters obtained from QELS should be 75–100 nm. The extrusion step can be omitted if ethanol is added very slowly under vigorous mixing to avoid high local concentrations of ethanol.

Protocol 7 continued

5   *Entrapment procedure.* Slowly add the oligonucleotide solution (1–2 mg ODN) with vortexing to the ethanolic liposome dispersion (10 mg lipid/ml), to give an ODN-to-lipid ratio of 0.1–0.2 mg/mg.

6   Incubate ethanolic ODN–lipid mixture at 40 °C for 1 h, and then dialyse for 2 h against 2 litres of citrate buffer to remove most of the ethanol, and twice against 2 litres of HBS. At pH 7.5 DODAP becomes charge-neutral and oligonucleotides bound to the external membrane surface are released from their association with the cationic lipid.

7   Remove unencapsulated ODNs by anion exchange chromatography on DEAE-Sepharose CL-6B columns (3–4 ml of DEAE-Sepharose per 1 ml of ODN–liposome dispersion) equilibrated in HBS pH 7.5.

8   *Determination of trapping efficiencies.* Solubilize SALP by addition of chloroform/methanol at a volume ratio of 1: 2.1: 1 chloroform/ methanol/ SALP. The oligonucleotide concentrations are determined from the absorbance at 260 nm on a Shimadzu UV160U spectrophotometer. If the solution is not completely clear after mixing, an additional 50–100 µl of methanol is added. Alternatively, the absorbance can be read after solubilization of the samples in 100 mM octylglucoside. The antisense concentrations are calculated according to c. $[\mu g/\mu l] = A_{260} \times 1\ OD_{260}$ unit $[\mu g/ml] \times$ dilution factor $[ml/\mu l]$, where the dilution factor is given by the total assay volume [ml] divided by the sample volume [µl]. OD_{260} units are calculated from pairwise extinction coefficients for individual deoxynucleotides, which take into account nearest neighbour interactions. 1 OD corresponds to 30.97 µg/ml anti-c-myc. Lipid concentrations are determined by the inorganic phosphate assay (Protocol 1) after separation of the lipids from the oligonucleotides by a Bligh and Dyer extraction (Protocol 4, step 6), for an initial aqueous volume of 250 µl (all volumes should be scaled accordingly).

References

1. Bangham, A. D. (1968). *Prog. Biophys. Mol. Biol.*, **18**, 29.
2. Sessa, G. and Weissmann, G. (1968). *J. Lipid Res.*, **9**, 310.
3. Hope, M. J., Bally, M. B., Mayer, L. D., Janoff, A. S., and Cullis, P. R. (1986). *Chem. Phys. Lipids*, **40**, 89.
4. Lichtenberg, D. and Barenholz, Y. (1988). *Methods Biochem. Anal.*, **33**, 337.
5. Mayer, L. D., Bally, M. B., and Cullis, P. R. (1990). *J. Liposome Res.*, **1**, 463.
6. Hope, M. J., Bally, M. B., Webb, G., and Cullis, P. R. (1985). *Biochim. Biophys. Acta*, **812**, 55.
7. Mayer, L. D., Hope, M. J., and Cullis, P. R. (1986). *Biochim. Biophys. Acta*, **858**, 161.
8. Mayer, L. D., Nayar, R., Thies, R. L., Boman, N. L., Cullis, P. R., and Bally, M. B. (1993). *Cancer Chemother. Pharmacol.*, **33**, 17.
9. Mayer, L. D., Tai, L. C., Ko, D. S., Masin, D., Ginsberg, R. S., Cullis, P. R., *et al.* (1989). *Cancer Res.*, **49**, 5922.
10. Webb, M. S., Harasym, T. O., Masin, D., Bally, M. B., and Mayer, L. D. (1995). *Br. J. Cancer*, **72**, 896.

11. Webb, M. S., Logan, P., Kanter, P. M., St-Onge, G., Gelmon, K., Harasym, T., *et al.* (1998). *Cancer Chemother. Pharmacol.*, **42**, 461.

12. Boman, N. L., Masin, D., Mayer, L. D., Cullis, P. R., and Bally, M. B. (1994). *Cancer Res.*, **54**, 2830.

13. Woodle, M. C., Newman, M. S., and Cohen, J. A. (1994). *J. Drug Target.*, **2**, 397.

14. Gabizon, A. and Papahadjopoulos, D. (1988). *Proc. Natl. Acad. Sci. USA*, **85**, 6949.

15. Allen, T. M., Hansen, C., Martin, F., Redemann, C., and Yau-Young, A. (1991). *Biochim. Biophys. Acta*, **1066**, 29.

16. Allen, T. M. (1994). *Trends Pharmacol. Sci.*, **15**, 215.

17. Allen, T. M. (1998). *Drugs*, **56**, 747.

18. Mayer, L. D., Bally, M. B., and Cullis, P. R. (1986). *Biochim. Biophys. Acta*, **857**, 123.

19. Madden, T. D., Harrigan, P. R., Tai, L. C., Bally, M. B., Mayer, L. D., Redelmeier, T. E., *et al.* (1990). *Chem. Phys. Lipids*, **53**, 37.

20. Cullis, P. R., Hope, M. J., Bally, M. B., Madden, T. D., Mayer, L. D., and Fenske, D. B. (1997). *Biochim. Biophys. Acta*, **1331**, 187.

21. Mayer, L. D., Bally, M. B., Cullis, P. R., Wilson, S. L., and Emerman, J. T. (1990). *Cancer Lett.*, **53**, 183.

22. Mayer, L. D., Bally, M. B., Loughrey, H., Masin, D., and Cullis, P. R. (1990). *Cancer Res.*, **50**, 575.

23. Chonn, A. and Cullis, P. R. (1995). *Curr. Opin. Biotechnol.*, **6**, 698.

24. Cheung, T. W., Remick, S. C., Azarnia, N., Proper, J. A., Barrueco, J. R., and Dezube, B. J. (1999). *Clin. Cancer Res.*, **5**, 3432.

25. Muggia, F. M. (2001). *Curr. Oncol. Rep.*, **3**, 156.

26. Burstein, H. J., Ramirez, M. J., Petros, W. P., Clarke, K. D., Warmuth, M. A., Marcom, P. K., *et al.* (1999). *Ann. Oncol.*, **10**, 1113.

27. Campos, S. M., Penson, R. T., Mays, A. R., Berkowitz, R. S., Fuller, A. F., Goodman, A., *et al.* (2001). *Gynecol. Oncol.*, **81**, 206.

28. Shields, A. F., Lange, L. M., and Zalupski, M. M. (2001). *Am. J. Clin. Oncol.*, **24**, 96.

29. Gokhale, P. C., Radhakrishnan, B., Husain, S. R., Abernethy, D. R., Sacher, R., Dritschilo, A., *et al.* (1996). *Br. J. Cancer*, **74**, 43.

30. Coukell, A. J. and Spencer, C. M. (1997). *Drugs*, **53**, 520.

31. Gordon, A. N., Granai, C. O., Rose, P. G., Hainsworth, J., Lopez, A., Weissman, C., *et al.* (2000). *J. Clin. Oncol.*, **18**, 3093.

32. Grunaug, M., Bogner, J. R., Loch, O., and Goebel, F. D. (1998). *Eur. J. Med. Res.*, **3**, 13.

33. Judson, I., Radford, J. A., Harris, M., Blay, J., van Hoesel, Q., le Cesne, A., *et al.* (2001). *Eur. J. Cancer*, **37**, 870.

34. Israel, V. P., Garcia, A. A., Roman, L., Muderspach, L., Burnett, A., Jeffers, S., *et al.* (2000). *Gynecol. Oncol.*, **78**, 143.

35. Northfelt, D. W., Dezube, B. J., Thommes, J. A., Miller, B. J., Fischl, M. A., Friedman-Kien, A., *et al.* (1998). *J. Clin. Oncol.*, **16**, 2445.

36. Gelmon, K. A., Tolcher, A., Diab, A. R., Bally, M. B., Embree, L., Hudon, N., *et al.* (1999). *J. Clin. Oncol.*, **17**, 697.

37. Millar, J. L., Millar, B. C., Powles, R. L., Steele, J. P., Clutterbuck, R. D., Mitchell, P. L., *et al.* (1998). *Br. J. Haematol.*, **102**, 718.

38. Tokudome, Y., Oku, N., Doi, K., Namba, Y., and Okada, S. (1996). *Biochim. Biophys. Acta*, **1279**, 70.

39. Webb, M. S., Harasym, T. O., Masin, D., Bally, M. B., and Mayer, L. D. (1995). *Br. J. Cancer*, **72**, 896.

40. Gill, P. S., Wernz, J., Scadden, D. T., Cohen, P., Mukwaya, G. M., Von Roenn, J. H., *et al.* (1996). *J. Clin. Oncol.*, **14**, 2353.

41. Pratt, G., Wiles, M. E., Rawstron, A. C., Davies, F. E., Fenton, J. A., Proffitt, J. A., *et al.* (1998). *Hematol. Oncol.*, **16**, 47.

42. Webb, M. S., Boman, N. L., Wiseman, D. J., Saxon, D., Sutton, K., Wong, K. F., *et al.* (1998). *Antimicrob. Agents Chemother.*, **42**, 45.

43. Bakker-Woudenberg, I. A., ten Kate, M. T., Guo, L., Working, P., and Mouton, J. W. (2001). *Antimicrob. Agents Chemother.*, **45**, 1487.

44. Tardi, P., Choice, E., Masin, D., Redelmeier, T., Bally, M., and Madden, T. D. (2000). *Cancer Res.*, **60**, 3389.

45. Mayer, L. D., Nayar, R., Thies, R. L., Boman, N. L., Cullis, P. R., and Bally, M. B. (1993). *Cancer Chemother. Pharmacol.*, **33**, 17.

46. Dvorak, H. F., Nagy, J. A., Dvorak, J. T., and Dvorak, A. M. (1988). *Am. J. Pathol.*, **133**, 95.

47. Brown, J. M. and Giaccia, A. J. (1998). *Cancer Res.*, **58**, 1408.

48. Boman, N. L., Mayer, L. D., and Cullis, P. R. (1993). *Biochim. Biophys. Acta*, **1152**, 253.

49. Bally, M. B., Mayer, L. D., Loughrey, H., Redelmeier, T., Madden, T. D., Wong, K., *et al.* (1988). *Chem. Phys. Lipids*, **47**, 97.

50. Hope, M. J. and Wong, K. F. (1995). In *Liposomes in biomedical applications* (ed. P. N. Shek), p. 121. Harwood Academic Publishers.

51. Maurer-Spurej, E., Wong, K. F., Maurer, N., Fenske, D. B., and Cullis, P. R. (1999). *Biochim. Biophys. Acta*, **1416**, 1.

52. Fenske, D. B., Wong, K. F., Maurer, E., Maurer, N., Leenhouts, J. M., Boman, N., *et al.* (1998). *Biochim. Biophys. Acta*, **1414**, 188.

53. Cheung, B. C. L., Sun, T. H. T., Leenhouts, J. M., and Cullis, P. R. (1998). *Biochim. Biophys. Acta*, **1414**, 205.

54. Semple, S. C., Klimuk, S. K., Harasym, T. O., Dos, S. N., Ansell, S. M., Wong, K. F., *et al.* (2001). *Biochim. Biophys. Acta*, **1510**, 152.

55. Semple, S. C., Klimuk, S. K., Harasym, T. O., and Hope, M. J. (2000). In *Methods in enzymology* (ed. M. I. Phillips). Vol. 313, p. 322. Academic Press, San Diego.

56. Maurer, N., Wong, K. F., Stark, H., Louie, L., McIntosh, D., Wong, T., *et al.* (2001). *Biophys. J.*, **80**, 2310.

57. Wheeler, J. J., Palmer, L., Ossanlou, M., MacLachlan, I., Graham, R. W., Zhang, Y. P., *et al.* (1999). *Gene Ther.*, **6**, 271.

58. Tam, P., Monck, M., Lee, D., Ludkovski, O., Leng, E. C., Clow, K., *et al.* (2000). *Gene Ther.*, **7**, 1867.

59. Mok, K. W., Lam, A. M., and Cullis, P. R. (1999). *Biochim. Biophys. Acta*, **1419**, 137.

60. Fenske, D. B., MacLachlan, I., and Cullis, P. R. (2001). In *Methods in enzymology* (ed. M. I. Phillips). Vol. 346, p. 36. Academic Press, San Diego.

61. Fiske, C. H. and Subbarow, Y. (1925). *J. Biol. Chem.*, **66**, 375.

62. Cullis, P. R. (2000). *J. Liposome Res.*, **10**, ix.

63. Batzri, S. and Korn, E. D. (1973). *Biochim. Biophys. Acta*, **298**, 1015.

64. Huang, C. (1969). *Biochemistry*, **8**, 344.

65. Mimms, L. T., Zampighi, G., Nozaki, Y., Tanford, C., and Reynolds, J. A. (1981). *Biochemistry*, **20**, 833.

66. Szoka, F. J. and Papahadjopoulos, D. (1978). *Proc. Natl. Acad. Sci. USA*, **75**, 4194.

67. Olson, F., Hunt, C. A., Szoka, F. C., Vail, W. J., and Papahadjopoulos, D. (1979). *Biochim. Biophys. Acta*, **557**, 9.

68. Mayer, L. D., Bally, M. B., and Cullis, P. R. (1986). *Biochim. Biophys. Acta*, **857**, 123.

69. Harrigan, P. R., Wong, K. F., Redelmeier, T. E., Wheeler, J. J., and Cullis, P. R. (1993). *Biochim. Biophys. Acta*, **1149**, 329.

70. Lasic, D. D., Ceh, B., Stuart, M. C., Guo, L., Frederik, P. M., and Barenholz, Y. (1995). *Biochim. Biophys. Acta*, **1239**, 145.

71. Lasic, D. D., Frederik, P. M., Stuart, M. C., Barenholz, Y., and McIntosh, T. J. (1992). *FEBS Lett.*, **312**, 255.

72. Cheung, B. C., Sun, T. H., Leenhouts, J. M., and Cullis, P. R. (1998). *Biochim. Biophys. Acta*, **1414**, 205.

73. Chonn, A., Semple, S. C., and Cullis, P. R. (1991). *Biochim. Biophys. Acta*, **1070**, 215.

74. Rottenberg, H. (1979). In *Methods in enzymology* (ed: S. Fleischer and L. Packer), Vol. 55, p. 547. Academic Press, San Diego.

75. Haran, G., Cohen, R., Bar, L. K., and Barenholz, Y. (1993). *Biochim. Biophys. Acta*, **1151**, 201.

76. Maurer, N., Wong, K. F., Hope, M. J., and Cullis, P. R. (1998). *Biochim. Biophys. Acta*, **1374**, 9.

77. Bligh, E. G. and Dyer, W. J. (1959). *Can. J. Biochem. Physiol.*, **37**, 911.

78. Wheeler, J. J., Veiro, J. A., and Cullis, P. R. (1994). *Mol. Membr. Biol.*, **11**, 151.

79. Fenske, D. B., MacLachlan, I., and Cullis, P. R. (2001). *Curr. Opin. Mol. Ther.*, **3**, 153.

80. Maurer, N., Mori, A., Palmer, L., Monck, M. A., Mok, K. W., Mui, B., *et al.* (1999). *Mol. Membr. Biol.*, **16**, 129.

81. Saravolac, E. G., Ludkovski, O., Skirrow, R., Ossanlou, M., Zhang, Y. P., Giesbrecht, C., *et al.* (2000). *J. Drug Target.*, **7**, 423.

82. Zhang, Y. P., Sekirov, L., Saravolac, E. G., Wheeler, J. J., Tardi, P., Clow, K., *et al.* (1999). *Gene Ther.*, **6**, 1438.

Chapter 7
Surface modification of liposomes

Vladimir P. Torchilin and Volkmar Weissig
Northeastern University, Bouve College of Health Sciences,
Department of Pharmaceutical Sciences, Boston, MA, USA.

Francis J. Martin
ALZA Corporation, Menlo Park, CA, USA.

Timothy D. Heath
University of Wisconsin, School of Pharmacy, Madison, WI, USA.

Roger R. C. New

1 Introduction

Modification of the liposome surface is a powerful approach to control liposome properties and biological behaviour. Attachment of certain specific ligands (such as antibodies, peptides, hormones, sugars) makes liposomes targeted; attachment of contrast agents converts liposomes into efficient diagnostic tools; coating liposomes with polymers, such as poly(ethylene glycol) imparts to them an ability to circulate long without being opsonized and recognized by cells of the reticulo endothelial system, etc.

Naturally, to couple all the substances mentioned and many others to the liposome surface, numerous chemical protocols were developed which enable liposome surface modification in reasonably simple and efficient ways. A vast number of such methods have been suggested within the last several years. It is impossible to give a detailed description of all these methods in a single chapter, thus, we will present here the most representative protocols, which have already been proven useful experimentally. Among those protocols, the reader will see variable chemistry for the attachment of antibodies, proteins, peptides, sugars, sterically protective synthetic polymers, and radiometals.

2 Protein and peptide attachment to the liposomal surface

Protein-conjugated liposomes have attracted a great deal of interest, principally because of their potential use as targeted drug delivery systems (1, 2) and in diagnostic applications (3–5). Antibodies are the most commonly conjugated proteins, although the techniques can be readily applied to other proteins such as *Staphylococcus aureus* protein A (2), plant lectins (6), and enzymes (7). Some early methods for conjugation used amino-reactive homobifunctional reagents such as glutaraldehyde and diethyl suberimidate (8). Water soluble carbodiimides have also been used to catalyse the formation of an amide linkage between amino groups (from phosphatidylethanolamine present in the liposome membrane) with carboxyl groups of proteins (9). However, as reviewed in detail elsewhere (10), these procedures are generally inefficient and are likely to bring about protein polymerization. The preferred methods are designed in such a way that the protein can react only with the liposome surface. The attachment of horseradish peroxidase to liposomes is one of the earliest examples of this approach (11). The carbohydrate on the enzyme is oxidized with sodium periodate to create reactive aldehydes after blocking the free amino groups with fluorodinitrobenzene. The enzyme is then coupled to liposomes by reaction of the aldehyde groups with the primary amino group of phosphatidylethanolamine present in low concentration in the liposome membrane. The bond is formed by reductive amination with sodium borohydride. The product, characterized biochemically and by electron microscopy, consists of intact liposomes with horseradish peroxidase attached to their outer surface.

During the 1980s, liposomal protein and peptide conjugation methodology was revolutionized by the development of three efficient and selective reactions. In the first of these reactions, activated carboxyl groups react with amino groups to produce an amide bond. In the second reaction, pyridyldithiols react with thiols to produce disulfide bonds. In the third reaction, maleimide derivatives react with thiols to produce thioether bonds. Most of the reactive lipid derivatives involved in these three techniques are now commercially available. In the following we introduce these three major conjugation techniques in detail.

2.1 Binding of proteins and peptides to liposomes via amino groups

Since the first description of conjugating proteins to liposomal surfaces via free amino groups in 1978 (8), numerous techniques were developed during the 1980s, which are based on the nucleophilic reactivity of free amino groups of the protein or peptide (summarized in ref. 12). In terms of selectivity, high-yield coupling, and preservation of the biological activity of the protein or peptide, a two-stage coupling procedure involving carboxyacyl derivatives of phosphatidyl-ethanolamine (or cardiolipin) proved to be superior. The lipidic free carboxylic group is first activated with water soluble carbodiimide [l-ethyl-3(3-dimethyl-aminopropyl) carbodiimide, EDC] at pH = pK_a – 1, where K_a is the ionization constant of the given carboxylic group. In the second stage, protein or peptide solutions are added with a simultaneous change to pH 8.0. This technique was introduced for the first time by Weissig et al. (13) and Kung and Redeman (14) (both submitted their papers in April 1986), and later improved and modified by Bogdanov et al. (15), by Holmberg et al. (16), and by Mori and Huang (17). Further, typical protocols are given covering all aspects of this universal applicable conjugation technique.

2.1.1 Synthesis of phospholipid carboxyacyl derivatives

The most commonly used N-glutaryl-phosphatidylethanolamine (NGPE, Figure 1) as well as the N-succinyl and N-dodecanoyl derivatives of PE are available from Avanti Polar Lipids, Inc., Alabaster, AL. For specific requirements in terms of the spacer length between the protein/peptide and the liposomal surface, the general protocol for derivatization of PE using the example of the sebacic derivative is given. Carboxyacyl derivatives of cardiolipin (Figure 2) are not commercially available.

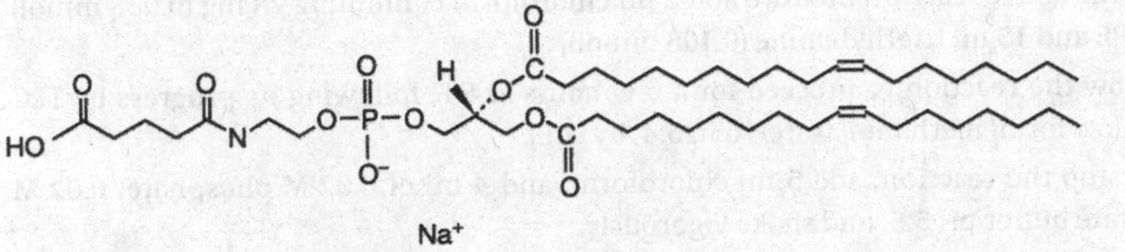

Figure 1 N-Glutaryl-phosphatidylethanolamine (NGPE).

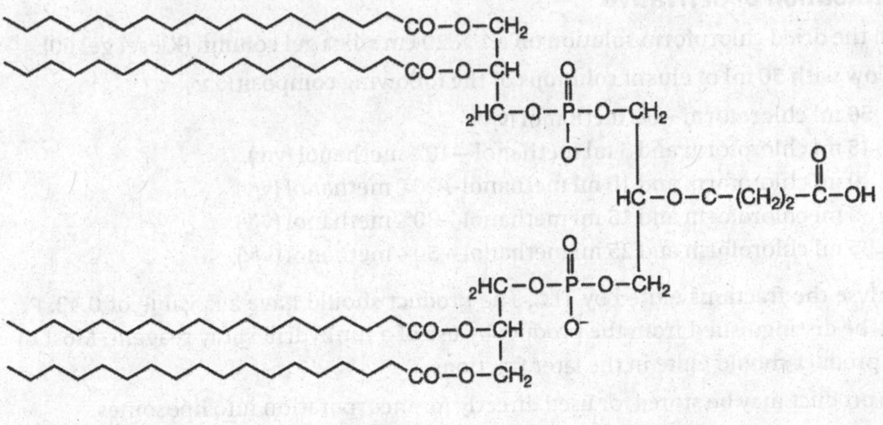

Figure 2 O-Succinyl cardiolipin (fatty acid residues are drawn schematically).

Protocol 1

PE derivatization with acid anhydride (14)

Equipment and reagents

- Glass screw-capped tubes
- Centrifuge
- 1 × 20 cm silica gel column (Kiesel gel 60)
- TLC equipment
- Sebacic acid
- Dicyclohexylcarbodiimide (DCCI)

- Methylene chloride
- PE, triethylamine
- Chloroform, methanol, water
- 0.02 M phosphate, 0.02 M citrate buffer: $Na_2HPO_4.7H_2O$, 5.4 mg/ml; $Na_3C_6H_6O_7.2H_2O$, 5.9 mg/ml; pH 5.5

A. Formation of sebacic anhydride

1   Dissolve 16.2 mg sebacic acid (0.08 mmol) and 8.7 mg (0.042 mmol) of dicyclo-hexylcarbodiimide (DCCI) in 2 ml methylene chloride in a 15–20 ml glass screw-capped tube.

2   Flush with nitrogen, cap tightly, and incubate the mixture for 48 h at room temperature (RT) with stirring. The anhydride formed may be used without further isolation.

B. Conjugation of PE

1   To the above reaction mixture add 2 ml chloroform containing 28 mg (0.038 mmol) of PE and 15 ml triethylamine (0.108 mmol).

2   Allow the reaction to proceed for a few hours at RT, following its progress by TLC (chloroform/ methanol/ water, 65:25:4, by vol.).

3   To stop the reaction, add 5 ml chloroform, and 4 ml of 0.02 M phosphate, 0.02 M citrate buffer pH 5.5, and shake vigorously.

4   Separate the two phases by low speed centrifugation (1000 g, for 10 min, at RT).

5   Discard the upper aqueous phase, and dry the organic phase over anhydrous sodium sulfate.

C. Purification of derivative

1   Run the dried chloroform solution on a 1 × 20 cm silica gel column (Kiesel gel 60).

2   Follow with 50 ml of eluant solutions of the following composition:
  (a) 50 ml chloroform—0% methanol (v/v).
  (b) 45 ml chloroform and 5 ml methanol—10% methanol (v/v).
  (c) 40 ml chloroform and 10 ml methanol—20% methanol (v/v).
  (d) 35 ml chloroform and 15 ml methanol—30% methanol (v/v).
  (e) 25 ml chloroform and 25 ml methanol—50% methanol (v/v).

3   Analyse the fractions eluted by TLC. The product should have a R_f value of 0.42. PE may be distinguished from the product by use of a ninhydrin spray reagent. Most of the product should elute in the later fractions.

4   The product may be stored, or used directly for incorporation into liposomes.

Protocol 2

Cardiolipin derivatization (18)

Equipment and reagents

- TLC equipment
- Succinic anhydride (or glutaric anhydride) and 4-dimethyl aminopyridine (DMAP) in anhydrous pyridine
- Cardiolipin (CL)
- 0.1 M NaHCO$_3$
- CHCl$_3$, CH$_3$OH, NH$_4$OH

Method

1 Dry 25 mg cardiolipin (CL) from an ethanolic solution using a nitrogen stream and vacuum.

2 Add a solution of 71.5 mg succinic anhydride (or 81.2 mg glutaric anhydride) and 6.5 mg 4-dimethyl aminopyridine (DMAP) in 3 ml anhydrous pyridine. Stir under nitrogen in the dark. Monitor the reaction by TLC (see below). After about 10–15 h the reaction is complete.

3 Evaporate the solvent, dissolve the residue in chloroform, and wash with 0.1 M NaHCO$_3$ to remove excess of anhydride.

4 Isolate the product by preparative TLC on silica gel plates of 0.5 mm thickness using CHCl$_3$/ CH$_3$OH/ 25% NH$_4$OH (130:64:15, by vol.) as a solvent system. Scrape the main phosphate-positive band off the plate and extract the CL derivative with CHCl$_3$/ CH$_3$OH (1:1, v/v).

5 The carboxyacyl derivative of cardiolipin can be stored in dry chloroform under nitrogen at –70 °C or used directly for incorporation into liposomes or hydro-phobization of proteins.

2.1.2 Hydrophobization of proteins or peptides prior to liposome formation

Since the protein is first coupled with the lipid in the absence of liposomal lipids, this method is compatible with different lipid compositions, which may be sensitive to the coupling reagent. Depending on the chosen liposome preparation technique, proteins and peptides can be conjugated to the lipid anchor either in the presence of or absence of a detergent. The addition of N-hydroxy-sulfo-succinimide (sulfo-NHS) to the reaction mixture during carbodiimide activation according to Bogdanov et al. (15) increases the yield of hydrophobized protein due to the avoidance of possible side reactions. The use of a four-tailed hydrophobic cardiolipin derivative instead of a two-tailed PE derivative allows a decrease of the number of amino groups involved in the conjugation reaction while maintaining the same degree of hydrophobicity. This results in an enhanced preservation of the biological activity of the hydrophobized and subsequently liposomal immo-bilized protein. For example, using the same liposome preparation procedure, the yield of liposomal immobilized chymotrypsin modified with two CL residues was in the same range as was obtained using chymotrypsin hydrophobized with five or six PE residues (13, 18). The introduction of eight hydrophobic acyl chains by covalent modification of only two amino groups by the CL derivative led to a loss of specific enzyme activity of only 25%, whereas the modification by the PE derivative reduced the activity to 46%.

Protocol 3

Hydrophobization of antibody with NGPE in the presence of detergent followed by incorporation in dialysis liposomes (17)

The antibody is first conjugated to NGPE (Figure 3) in the presence of detergent and then mixed with lipid detergent mixture. Upon removal of the detergent by dialysis, liposomes are formed with membrane-anchored antibody.

Equipment and reagents

- Dialysis equipment
- 0.4 and 0.2 μm Nucleopore membranes
- NGPE

- Octylglucoside
- EDC, sulfo-NHS
- Antibody in 0.1 M HEPES pH 7.5

Method

1. Prepare a dry film of 0.3 mg NGPE dissolved in chloroform by evaporating the solvent with a stream of nitrogen.

2. Solubilize the dry NGPE with 0.5 ml of 0.016 M octylglucoside in 50 mM MES pH 5.5.

3. Add to the solution 12 mg EDC and 15 mg sulfo-NHS, mix, and incubate for 5 min at RT.

4. Add to the solution 2 ml antibodies (about 1 mg/ml) in 0.1 M HEPES pH 7.5.

5. Adjust to pH 8.0 by adding about 20 μl of 0.1 M NaOH and incubate the mixture overnight at 4 °C with slight shaking.

6. For liposome preparation, solubilize a dry film of phospholipids with 100 mM octylglucoside in PBS pH 7.4. The molar ratio of lipid to octylglucoside is usually 1:5.

7. Add the desired amount of NGPE-conjugated antibody, mix vigorously, and remove all detergent by dialysis against PBS.

8. Extrude the resulting antibody-bearing liposomes several times through stacked 0.4 and 0.2 μm Nucleopore membranes to generate lipsomes with an average diameter of 200–300 nm.

9. Remove unbound antibody by column chromatography (BioGel A 1.5M or others).

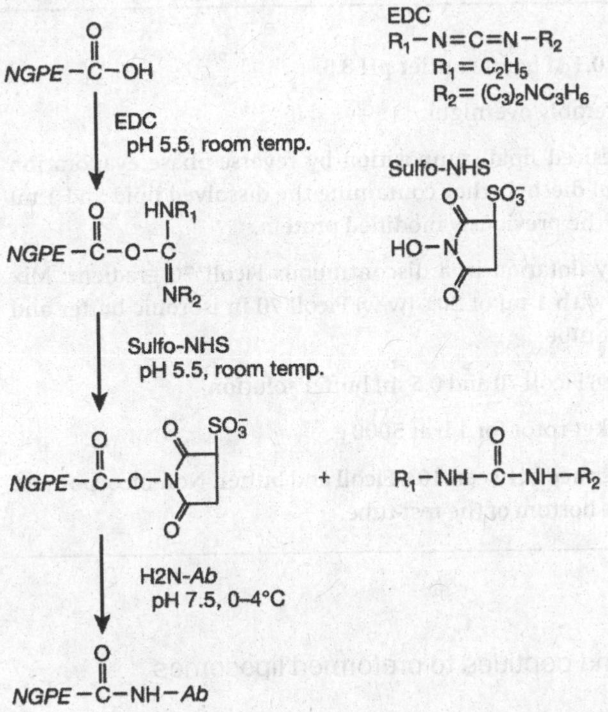

$NGPE-\overset{\overset{\displaystyle O}{\|}}{C}-OH$

EDC
$R_1-N=C=N-R_2$
$R_1 = C_2H_5$
$R_2 = (C_3)_2NC_3H_6$

EDC
pH 5.5, room temp.

$NGPE-\overset{\overset{\displaystyle O}{\|}}{C}-O-\overset{\overset{\displaystyle HNR_1}{\|}}{\underset{NR_2}{C}}$

Sulfo-NHS
$HO-N$ with SO_3^- and two C=O groups

Sulfo-NHS
pH 5.5, room temp.

$NGPE-\overset{\overset{\displaystyle O}{\|}}{C}-O-N$ (with SO_3^- and two C=O groups) $+$ $R_1-NH-\overset{\overset{\displaystyle O}{\|}}{C}-NH-R_2$

H2N-Ab
pH 7.5, 0–4°C

$NGPE-\overset{\overset{\displaystyle O}{\|}}{C}-NH-Ab$

Figure 3 Coupling reaction of NGPE with antibody in the presence of water soluble carbodiimide and N-hydroxy-sulfosuccinimide (17).

Protocol 4

Hydrophobization of proteins with carboxyacyl derivatives of PE or CL in the absence of detergent followed by incorporation in REV liposomes (13)

Equipment and reagents

- Centrifuge
- NGPE (or 0-glutaryl-CL)
- EDC

- Protein solution in 0.1 M borate buffer pH 8.5
- Ficoll 70

Method

1 Suspend the desired amount (2–20 mg) of dry NGPE (or 0-glutaryl-CL) in 150 μl DMSO and mix via brief sonication with 2 ml of 0.15 M NaCl solution.

2 Adjust the pH to about 3.5 with 0.01 N HCl and add, depending on the amount of NGPE used, between 3–30 mg EDC. Incubate for 5 min at RT.

Protocol 4 continued

3 Add 1 ml protein solution in 0.1 M borate buffer pH 8.5.

4 Incubate for at least 2 h, preferably overnight.

5 Prepare liposomes of the desired lipid composition by reverse-phase evaporation (19) from an emulsion of 3 ml diethyl ether containing the dissolved lipid and 1 ml aqueous solution containing the previously modified protein.

6 Remove unbound protein by flotation in a discontinuous Ficoll 70 gradient: Mix 0.5 ml liposome suspension with 1 ml of 20% (w/w) Ficoll 70 in isotonic buffer and layer it at the bottom of a test-tube.

7 Overlay with 5 ml of 10% (w/w) Ficoll 70 and 0.5 ml buffer solution.

8 Centrifuge in a swinging-bucket rotor for 1 h at 5000 g.

9 Pipette liposomes off the interface between 10% Ficoll and buffer. Non-incorporated protein is concentrated at the bottom of the test-tube.

2.1.3 Binding of proteins and peptides to preformed liposomes

Protocol 5

Immobilization of protein on the surface of preformed liposomes containing incorporated NGPE (15)

Equipment and reagents

- Sepharose CL-6B or CL-4B column
- Liposomes
- 5 mM MES, 0.15 M NaCl pH 5.5
- 50 mM borate buffer, 0.1 M NaCl pH 7.5
- EDC, sulfo-NHS
- Protein solution

Method

1 Prepare liposomes in 5 mM MES, 0.15 M NaCl pH 5.5, with up to 10 mol% incorporated NGPE (all common liposome preparation procedures are applicable).

2 Solubilize the protein in 50 mM borate buffer, 0.1 M NaCl pH 7.5.

3 Add 20 μl EDC (0.25 M in water) and 20 μl of 0.1 M sulfo-NHS to 200 μl of liposomes (1 μmol lipids) and incubate for 10 min.

4 Mix with 200 μl of protein solution (about 1 mg/ml protein) and incubate for 3 h.

5 Separate liposomes from unbound protein on Sepharose CL-6B or CL-4B (depending on liposome size). Pre-saturation of the column with lipid and BSA is recommended.

Protocol 6

Covalent coupling of water soluble peptides to dehydration–rehydration vesicles (12, 20)

As an example, the covalent binding of two synthetic poliovirus peptides is described (3-VP2, CFNKDNAVTSPKREFC sequence and 1-VP2, CFTPDDNQTSPARRFC sequence, both synthesized by M. Ferguson, Hertfordshire, UK). In immunization experiments it was shown that NGPE surface-linked peptides elicit more rapid rise in antibody level (IgG) as compared to liposomally entrapped peptide (21).

Equipment and reagents

- Centrifuge
- Probe sonicator
- PC, Chol, NGPE
- NaCl, EDC
- Peptide in borate buffer

Method

1. Prepare SUV consisting of 16 μmol PC, 16 μmol Chol, and the appropriate amount of NGPE (usually 4.5 μmol) in 1 ml distilled water by probe sonication. Centrifuge at 100 000 g for 1 h to remove metal traces and larger liposomes.

2. Transform the SUV into multilamellar liposomes according to the dehydration–rehydration method (DRV) (22). Mix 1 ml SUV with 1 ml of 1:10 diluted 0.15 N NaCl and lyophilize. Rehydrate the lyophilized material with 0.1 ml of distilled water followed by addition of 0.9 ml of 0.15 N NaCl.

3. Adjust 1 ml suspension of DRV with 0.01 N HCl to pH 3.5, mix with 15 mg EDC added as dry crystals, and incubate at RT for 5 min.

4. Add 1 ml of 0.1 M borate buffer pH 8.5, containing 200 μg peptide and incubate for at least 2 h, preferably overnight.

5. To remove unbound peptide, precipitate the DRV by centrifugation at 100 000 g for 1 h and wash repeatedly with borate buffer.

6. The amount of bound peptide can be determined indirectly by measuring the non-bound peptide in the pooled supernatant.

The yield of bound peptide is shown in Table 1. The numbers in parentheses denote values of control experiments carried out without the carbodiimide activation step. The amount of bound peptide varies (table shows best results obtained) and seems to be independent on the % of incorporated NGPE.

2.1.4 Protein binding to liposomes via reductive amination

The coupling of proteins to liposomes can also be carried out utilizing the reaction of a Schiff base with primary or secondary amino groups (Figure 4). Since the endogenous amino groups of the protein can be used without modification,

Table 1 Covalent binding of peptides to the surface of DRV liposomes via NGPE

PC: Ch: NGPE	Peptide bound [%]		Mol peptide bound/mol lipid × 10^4	
	3-VP2	1-VP2	3-VP2	1-VP2
1: 1: 0.11	70 (13)	52 (9)	9.7 (1.8)	7.0 (1.2)
1: 1: 0.28	65 (8)	63 (7)	8.4 (1.0)	7.8 (0.9)

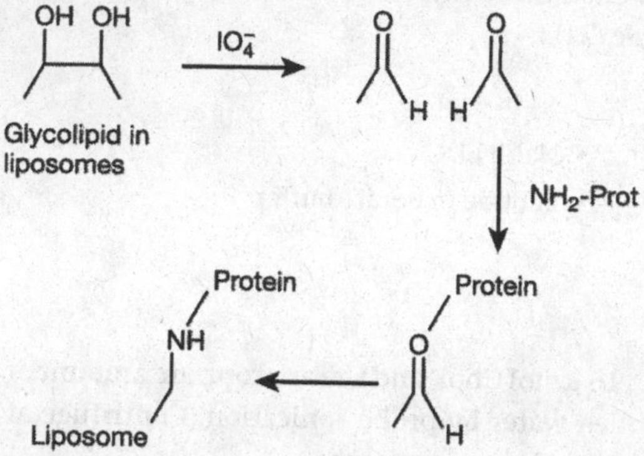

Figure 4 Linkage of liposome-bound sugars to proteins via Schiff base. Glycolipids such as cerebrosides or gangliosides incorporated into the liposome membrane can be used to link liposomes to proteins. Membrane-bound sugars containing two adjacent (vicinal) hydroxyl groups can be oxidized by periodate to aldehyde functional groups, which then react readily with the amino groups in proteins. Unreacted aldehyde functions, and the newly formed imine linkage, can be converted to unreactive species by reduction with sodium cyanoborohydride.

and liposome-bound glycolipids can be oxidized *in situ* without destroying the integrity of the liposomes, conjugation can be performed in a simple two-step reaction. Liposomes containing 50 mol% cholesterol and 10 mol% lactosyl ceramide, 20 mol% galactose cerebroside, or 5 mol% gangliosides have been employed successfully. Use of sucrose stearate-palmitate (23) and phosphatidylinositol (24) has also been reported. A protocol for periodate coupling of liposomes is given below (25).

Protocol 7

Periodate coupling of liposomes

Equipment and reagents

- Dialysis or minicolumn chromatography equipment
- Borate-buffered saline
- Glycolipid liposome suspension
- Sodium periodate
- IgG in borate-buffered saline
- Sodium cyanoborohydride

Protocol 7 continued

Method

1 Prepare borate-buffered saline containing 20 mM borate ($Na_2B_4O_7.10H_2O$, 7.6 mg/ml) and 120 mM NaCl (7 mg/ml) adjusted to pH 8.4.

2 To 1 ml of glycolipid liposome suspension, containing approx. 5 mg/ml of total lipid in borate-buffered saline, add 200 μl of 0.6 M sodium periodate ($NaIO_4$, 128 mg/ml distilled water) with stirring.

3 Incubate at RT in the dark for 30 min.

4 Remove free periodate either by dialysis overnight, or by minicolumn chromatography.

5 To 1 ml of oxidized liposomes, add 0.5 ml of the protein solution, containing 10–30 mg of IgG in borate-buffered saline pH 8.4.

6 Add 10 μl of 2 M sodium cyanoborohydride (125 mg/ml) per ml reaction mixture and leave overnight at 4 °C.

7 Separate free protein from liposomes by column chromatography or centrifugal flotation.

Although the optimal pH for periodate oxidation is pH 5.5, this reaction is carried out at higher pH values here to avoid increase in the permeability of the liposome membrane, and resultant loss of contents due to leakage at low pH. Also, at low pH, neutral liposomes are permeable to periodate, leading to oxidation of internal contents as well as surface glycolipids. Negatively-charged liposomes, however, are impermeable to periodate at low pH. If desired, periodate oxidation may be carried out at low pH provided the final periodate concentration is reduced to 10 mM or less. The incubation mixture may then be left overnight. Sodium cyanoborohydride is less reactive than sodium borohydride, but is used in preference since it is stable around pH 8.0 or lower (i.e. it does not require pH 9 as when $NaBH_4$ is used) and will not attack the disulfide bridges of proteins. The protein/lipid ratio is increased with increasing protein concentration, while the total protein bound is higher when the lipid concentration is higher. Under optimal conditions, approximately 20% of the initial protein can be bound, and about 40% of the theoretical available space on the liposome surface can be filled. With small sonicated liposomes, coupling at high concentration of both lipid and protein can lead to the aggregation by crosslinking of adjacent liposomes with proteins; this behaviour is not displayed with larger liposome (e.g. REVs). It is important to note that with glycolipids such as galactocerebroside, good coupling is not observed at concentrations less than 20 mol%, presumably because only one sugar residue is available for oxidation per molecule. Linkage with PO appears to be difficult, possibly because of steric considerations.

2.2 Binding of proteins to liposomes via sulfhydryl groups

The two methods we introduce here have been used by several laboratories for the conjugation of proteins to liposomes. They rely upon the reaction of thiol-reactive phospholipid derivatives included in the liposome with thiol groups of the proteins to be conjugated. Both reactive phospholipids, N-PDP-PE and N-MPB-PE, have been made commercially available during the last decade. However, the routine protocol of their preparation shall be described. The thiol-reactive lipids are synthesized using the reagents N-succinimidyl pyridyl dithio propionate (SPDP) and N-succinimidyl-(4-[p-maleimidophenyl]) butyrate (SMPB) (Figure 5). The former approach results in the reversible coupling of protein via a disulfide bond while the latter produces an irreversible thioether linkage. Because both methods are similar or identical in a number of steps, only the SPDP method will be given in detail, and modifications relevant to SMPB will be noted at the end. The basis of the methods is outlined in Figure 6.

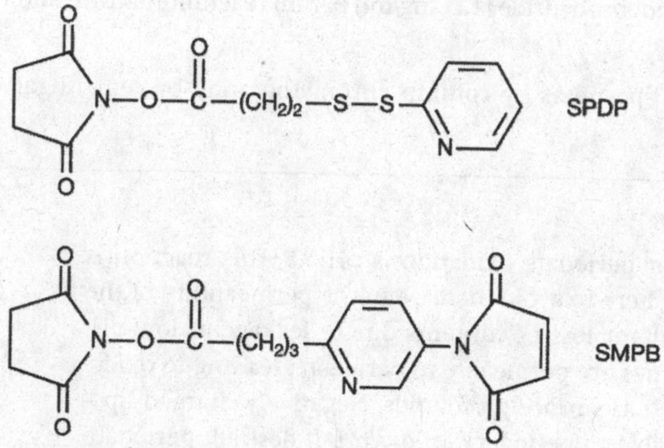

Figure 5 Structures of the two compounds most widely used for introducing thiol groups into moieties containing amino groups. SPDP, N-succinimidyl pyridyl dithiopropionate; SMPB, N-succinimidyl-(-4-[p-maleimidophenyl]) butyrate.

2.2.1 SPDP method of linking proteins to liposomes

Protocol 8

Synthesis of N-PDP-PE

Equipment and reagents

- Column chromatography: using silicic acid in chloroform in a 10 ml plastic syringe barrel plugged with glass fibre
- Rotary evaporator
- TLC using silica gel plates
- PE, TEA, SPDP
- Chloroform, methanol, water

Protocol 8 continued

Method

1 Dry down 15 mg of PE (approx. 20 μmol) in a 5 ml glass bottle.

2 Redissolve in 2 ml of dry chloroform (dried over a molecular sieve type 3a).

3 Add 30 μmol of TEA (3 mg), followed by 30 μmol of SPDP (approx. 10 mg) in 1 ml of dried methanol.

4 Stir the mixture at room temperature under nitrogen for 1–2 h until the reaction is complete.

5 While the reaction is proceeding, prepare a chromatography column of 2 g of silicic acid in chloroform. (Dissolve the silicic acid in 10 ml chloroform and pour the contents into a 10 ml plastic syringe barrel plugged with glass fibre. Allow the surplus to drain out and fit the syringe barrel with a plastic disposable three-way tap.)

6 Check the progress of the reaction by TLC using silica gel plates developed with chloroform/ methanol/ water (65:25:4, by vol.). The derivative runs faster than free PE. Visualize the spots using phosphomolybdate or iodine.

7 If the reaction has not gone to completion, add another 1 mg of TEA and continue stirring.

8 When the reaction is complete (i.e. no more free PE on the TLC plate), dry down the mixture on a rotary evaporator.

9 Resuspend the dried lipids in chloroform, and apply immediately to the top of the silicic acid column. (Note: it is not advisable to leave the lipids in contact with TEA for a long period of time, since the TEA appears to cause hydrolysis of ester linkages, leading to the formation of lyso-compounds. If it is necessary to wait before removing the TEA chromatographically, connect the flask with dried lipids to a lyophilizer, and keep under high vacuum overnight.)

10 Wash the column with 4 ml chloroform, then elute with 4 ml portions of a series of chloroform/methanol mixtures, first 4:0.25 (v/v) followed by 4:0.5 (v/v), 4:0.75 (v/v), and finally 4:1 (v/v). Collect 2 ml fractions and locate the pure derivative by TLC.

11 Pool the fractions containing the desired product and concentrate by evaporation at reduced pressure in a rotary evaporator.

12 Recheck for purity by TLC. The purity can also be confirmed by determining whether the phosphate/2-thiopyridine ratio is unity. Measure phosphorus by the Bartlett assay; 2-thiopyridine may be measured spectrophotometrically after reduction with dithiothreitol (the molar extinction coefficient of 2-thiopyridine at 343 nm is 8300).

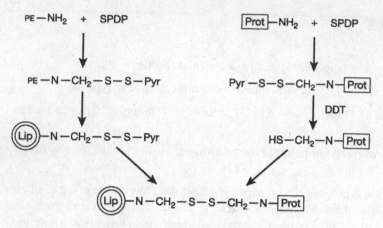

Figure 6 Use of SPDP for conjugation of proteins to liposomes. In this method, a potential sulfhydryl (SH)-forming residue is introduced into each of the components to be linked together by reaction of both of the individual components separately with SPDP. In the case of the protein, this can be carried out in aqueous solution at neutral pH; the lipid reaction takes place in organic solvent at high pH. Both derivatized products can be stored for long periods of time. In order to link the protein to liposomes, liposomes are prepared which contain the lipid derivative (PDP-PE) in the membrane. At the same time, the disulfide bond (–S–S–) in the derivatized protein (PDP–protein) is reduced by reaction with dithiothreitol (DTT) at pH 5.5 for 30 min. After removal of the DTT (e.g. by column chromatography) the liposomes and the protein solution are mixed together at neutral pH for 18 h, during which time the less stable aromatic pyridyl sulfhydryl group (–S–Pyr) is displaced from the disulfide bond by the aliphatic –SH group of the reduced protein, resulting in linkage of the protein to liposomes via a disulfide bridge. Because the two components to be conjugated contain sulfur residues in two different oxidation states (i.e. oxidized as a disulfide bond, or reduced as a sulfhydryl group), there is little chance of crosslinking of the homologous reagents with themselves, so that protein–protein and liposome–liposome crosslinking does not occur.

Store the product at –20 °C or below under nitrogen in chloroform solution, preferably sealed in glass ampules. Completion of the reaction and purity of the product can also be checked by staining with ninhydrin spray after TLC. The spray is made up by dissolving 0.25 g of ninhydrin in 100 ml of acetone/lutidine (9:1, v/v lutidine is dimethyl pyridine). Lipids such as PE, which contain free amino groups, stain blue after 5–10 min although weaker spots may take longer; PDP-PE gives no coloration at all. Ninhydrin spray seems to interfere with iodine staining, so it is advisable to run two samples side by side and mask one lane during spraying.

Protocol 9

Protein thiolation (illustrated using IgG)

Equipment and reagents

- Hamilton syringe
- IgG solution in phosphate buffer
- SPDP
- Sephadex G-50

Protocol 9 continued

Method

1 Prepare 5 ml of IgG solution in 0.1 M phosphate buffer pH 7.5 at a concentration of 5 mg/ml.

2 Prepare SPDP solution at a concentration of 20 mmol/ml (6 mg/ml) in ethanol.

3 Add 150 μl SPDP solution slowly to 5 ml of the stirred protein solution with a Hamilton syringe to give a molar ratio of SPDP to protein of 15:1. The ethanol concentration should not exceed 5% or protein denaturation may occur. Allow the mixture to react for 30 min at room temperature (approx. 20 °C).

4 Separate the protein from reactants by gel chromatography on Sephadex G-50 equilibrated with 0.05 M sodium citrate ($Na_3C_6H_5O_7.2H_2O$, 19.7 g), 0.05 M sodium phosphate ($Na_2HPO_4.7H_2O$, 13.4 g), 0.05 M sodium chloride (2.9 g) pH 7.0.

The product is characterized by measuring the number of pyridyl thiols per molecule as described earlier, in which a sample of the protein is treated with 50 mM DTT to release free thiopyridone, whose absorbance is measured at 343 nm. Typically, these conditions yield three to five pyridyl thiols per IgG molecule. If measuring the concentration of protein by absorbance at 280 nm, allowance must be made for the fact that bound thiopyridone also absorbs at this wavelength. The product can be stored for long periods at 4 °C provided it is sterilized by filtration, or by the addition of azide (10 mg/ml). Note: the examples given here are typical thiolation procedures for monoclonal mouse IgG and rabbit Fab' fragments. It should be remembered that if proteins other than immunoglobulins (or their binding fragments) are to be used, the number of thiols required may be different. An example of this is given in Shek and Heath (7), where bovine serum albumin required 15 thiols per molecule for efficient conjugation to liposomes.

Protocol 10

Effecting the coupling reaction

Equipment and reagents

- Column chromatography equipment
- Sephadex G-50
- Liposome preparation
- DTT

A. Liposome preparation

1 Prepare liposomes suspended in pH 7.0 buffer by any of the methods described earlier. A suitable lipid composition is PC/ Chol/ PG/ PDP-PE molar ratio 8:10:1:1. The concentration range of PDP-PE can be 1–10 mol per 100 mol total lipid.

Protocol 10 continued

B. Reduction of derivatized protein

1 Titrate the pyridyl dithio-protein solution in citrate-phosphate buffer to pH 5.5 by addition of 1 M HCl.

2 Make up a solution of 2.5 M dithiothreitol (DTT, 380 mg/ml) in 0.2 M acetate buffer pH 5.5 (165 mg of sodium acetate in 10 ml).

3 Add 10 μl DTT solution for each ml of protein solution.

4 Allow to stand for 30 min.

5 Separate the protein from the DTT by chromatography on a Sephadex G-50 column equilibrated with a buffer at pH 7.0. Note: care should be taken to exclude oxygen from the reaction mixture since thiols are rather unstable and prone to oxidation. Therefore, bubble nitrogen through all buffers to remove oxygen, and collect the protein fractions under nitrogen.

C. Conjugation of components

1 Mix liposomes with protein, and allow to stand overnight, with stirring, at RT. Separation of liposomes from free protein may be carried out using the flotation methods described earlier.

Aromatic dithiols are much more susceptible to cleavage by free sulfydryl groups than are aliphatic disulfide bridges. Consequently, in the presence of reduced protein, the PDP moiety is readily broken down, the thiopyridine being replaced by the protein thiol forming a disulfide bridge, which is resistant to further attack. If desired, unreacted residues may be blocked or destroyed. Thiols may be blocked with Ellman's reagent (27), or may be reacted with alkylating reagents such as N-ethylmaleimide or iodoacetamide. Maleimide residues may be reacted with thiol-containing reagents, such as DTT, mercaptoethanol, or cysteine. Residual pyridyl dithiols could theoretically be eliminated by reduction at pH 4.5, with subsequent alkylation of the thiols generated. To date, no investigators have considered this process necessary.

i. Use of endogenous thiol residues

In the method described above, SPDP has been used to introduce extra reactive groups into the protein. In certain cases, however, it is possible to use as precursors for free thiol groups the disulfide bridges already present in the protein, which after reduction by DTT, are converted to cysteine residues which are then available for linking to the derivatized PE on the liposome surface. Such an approach is particularly convenient for IgG which may be converted to F(ab')$_2$ fragments by pepsin digestion, followed by reduction with 20 mM DTT (final concentration) at pH 5 for an hour (Figure 7). DTT removal and handling of protein are carried out exactly as before.

2.2.2 Modifications of the SPDP method when using SMPB

With regard to the protein component of conjugation, the method using SMPB is identical to that described above. Free thiol groups are introduced into the protein either by reaction with SPDP, or by conversion of endogenous disulfide linkages. The difference between the two methods is in the derivatization of the PE, where SPDP is replaced by SMPB (Figure 8), but otherwise exactly the same protocol is followed. The product of derivatization, 4-(p-maleimidophenyl)butyryl phosphatidylethanolamine (MPB-PE) has a R_f of 0.52 in the TLC solvent system given above. In the final conjugation step (Figure 8) one should be aware that the maleimide residue of MPB-PE is rather unstable, particularly at pH values greater than pH 7.0. Liposomes containing MPB-PE should be prepared at pH 6.0–6.8 not more than a few hours before their conjugation to the protein. The stability of

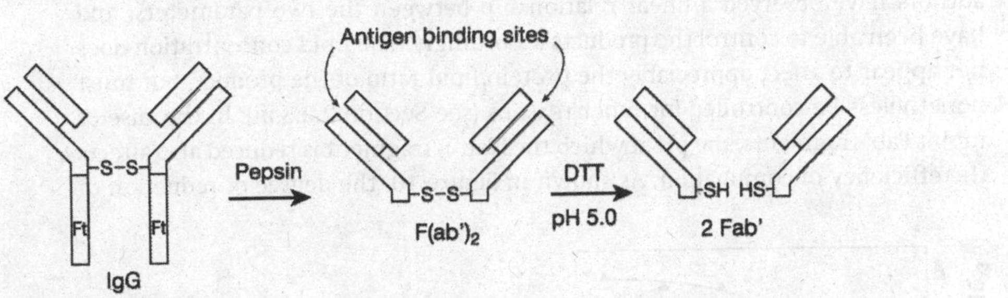

Figure 7 Conversion of IgG to Fab' fragments containing free endogenous thiol groups. The Fab' fragments formed in this way contain free sulfhydryl groups which can react directly with liposomes containing PDP-PE, without the need for introduction of PDP residues into the protein.

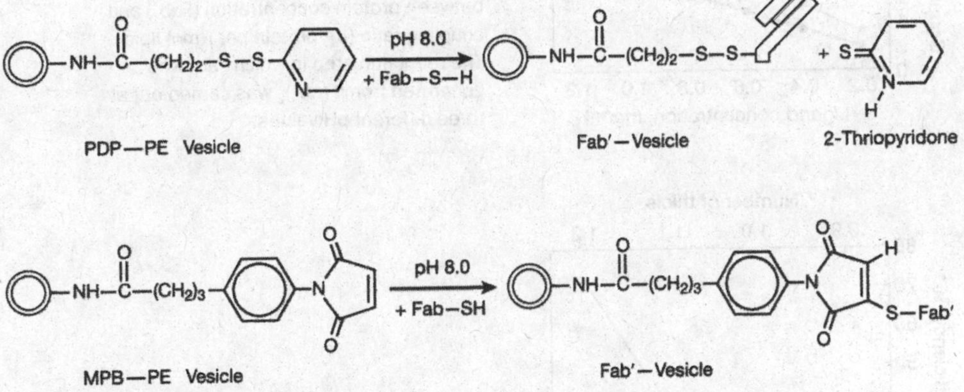

Figure 8 Comparison of SMPB and SPDP. This figure shows the difference in reaction conditions and the type of linkage finally obtained when using MPB-PE rather than PDP-PE as the liposomal conjugating agent. In both cases, the reaction is illustrated using Fab' protein subunits bearing endogenous thiol residues. The pH tolerance for the PDP reaction (pH 6.0–8.0) is much wider than for the MPB reaction (pH 6.0–6.8). The product of linkage via the PDP group is a disulfide bridge, which may be easily cleaved under certain conditions, whereas the MPB method gives rise to a very stable thioether linkage.

MPB-PE is sufficient to allow gel filtration and other manipulations prior to conjugation. The pH range for conjugation of MPB-PE (pH 6.5–6.8) is considerably narrower than that permissible for SPDP (pH 6.0–8.0) to allow reaction while avoiding excessively rapid degradation of the maleimide residue. Often the reaction is allowed to proceed overnight (12–16 h) with stirring, although 6 h is sufficient time for protein conjugation to MPB-PE liposomes.

2.2.3 Factors affecting conjugation efficiency

i. Conjugation of reduced protein and lipid

Conjugation is most easily regulated by adjustment of the protein and liposome concentrations. For the most part, the protein concentration in the conjugation mixture determines the protein-to-lipid ratio of the product (Figure 9). The authors have observed a linear relationship between the two parameters, and have been able to control the products accordingly. The lipid concentration does not appear to affect appreciably the protein/lipid ratio of the product, but must nonetheless be controlled for other reasons (see Section 2.2.3.iii). In the case of rabbit Fab' fragments, the pH at which the F(ab')$_2$ fragment is reduced also affects the efficiency of conjugation. As shown in Figure 10, the degree of reduction of

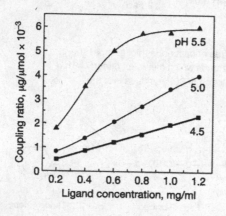

Figure 9 Relationship between Fab' concentration and coupling ratio (expressed as μg Fab' per μmol lipid). Relationship between protein concentration (Fab') and coupling ratio (μg protein per μmol lipid). The reduction step in which Fab' was generated from F(ab')$_2$ was carried out at three different pH values.

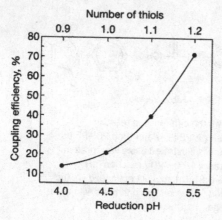

Figure 10 Relationship between reduction pH, number of thiols, and coupling efficiency, expressed as a percentage of the total added Fab' fragments coupled to liposomes.

the F(ab')$_2$ fragment by DTT is a function of the pH and ranges from 0.9 thiols per monomer at pH 4.0 to 1.2 thiols at pH 5.5. As expected, the degree of conjugation of these fragments to liposomes containing thiol-reactive groups increases with increasing number of thiols per fragment. Figure 10 also demonstrates that the coupling efficiency improves from about 15% for fragments reduced at pH 4.0 to 75% at pH 5.5.

ii. Presence of cholesterol in the liposome membrane

As shown in Table 2, cholesterol appears to be required for efficient coupling of Fab' fragments to MPB-PE-containing liposomes. Liposomes containing no cholesterol fail to couple the fragments above control levels. The inclusion of up to 30 mol% of cholesterol produces a dramatic increase in the coupling efficiency.

iii. Aggregation during conjugation

In some circumstances, protein can induce aggregation of liposomes. Such aggregation can be particularly prevalent with small liposomes, and is best controlled by minimizing the liposome concentration and keeping the protein concentration to a level which does not induce aggregation (11, 28). Aggregation may be due either to the covalent crosslinking of liposomes via a protein bridge, or to the clumping of the protein-bearing liposomes as a result of reduction in the number of mutually repulsive surface charges. This phenomenon has not been extensively investigated, although a recent report has suggested that it may be controlled by minimizing the number of thiols on the protein molecule (29). Inclusion of charged lipids such as PG or PS has also been used to reduce aggregation by providing electrostatic repulsive forces among the suspended liposomes, limiting close approach and thereby inhibiting aggregate formation (30). As shown in Figure 11, the ionic strength of the suspending medium also affects aggregation behaviour. In general, a balance must be struck between the tendency of the protein-conjugated liposomes to aggregate (manifesting visibly as flocculation) and the electrostatic repulsive forces engineered into the system.

2.2.4 Comparison of protein thiolation methods

The method employed for thiolating proteins depends to a large extent on the protein one wishes to use. If the protein has endogenous disulfide bridges which

Table 2 Effect of cholesterol on ligand conjugation

| PC | Liposome composition | | Coupling ratio (mg/mmol) |
	Cholesterol	MPB-BE	
10.0	0	1.0	< 25
10.0	1.0	1.0	62
10.0	2.5	1.0	146
10.0	5.0	1.0	168
10.0	10.0	1.0	174

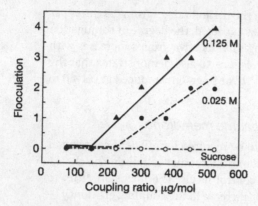

Figure 11 Effect of ionic strength of the medium and coupling ratio on flocculation (aggregation) behaviour of liposomes. Liposomes were suspended either on 0.3 M sucrose solution, in 0.025 M NaCl, or in isotonic saline (0.125 M). The extent of aggregation (flocculation) was assessed qualitatively on a score of one to four by microscopic examination.

can be broken without destroying essential enzymic, binding, or immunogenic properties of the molecule, then this approach is to be preferred, since it appears that endogenous free thiols are often more reactive than those introduced as thiopropionyl derivatives, so that one may expect the rate of reaction, and the efficiency of conjugation to be increased.

While the most widely used method for introduction of exogenous thiols employs SPDP, one disadvantage of using this reagent is the large number of purifications, which have to be carried out at each stage—one to separate unreacted SPDP from protein, and one to remove DTT, with concomitant loss of the protein on columns, etc. Hashimoto *et al.* (31) have pointed out that one separation step can be avoided by using the reagent SAMSA instead (*S*-acetyl mercaptosuccinic anhydride) to introduce thiol groups (again employing an *N*-hydroxy succinimide ester). In this case, the sulfur atom is introduced not as part of a disulfide bridge, but as a thioester, which is easily unblocked with hydroxylamine. Since the presence of hydroxylamine (unlike DTT) does not compete, or otherwise interfere, with the subsequent formation of either disulfide or thioether linkages, the two reactions (unblocking and conjugation) can be carried out in the same vessel without the need for removal of the hydroxylamine before addition of the protein to liposomes (see Figure 12). One difficulty with SAMSA is that upon binding to the amino group of the protein, a free carboxyl group is revealed, which is retained as part of the linker molecule, thus changing the net charge of the protein radically after only a few substitutions. Such alterations, while sometimes being innocuous, may easily lead to increased aggregation, or non-specific binding to cells. This problem is overcome with SATA (succinimidyl-*S*-acetyl thioacetate) which works in the same way as SAMSA, but releases the free carboxy moiety into the bulk medium (see Figure 12). Protocol 11 has been developed for using these reagents (32, 33).

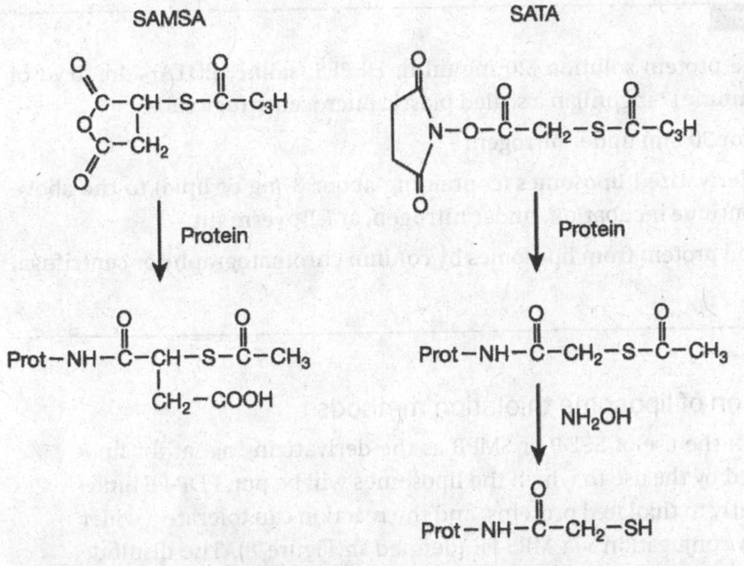

Figure 12 Introduction of thioacetate groups into proteins. SAMSA, S-acetyl mercaptosuccinic anhydride; SATA, succinimidyl-S-acetyl thioacetate. Reaction of SAMSA with proteins results in the introduction of an extra carboxy function, in addition to the thioacetate group. Use of SATA avoids this complication. Proteins derivatized with either agent can yield a free sulfhydryl group upon incubation with hydroxylamine, as shown here for the SATA derivative.

Protocol 11

SAMSA/SATA modification of proteins

Equipment and reagents

- Dialysis or column chromatography equipment
- HEPES, saline, EDTA buffer
- IgG solution
- SAMSA/SATA
- Hydroxylamine

Method

1 Prepare buffer containing 145 mM NaCl, 2 mM EDTA, 10 mM HEPES– NaOH pH 7.6 by dissolving 2.4 g HEPES, 8.4 g NaCl, and 0.75 g EDTA disodium salt in a litre of distilled water. Bring to pH 7.4 with about 1 ml of 5 M NaOH.

2 Prepare 2 ml IgG solution (5 mg/ml in phosphate-buffered saline).

3 To the stirred solution of IgG add 40 µl of SAMSA/SATA (1 mg) at a concentration of 25 mg/ml in dimethylformamide.

4 Incubate at room temperature under nitrogen for 30 min.

5 Remove unreacted reagent by dialysis or column chromatography. Equilibrate with HEPES, saline, EDTA buffer. The protein may be concentrated and stored at –20 °C until required.

Protocol 11 continued

6 To 100 μl of the protein solution (20 mg/ml in HEPES, saline, EDTA) add 10 μl of 0.1 M hydroxylamine (7 mg/ml) in a sealed plastic microcentrifuge tube.

7 Incubate at RT for 30 min under nitrogen.

8 Add 100 μl of derivatized liposomes (containing about 3 mg of lipid) to the above mixture, and continue incubation, under nitrogen, at RT overnight.

9 Remove unbound protein from liposomes by column chromatography or centrifugal flotation.

2.2.5 Comparison of liposome thiolation methods

The choice between the use of SPDP or SMPB as the derivatizing agent for liposomes is determined by the use to which the liposomes will be put. PDP-PE binds rapidly and efficiently to thiolated proteins, and the reaction can tolerate a wider pH range than can conjugation via MPB-PE (defined in Figure 8). The disulfide linkage formed, however, is a reversible one, and can easily be broken in the presence of thiols such as glutathione, which is present in high concentration in biological tissues. For *in vivo* use, therefore, SPDP derivatization may be inadvisable, except in cases where dissociation of the protein from liposomes is particularly desired. The MPB reaction, on the other hand, results in a thioether linkage which is very stable in biological environment (see Figure 8).

One objection to the use of SMPB is the possibility that the large maleimido benzoyl residue may act as an immunogenic determinant in its own right (especially if conjugated with small proteins or haptens), and may interfere with the stimulation of immune responses by liposomes, or create difficulties in interpretation of the results of immunological experiments. It has been proposed (31) that the introduction of iodoacetate residues onto the liposome surface (via N-hydroxysuccinimido-iodoacetate, NHSIA) may be a suitable alternative (Figure 13). However, one group of workers found that the iodoacetate resulted in a very low efficiency of protein binding (34) while others found that the use of a spacer group was necessary to overcome steric hindrances (31). MPB is already large enough not to need an extra spacer group.

Other approaches to effecting the coupling reaction between protein and liposomes have been to employ sandwich techniques in which the methods described above are used to bind staphylococcal protein A (2), avidin (35), or biotin to the liposomes (Figure 14), which are then able to bind a whole range of IgG molecules of varying specificities, or biotinylated proteins. Avidin precipitation of biotin liposomes has also been used as a means of purification of liposomes from unassociated protein (31).

2.2.6 Thiolation of preformed liposomes

In the methods described so far, lipophilic thio-derivatives have been synthesized prior to their incorporation, during formation of liposomes, into the bilayer

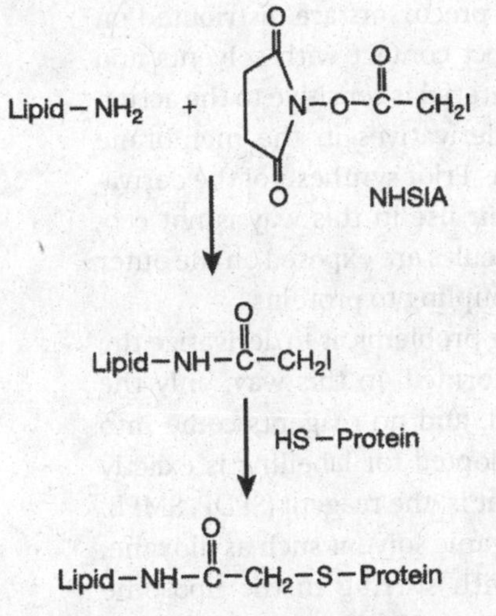

Lipid—NH$_2$ +

NHSIA

Lipid—NH—$\overset{\text{O}}{\overset{\|}{C}}$—CH$_2$I

HS—Protein

Lipid—NH—$\overset{\text{O}}{\overset{\|}{C}}$—CH$_2$—S—Protein

Figure 13 Conjugation of iodoacetate to PE using NHSIA.

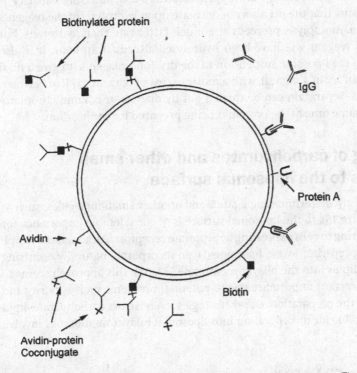

Figure 14 Sandwich techniques for binding proteins to 'multipurpose' liposomes. The use of non-covalent methods for linking proteins to liposomes opens up the possibility of attaching several different types of protein to the same liposome, or of producing different populations of liposomes, each bearing a different protein ligand, but otherwise absolutely identical with respect to membrane composition and aqueous contents. The concept is illustrated here for avidin and biotin, and for protein A-mediated binding of IgG.

membrane. Under these circumstances, the thiol precursors are distributed on both sides of the membrane, and come into direct contact with solvents and entrapped solute. In cases where the entrapped material is sensitive to the action of these precursors, the presence of such thio-derivatives in the membrane during liposome manufacture is clearly undesirable. Prior synthesis of the derivatives is also tedious and time-consuming, and their use in this way is not economical, since only a proportion of the ligand molecules are exposed on the outer surface of the liposome membrane, available for coupling to proteins.

An alternative approach, which overcomes these problems, is to derivatize the PE or other lipid after the liposomes have been formed. In this way, only the residues on the outer membrane are transformed, and no reagents come into contact with entrapped materials. The method adopted for labelling is exactly the same as is employed for protein molecules—that is, the reagent (SPDP, SMPB, NHSIA) is dissolved in concentrated form in an organic solvent such as dioxane, dimethylformamide, or ethanol, and is added with stirring to the liposome suspension. In the case of liposomes containing 50 mol% cholesterol, the concentration of solvent added to the suspension can be tolerated up to a value of 5% without causing leakage of entrapped solutes. Good buffering capacity is required to ensure that the pH does not decrease upon hydrolysis of the reagents to the free acid. Aminolysis proceeds at a much faster rate than hydrolysis, but any unreacted reagent will have been hydrolysed after half an hour. It is also possible to add the liposome suspension to the dry solid reagents (to give a final concentration of about 1 mg/ml), with a molar excess of reagent to PE of between 10- and 20-fold. Separation can be carried out by dialysis or column chromatography at the same time as the protein is being prepared for conjugation.

3 Binding of carbohydrates and other small molecules to the liposomal surface

Attachment of glycon-terminating ligands and of other small molecules, such as folate (36) (Figure 15), to the liposomal surface is of considerable importance for liposome targeting to cells expressing appropriate receptors. Although the simplest method of preparing 'sweet liposomes' is to incorporate naturally occurring bacterial glycolipids into the bilayer membrane (37, 38), this approach seems to be of limited practical importance due to potential problems such as purity and anitgenicity of the preparation. Other strategies to construct carbohydrate–lipid conjugates suitable for incorporation into liposomal bilayer membranes involve

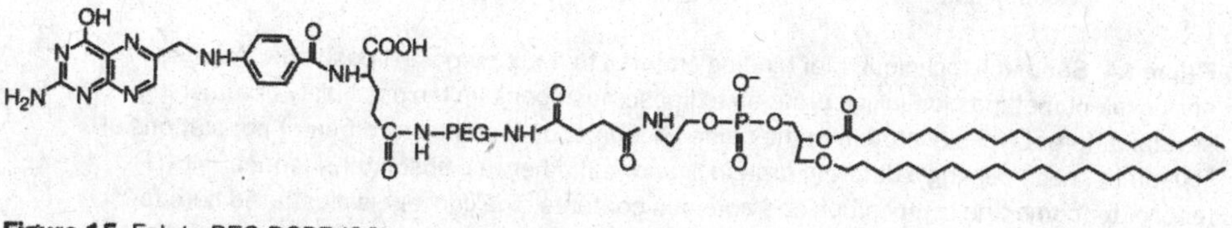

Figure 15 Folate-PEG-DSPE (36).

several synthetic steps, confining their application to only a few laboratories. Sunamoto and colleagues have hydrophobized several polysaccharides with either palmitoyl chains or cholesterol derivatives (summarized in ref. 39). Schuber and co-workers (40, 41) have developed a strategy to bind sugar residues to liposomal MPB-PE. They use either thiomannosyl or aminophenylmannosyl derivatives substituted with a hydrophilic spacer arm and functionalized with a sulfhydryl group. Kempen et al. (42) prepared a triantennary galactose-terminated cholesterol derivative by coupling tris-(galactosyloxymethyl)-aminomethane to cholesterol, using glycyl and succinyl as intermediate hydrophilic spacer moieties. The following protocol describes a simple procedure for the liposomal coupling of sugar molecules without requiring the synthesis of any sugar or lipid derivative. It is based on p-aminophenyl-sugar derivatives which are commercially available from Sigma for a wide variety of different carbohydrates. Gosh et al. (43) have described the covalent coupling of p-aminophenyl-sugar derivatives to PE containing liposomes by the use of glutaraldehyde. A drawback of this and other homo-crosslinking reagents is the formation of crosslinking products. Aminophenyl carbohydrates sandwiched between the phospholipid molecules of the liposomal lamellae, as described by Umezawa et al. (44) may have their glycon moiety positioned too near the bilayer surface for effective recognition by the receptor. The use of NOPE avoids crosslinking products and provides for a spacer arm between the sugar and the liposomal surface. The liposomal integrity during the coupling reaction is preserved as assayed by measuring the bilayer permeability to aqueous fluorescence markers (45).

Protocol 12

Covalent coupling of sugar derivatives to preformed liposomes containing NGPE (45, 46)

Equipment and reagents

- See Protocol 6
- NGPE
- p-Aminophenyl sugar derivative

Method

1 Prepare DRV liposomes with incorporated NGPE as described for the peptide in Protocol 6, steps 1 and 2.

2 Adjust 1 ml suspension of DRV with 0.01 N HCl to pH 3.5, mix with 15 mg EDC added as dry crystals, and incubate at RT for 5 min.

3 Supplement the mixture with 1 ml of 0.1 M borate buffer pH 8.5, containing approx. a four-fold molar excess of p-aminophenyl sugar derivative over liposomal NGPE and incubate overnight.

4 Separate the sugar coated DRV liposomes from non-bound sugar by centrifugation at 100 000 g for 1 h and wash the liposomal pellet repeatedly with isotonic buffer.

Protocol 13

Quantitative assay for liposomal bound sugar (from refs 45 and 47)

As this sugar assay is interfered with in the presence of phospholipids, the amount of the liposomal bound sugar is estimated indirectly by measuring the sugar in the pooled supernatants.

Equipment and reagents

- Spectrophotometer
- Liposomal sample

- HCl, phenol, H_2SO_4

Method

1 Mix 200 μl supernatant containing 5–25 μg *p*-aminophenyl sugar with 200 μl concentrated HCl and incubate at 80 °C for 1 h.

2 Lyophilize, add 400 μl of 2% phenol in water, and 1 ml concentrated H_2SO_4.

3 Measure absorbance at 485 nm after 30 min.

Table 3 Covalent binding of mannose to the surface of DRV liposomes via NGPE

Liposomal NGPE [μmol]	Aminophenylmannose (initial) [μmol]	Aminophenylmannose bound [~mol] [μmol mannose / μmol NGPE][a]
1.2	1.2	0.15
1.2	2.4	0.30
1.8	3.6	0.36
4.5	4.5	0.15
4.5	18.0	0.52

[a] Values of bound mannose were calculated after the subtraction of values for controls, i.e. the sugar bound in the absence of carbodiimide, from those measured in the presence of the carboxylic group activating reagent.

Table 3 shows results for the binding of mannose (45). Under optimal conditions, about 0.5 mol sugar/mol NGPE is bound. Assuming a nearly symmetrically distribution of NGPE between the inner and the outer liposomal monolayer, all available anchor molecules seem to have reacted with the sugar derivative.

4 Attachment of diagnostically significant reporter metal atoms to the liposome surface

The use of liposomes for the delivery of imaging agents has quite a long history (48). The ability of liposomes to entrap different substances into both the aqueous phase and the liposome membrane compartment made them suitable for carrying the diagnostic moieties used with all imaging modalities: gamma-scintigraphy, magnetic resonance (MR) imaging, computed tomography (CT) imaging, and even sonography. However, the binding of the diagnostic moieties with the liposome surface is of particular importance for gamma- and MR imaging, since both require that a sufficient quantity of radionuclide or paramagnetic metal is associated with the liposome. Two approaches have been tried to prepare liposomes for gamma- and MR imaging. In the first approach, metal was chelated into the appropriate chelate (for example, diethylene triamine pentaacetic acid or DTPA) and then introduced into the aqueous interior of a liposome. Alternatively, DTPA or other chelators may be chemically derivatized by the incorporation of a hydrophobic group, which can anchor the chelating moiety on the liposome surface during or after liposome preparation. The second approach clearly falls into the scope of our chapter, since in this case reporter metal atoms are attached to the liposome surface via chelating groups.

Different chelators and different hydrophobic anchors were successfully used for the preparation of 111-indium (^{111}In)-, 99(metastable)-technetium (^{99m}Tc)-, manganese (Mn)-, and gadolinium (Gd)-containing liposomes (review in refs 48 and 49). Later, it was suggested that amphiphilic polychelating polymers could be used for the same purpose (50). The advantage of the latter approach is that one phospholipid anchor can carry a polymer molecule with multiple chelating side-groups on the liposome surface, i.e. carry an increased number of metal atoms.

4.1 Conjugation of low molecular weight chelate DTPA with lipid for incorporation into the liposomal membrane

There are quite a few protocols for preparation of amphiphilic derivatives of low molecular weight chelating agents, such as DTPA, for incorporation into the liposomal membrane. Here, we will describe only some of them.

Protocol 14

Preparation of DTPA distearylester (51)

Equipment and reagents

- Reflux equipment
- Stearyl alcohol
- Pyridine
- DTPA dianhydride
- Ethanol, dimethylformamide

Method

1 Dissolve 2.5 g (9.25 mmol) of stearyl alcohol in 50 ml of dry pyridine under nitrogen atmosphere.

2 Add to the solution 1.32 g (3.7 mmol) of DTPA dianhydride.

3 Heat until a solution is formed and then reflux for 4 h.

4 After removal of the solvent, stir crude solid in 50 ml of ethanol to dissolve the excess stearyl alcohol.

5 Collect the residual, solid DTPA diester by vacuum filtration.

6 Recrystallize from dimethylformamide. The product is a white powder with a melting point at 194–196 °C.

Protocol 15

Preparation of DTPA distearylthioester (51)

Equipment and reagents

- Reflux equipment
- Octadecanthiol
- Pyridine
- DTPA dianhydride
- Dimethylformamide

Method

1 Dissolve 6.42 g (22.4 mmol) of octadecanthiol in 50 ml of dry pyridine under nitrogen atmosphere.

2 Add to the solution 1.0 g (2.8 mmol) of DTPA dianhydride.

3 Heat until a solution is formed and then reflux for 4 h.

4 Remove the solvent and stir crude solid in 50 ml of dimethylformamide to dissolve the excess octadecanthiol.

5 Collect the residual, solid DTPA dithioester by vacuum filtration.

6 Recrystallize from dimethylformamide. The product is a white powder with a melting point at 179–181 °C.

Protocol 16

Preparation of DTPA distearylamide (as done in V. P. T.'s laboratory)

Equipment and reagents

- Reflux equipment
- Rotary evaporator
- Centrifuge
- Stearylamine
- DTPA anhydride
- Chloroform
- Triethylamine
- HCl, methanol

Method

1 Mix 1.55 g of stearylamine and 2.5 g of DTPA anhydride with 250 ml of dry chloroform.

2 Reflux the mixture for 1 h, with the top outlet of the system closed with foil.

3 Then add 3 ml of triethylamine and reflux the mixture for additional 48 h.

4 Remove chloroform on a rotary evaporator.

5 Add 100 ml of 0.1 N HCl to a dry product, stir the mixture at 80 °C for 10 min, and then overnight at room temperature.

Protocol 16 continued

6　Separate the precipitate by centrifugation, wash it three times with 0.1 N HCl with stirring, and lyophilize.

7　Wash the lyophilized product twice with 100 ml methanol at room temperature.

8　Recrystallize the product from boiling methanol and dry.

Protocol 17

Preparation of DTPA phosphatidylethanolamine (DTPA-PE) (52)

Equipment and reagents

- Reflux equipment
- Rotary evaporator
- Silica gel column (3 × 50 cm; Bio-Sil A silicic acid 100–200 mesh)

- Dipalmitoyl-PE
- Pyridine
- DTPA anhydride
- Chloroform, methanol, water, formic acid

Method

1　For the covalent attachment of DTPA to the amino group of PE, add 1 g of dipalmitoyl-PE to 100 ml of anhydrous pyridine (dried over CaH_2) in a 500 ml round-bottom flask fitted with a reflux condenser and drying tube.

2　Heat the mixture until the lipid dissolves, resulting in a clear solution.

3　In a separate flask warm 5 g of DTPA anhydride (ten-fold molar excess relative to PE) with 100 ml of anhydrous pyridine until dissolved.

4　Add the solution of DTPA anhydride via a sidearm to a vigorously stirred lipid solution.

5　Following addition, heat the reaction mixture to reflux for 70 min, during which time an orange tint disappears but the solution remains clear.

6　Then add to the reaction mixture 50 ml of water and continue refluxing for another 70 min to hydrolyse remaining anhydride linkages.

7　Cool the mixture to RT and rotary evaporate to dryness.

8　Dissolve the reaction mixture in 150 ml of chloroform/methanol/ water/ formic acid (65:25:4:1, by vol.) solvent mixture (leaving a small solid residue).

9　Purify the product by chromatography of the soluble portion on a silica gel column (3 × 50 cm; Bio-Sil A silicic acid 100–200 mesh) eluting with a solvent mixture from step 8.

10　Evaporate the solvent and store the material as a stock solution in 1:1 chloroform/ methanol mixture.

Protocol 18

Alternative preparation of DTPA-PE (as done in V. P. T.'s laboratory)

Equipment and reagents

- Dialysis equipment
- Rotary evaporator
- PE, triethylamine

- Pyridine
- DTPA anhydride, DMSO
- Chloroform, methanol, water

Method

1   Make a solution of 100 mg of PE in 4 ml chloroform containing 30 μl triethylamine.

2   Make a solution of 400 mg of DTPA anhydride in 20 ml DMSO.

3   Add the PE solution to the DTPA anhydride solution slowly and dropwise. The reaction proceeds at RT with stirring for 3 h. Check the completion of the reaction with ninhydrin.

4   Place the reaction mixture in a regular dialysis bag (DTPA-treated, 12 kDa MWCO), and dialyse against deionized water for 48 h at 4 °C with several changes.

5   Remove the traces of chloroform on a rotary evaporator and freeze-dry the solid white residue.

6   Purity control by TLC in chloroform/methanol/water mixture (65:25:4, by vol.) shows a spot with $R_f = 0.4$.

In order to significantly increase the liposome load of diagnostically important metals for MR or gamma-imaging, amphiphilic polychelators were suggested (50). In these compounds, the lipid residue is attached not to a single chelating group, but to a certain polymeric chain which contains numerous chelating groups as side substitutes. To build such a polymeric chain, polylysine is often used, since every individual unit in this polymer contains a free ε-amino group which can be easily derivatized by a low molecular weight chelator, such as DTPA. Protocol 19 presents the preparation of polylysine substituted with multiple DTPA residues and containing terminal phospholipid group (for anchoring into liposome) derived from commercially available *N*-glutaryl-phosphatidyl-ethanolamine (NGPE) (see also Figure 16).

Protocol 19

Preparation of polychelating polymers

Equipment and reagents

- Dialysis equipment
- NGPE, N',N'-carbonyldiimidazole, chloroform, N-hydroxysuccinimide
- e,N-carbobenzoxy-poly-L-lysine (CBZ-PLL, MW 3000)
- Triethylamine
- HBr, glacial acetic acid, ethyl ether
- Chloroform, methanol, methylsulfoxide

Method

1 React 25 mg of NGPE with 25 mg of N',N'-carbonyldiimidazole in 5 ml chloroform in the presence of 11.4 mg of N-hydroxysuccinimide for 16 h at RT.

2 Add 100 mg of ε,N-carbobenzoxy-poly-L-lysine (CBZ-PLL, MW 3000) and 10 µl triethyl-amine to the initial mixture and allow reaction to proceed for another 5 h at RT with stirring.

3 Precipitate the product, CBZ-PLL-NGPE, with water, wash, and lyophilize.

4 To remove the protecting CBZ groups, dissolve 67.4 mg of CBZ-PLL-NGPE in 3 ml of a 30% HBr in glacial acetic acid and allow deprotection reaction to proceed for 2 h at RT.

5 Precipitate deprotected amphiphilic PLL-NGPE with dry ethyl ether, wash with ether, and freeze-dry.

6 For substitution of free amino groups in PLL-NGPA with DTPA residues, suspend 37 mg of PLL-NGPE in a chloroform/methanol (1:1, v/v) mixture.

7 Add 100 mg of DTPA anhydride in 2 ml methylsulfoxide and then 5 µl triethylamine, and allow reaction to proceed for 16 h at RT with stirring.

8 After that, add 100 mg of succinic anhydride in 0.2 ml methylsulfoxide to block any remaining amino groups in PLL.

9 Purify obtained DTPA-PLL-NGPE from any water soluble impurities by dialysis against the deionized water and then freeze-dry. Store the product in a freezer.

4.2 Loading liposome-associated chelates with metals

As was mentioned above, chelate-modified liposomes can be loaded with both radioactive and paramagnetic metal atoms for gamma- and MR imaging, respectively. The labelling of chelates with an appropriate metal can be performed both before their addition to a lipid mixture and after liposomes are already prepared. Since, in certain cases, short-living isotopes are used to label liposomes (such as ^{99m}Tc), the last step of the preparation of contrast liposomes for gamma-imaging normally takes place directly prior to the application moment. The majority of known protocols deal with the loading of metals onto already prepared liposomes, which reduces the time required for liposome preparation. With this in mind, liposomes have to be prepared which can be sufficiently loaded with a contrast label by applying a simple and fast labelling protocol. Some of those protocols are described below. Chelate-containing liposomes may be prepared by any appropriate method.

For the preparation of MR-contrast Gd-loaded liposomes, however, loading with Gd is often performed with lipid-conjugated chelates, which are then added in required quantities to a lipid mixture for liposome preparation. Some of those protocols are also presented. Amphiphilic polymeric chelates are loaded with

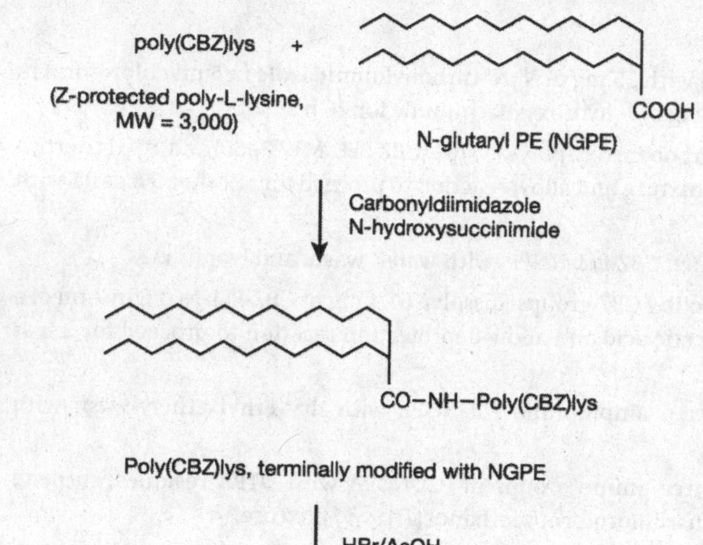

Figure 16 Synthesis of DTPA-polylysine-NGPE.

radiometals or paramagnetic metals in the same fashion as amphiphilic mono-meric chelates, just all reactant quantities are calculated per single chelating group.

Protocol 20

Loading of DTPA stearylamide (DTPA-SA) with Gd (51)

Equipment and reagents

- Reflux equipment
- Desiccator
- GdCl$_3$ hexahydrate
- DTPA-SA
- Ethanol

Method

1 Dissolve 0.091 g (0.245 mmol) of GdCl$_3$ hexahydrate in 1 ml water.

2 Add the solution obtained dropwise to a solution of 0.20 g (0.233 mmol) of DTPA-SA in 20 ml hot ethanol.

3 Reflux the resulting mixture for 30 min.

4 Concentrate the solution to one-third volume and cool to 0 °C.

5 Collect resulting solid by vacuum filtration, wash with water, and dry in a desiccator under vacuum.

Protocol 21

Loading of DTPA stearylester (DTPA-SE) with Gd (51)

Equipment and reagents

- Desiccator
- GdCl$_3$ hexahydrate
- DTPA-SE
- Pyridine

Method

1 Dissolve 0.091 g (0.245 mmol) of GdCl$_3$ hexahydrate in 1 ml water.

2 Add the solution obtained dropwise to a solution of 0.20 g (0.24 mmol) of DTPA-SE in 20 ml pyridine.

3 Stir the resulting solution for 30 min at 25 °C.

4 After solvent removal, stir the solid residue in 10 ml water to dissolve the excess of gadolinium chloride.

5 Collect the remaining solid by vacuum filtration, wash with water, and dry in a desiccator under vacuum.

Protocol 22

Loading of DTPA-PLL-NGPE with Gd (V. P. T.'s laboratory)

Equipment and reagents

- Dialysis equipment
- DTPA-PLL-NGPE
- Pyridine
- Gadolinium hydrochloride hexahydrate
- 0.1 M citrate pH 5.3

Method

1 Suspend 25 mg of dry DTPA-PLL-NGPE in 2 ml of dry pyridine.

2 Add 150 mg of $GdCl_3$ hexahydrate on 0.25 ml of 0.1 M citrate pH 5.3.

3 Incubate the mixture for 2 h at RT with stirring.

4 Dialyse the reaction mixture against deionized water and freeze-dry to obtain Gd-DTPA-PLL-NGPE. Store frozen.

Protocol 23

Loading of DTPA-containing liposomes with Gd (52)

Equipment and reagents

- Dialysis equipment
- Gadolinium hydrochloride
- Saline solution
- Liposome suspension

Method

1 Prepare solution of required concentration of $GdCl_3$ in 0.15 N saline.

2 Add 100 µl of this stock solution in 10 µl aliquots to 1 ml of liposome suspension while vortexing vigorously.

3 Purify liposome suspension by dialysis against saline.

Protocol 24

Loading of DTPA-containing liposomes with ^{99m}Tc (53)

Equipment and reagents

- 1 ml minicolumns with Bio-Gel A15M, 100–200 mesh
- Pertechnetate
- DTPA-containing liposomes
- Stannous chloride
- Saline solution

Protocol 24 continued

Method

1. Add 300 MBq of pertechnetate used within 3 h of elution from a commercial molybdenum generator to 0.5 ml of DTPA-containing liposomes (20 μmol total lipid/ml).

2. Prepare a fresh solution of 6.7 mg of stannous chloride in 1 ml of degassed 0.9% saline.

3. Quickly add 10 μl of stannous chloride to a solution with liposomes and pertechnetate.

4. Allow the mixture to stand for 10–30 min at RT.

5. Separate liposome-associated, free, and colloidal forms of Tc by chromatography on 1 ml minicolumns with Bio-Gel A15M, 100–200 mesh, washed with 0.9% saline.

Protocol 25

Labelling of chelate-containing liposomes with ^{111}In (V. P. T.'s laboratory)

Equipment and reagents

- Dialysis equipment
- ^{111}InCl$_3$/HCl commercial sample
- 0.1 M citrate buffer pH 3.0
- Chelate-containing liposomes

Method

1. Prepare a solution of fresh ^{111}InCl$_3$/HCl commercial sample in 0.1 M citrate buffer pH 3.0, at a concentration of about 0.5 mCi of ^{111}In/ml.

2. Add 0.1 mCi of ^{111}In to 2 ml of chelate-containing liposomes (10 mg/ml total lipid) with careful vortexing.

3. Incubate for 1 h at RT.

4. Remove non-bound ^{111}In by overnight dialysis against HBS. Usual binding yield is c. 80%.

References

1. Heath, T. D., Montgomery, J. A., Piper, J. R., and Papahadjopoulos, D. (1983). *Proc. Natl. Acad. Sci. USA*, **80**, 377.
2. Leserman, L. D., Machy, P., and Barbet, J. (1981). *Nature*, **293**, 226.
3. O'Connell, J., Campbell, R., Fleming, B., Mercolino, T., Johnson, M., and McLaurin, D. (1985). *Clin. Chem.*, **31**, 1424.
4. Kung, V. T., Maxim, P., Veltri, R., and Martin, F. (1985). *Biochim. Biophys. Acta*, **839**, 105.
5. Kung, V. T., Vollmer, Y., and Martin, F. (1986). *J. Immunol. Methods*, **90**, 189.
6. Martin, F. and Kung, V. T. Unpublished results.
7. Shek, P. S. and Heath, T. D. (1983). *Immunology*, **50**, 101.

8. Torchilin, V. P., Goldmacher, V. S., and Smirnov, V. N. (1978). *Biochem. Biophys. Res. Commun.*, **85**, 983.

9. Dunnick, J. K., McDougall, R., Aragon, S., Goris, M., and Kriss, J. (1975). *J. Nucl. Med.*, **16**, 483.

10. Heath, T. D. and Martin, F. J. (1986). *Chem. Phys. Lipids*, **40**, 347.

11. Heath, T. D., Robertson, D., Birbeck, M. S. C., and Davies, A. J. S. (1980). *Biochim. Biophys. Acta*, **599**, 42.

12. Weissig, V. and Gregoriadis, G. (1992). In *Liposome technology*, 2nd edn (ed. G. Gregoriadis), Vol. III, pp. 231–48. CRC Press Inc., Boca Raton, FL.

13. Weissig, V., Lasch, J., Klibanov, A. L., and Torchilin, V. P. (1986). *FEBS Lett.*, **202**, 86.

14. Kung, V. T. and Redemann, C. T. (1986). *Biochim. Biophys. Acta*, **862**, 435.

15. Bogdanov, Jr, A. A., Klibanov, A. L., and Torchilin, V. P. (1988). *FEBS Lett.*, **231**, 381.

16. Holmberg, E., Maruyama, K., Litzinger, D. C., Wright, S., Davis, M., Kabalka, G. W., *et al.* (1989). *Biochem. Biophys. Res. Commun.*, **165**, 1272.

17. Mori, A. and Huang, L. (1992). In *Liposome technology*, 2nd edn (ed. G. Gregoriadis), Vol. III, pp. 153–62. CRC Press Inc., Boca Raton, FL.

18. Niedermann, G., Weissig, V., Sternberg, B., and Lasch, J. (1991). *Biochim. Biophys. Acta*, **1070**, 401.

19. Szoka, F. and Papahadjopoulos, D. (1978). *Proc. Natl. Acad. Sci. USA*, **75**, 4194.

20. Weissig, V., Lasch, J., and Gregoriadis, G. (1990). *Pharmazie*, **45**, 849.

21. Tan, L., Weissig, V., and Gregoriadis, G. (1991). *Asian Pacific J. Allergy Immunol.*, **9**, 25.

22. Kirby, C. and Gregoriadis, G. (1984). *Biotechnology*, **2**, 979.

23. Bogdanov, A. A., Klibanov, A. L., and Torchilin, V. P. (1984). *FEBS Lett.*, **175**, 178.

24. Torchilin, V. P., Klibanov, A. L., and Smirnov, V. N. (1982). *FEBS Lett.*, **138**, 117.

25. Heath, T. D., Macher, B. A., and Paphadjopoulos, D. (1981). *Biochim. Biophys. Acta*, **640**, 66.

26. Carlsson, J., Drevin, H., and Axen, R. (1978). *J. Biochem.*, **173**, 723.

27. Ellman, G. L. (1959). *Arch. Biochem. Biophys.*, **82**, 70.

28. Matthay, K. K., Heath, T. D., and Papahadjopoulos, D. (1984). *Cancer Res.*, **44**, 1880.

29. Jou, Y. H., Jarlinski, S., Mayhew, E., and Bankert, R. B. (1984). *Fed. Proc.*, **43**, 3218.

30. Martin, F. and Kung, V. T. (1985). *Ann. NY Acad. Sci.*, **446**, 443.

31. Hashimoto, K., Loader, J. E., and Kinsky, S. C. (1986). *Biochim. Biophys. Acta*, **856**, 556.

32. Rector, E. S., Schwenck, R. J., Tse, K. S., and Sehon, A. H. (1978). *J. Immunol. Methods*, **24**, 321.

33. Derksen, J. T. P. and Scherphof, G. L. (1985). *Biochim. Biophys. Acta*, **841**, 151.

34. Wolff, B. and Gregoriadis, G. (1984). *Biochim. Biophys. Acta*, **802**, 259.

35. Urdal, D. L. and Hakomori, S. (1980). *J. Biol. Chem.*, **255**, 10509.

36. Lee, R. J. and Low, P. S. (1995). *Biochim. Biophys. Acta*, **1233**, 134.

37. Szoka, F. and Mayhew, E. (1983). *Biochem. Biophys. Res. Commun.*, **110**, 140.

38. Barratt, G., Tenu, J. P., Yapo, A., and Petit, J. F. (1986). *Biochim. Biophys. Acta*, **862**, 153.

39. Sato, T. and Sunamoto, J. (1992). In In *Liposome technology*, 2nd edn (ed. G. Gregoriadis), Vol. III, pp. 179–98. CRC Press Inc., Boca Raton, FL.

40. Muller, C. D. and Schuber, F. (1989). *Biochim. Biophys. Acta*, **986**, 97.

41. Barratt, G. and Schuber, F. (1992). In *Liposome technology*, 2nd edn (ed. G. Gregoriadis), Vol. III, pp. 199–218. CRC Press Inc., Boca Raton, FL.

42. Kempen, H. J. M., Hoes, C., Van Boom, J. H., Spanjer, H. H., De Lange, J., Langendoen, A., *et al.* (1984). *J. Med. Chem.*, **27**, 1306.

43. Gosh, P. and Bachhawat, B. K. (1980). *Biochim. Biophys. Acta*, **632**, 562.

44. Umezawa, F. and Eto, Y. (1988). *Biochem. Biophys. Res. Commun.*, **153**, 1038.

45. Weissig, V., Lasch, J., and Gregoriadis, G. (1989). *Biochim. Biophys. Acta*, **1003**, 54.

46. Gregoriadis, G., Weissig, V., Tan, L., and Xiao, Q. (1989). *Biochem. Soc. Trans.*, **17**, 128.

47. Dubois, M., Gilles, K. A., Hamilton, J. K., Rebers, P. A., and Smith, F. (1956). *Anal. Chem.*, **28**, 350.

48. Torchilin, V. P. (1995). *J. Liposome Res.*, **5**, 795.

49. Torchilin, V. P. (1997). *Adv. Drug Deliv. Rev.*, **24**, 301.

50. Torchilin, V. P. (2000). *Curr. Pharm. Biotech.*, **1**, 183.

51. Kabalka, G. W., Davis, M. A., Moss, T. H., Buonocore, E., Hubner, K., Holmberg, E., *et al.* (1991). *Magn. Res. Med.*, **19**, 406.

52. Grant, C. W. M., Karlik, S., and Florio, E. (1989). *Magn. Res. Med.*, **11**, 236.

53. Ahkong, Q. F. and Tilcock, C. (1992). *Nucl. Med. Biol.*, **19**, 831.

Chapter 8
Long-circulating sterically protected liposomes

Alexander L. Klibanov
University of Virginia Cardiovascular Division, Charlottesville, VA, USA.

Vladimir P. Torchilin
Northeastern University, Bouve College of Health Sciences,
Department of Pharmaceutical Sciences, Boston, MA, USA.

Samuel Zalipsky
ALZA Corporation, Menlo Park, CA, USA.

1 Introduction

Soon after liposomes were proposed as vehicles for drug delivery and targeting, their major disadvantage was discovered: Typical liposome compositions rapidly exited the bloodstream and accumulated in the Kupffer cells in the liver, as well as in spleen macrophages (RES) (1). Various approaches to overcome this problem have been tested. Initially, the simple approach of blocking RES cells by administering an excess of 'empty' liposomes, a colloid dispersion or dextran sulfate was tested (2, 3). However, blocking RES is not the most appropriate approach for human therapy. On the other hand, to target liposomal pharmaceuticals to organs other than the liver and spleen, liposomes have been modified with specific targeting moieties, e.g. antibodies. However, immunoliposomes also do not exhibit prolonged circulation times and fail to accumulate sufficiently in the targets with limited blood supply and/or low antigen concentration (i.e. tissues and organs that require increased circulation times for liposome-to-target interaction). It is evident that a longer circulation time increases the probability that the liposomes will interact with the target tissue, yielding better targeting. Therefore, numerous attempts have been made to prolong the circulation time by varying liposome properties.

Several parameters were studied, some with reasonable success. When small liposomes (<100 nm) containing gel-state phospholipids (such as DSPC) and cholesterol were tested, their circulation time was extended considerably (4). Perhaps most interesting and successful were the efforts to modify the surface of the liposomes, for example, with proteins, carbohydrates, charged molecules, or polymers. The circulation time of antibody-coated liposomes with sialoglycoprotein fetuin was extended (5), possibly because sialiylated glycolipids and glycoproteins are used in natural systems (e.g. to protect circulating red blood cells from undesired capture by macrophages). Other experiments were performed using a monosialoglycolipid, ganglioside G_{M1} (6). Addition of this material or phosphatidylinositol (7), increased the circulation time by more than an order of magnitude. Uptake of these liposomes by the liver and spleen decreased. The exact mechanism of this effect of sialoglycolipids still remains unclear. One hypothesis is based on its structure and a possible role of the negative charge located below a carbohydrate unit which itself lacked available receptors for RES cells or other cells in the liver (e.g. mannose or galactose). Interestingly, a much simpler structure—an *N*-acyl phosphatidylethanolamine derivative of a dicarboxylic acid (e.g. glutaric acid)—also improved liposome circulation time. This structure has two negative charges, one from the outer carboxyl, and one from the PE phosphate group (8).

The real breakthrough, however, was achieved with the discovery of polymer-modified long-circulating liposomes (9). Among other polymers, dextran derivatives have been immobilized on the liposome surface in an attempt to prolong circulation time (see ref. 10 for review). Still, the most popular method of preparing such liposomes involves coating of liposome with linear poly(ethylene glycol) or PEG. The success of PEG in extending the circulation time of polystyrene latex particles (11) was the basis for the suggestion to attach PEG to the liposome surface as well (12–15). Explanations of the phenomenon of long-circulating PEG-coated (PEGylated) liposomes involve the role of surface charge and hydrophilicity of PEGylated liposomes (16), the role of PEG in the repulsive interactions between PEG-grafted membranes and another particles (17), the formation of a dense 'conformational cloud' by flexible liposome-grafted polymers over the liposome surface (18), and more generally, the decreased rate of plasma protein adsorption on the hydrophilic surface of PEGylated liposomes (19).

Although some other polymers have been successfully tested as steric protectors for liposomes (20–23), PEG remains the golden standard for preparing long-circulating liposomes, and the majority of this chapter is devoted to the preparation of PEGylated liposomes.

2 Attachment of sterically protecting polymer (PEG) to liposomes

2.1 Incorporation of PEG into liposomes

For incorporation into the liposomal membrane, PEG with a molecular weight of 1–10 kDa is modified at one end with hydrophobic group, such as phospholipid residue (12) (see the reaction scheme in Figure 1). Although some hydrophobic derivatives of PEG (usually, PEG-PE) are commercially available, the routine protocol of their preparation as well as certain alternative protocols deserve to be described here.

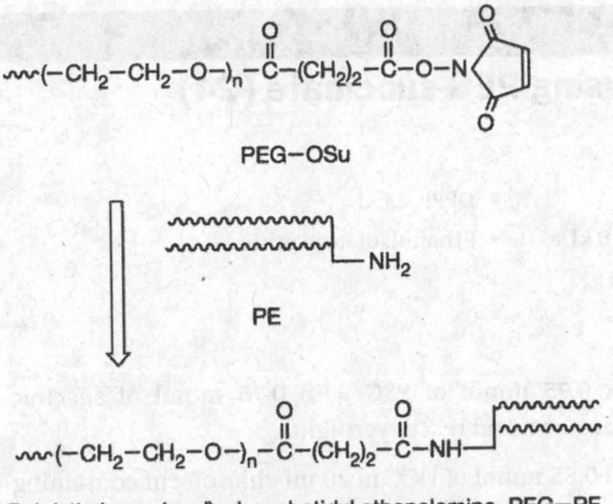

Figure 1 The reaction scheme for preparation of PEG-PE.

Protocol 1

Preparation of PEG-PE using PEG hydroxysuccinimide ester (12)

Equipment and reagents

- Bio-Gel A-15m column
- Dialysis equipment
- PEG hydroxysuccinimide ester (PEG-OSu)
- Chloroform

- PE
- Triethylamine
- NaCl

Method

1. To prepare PEG-PE, first add an aliquot of PEG-OSu in chloroform to a solution of PE in chloroform and then immediately add triethylamine at a PEG-OSu/PE/triethylamine 3:1:3.5 molar ratio.

2. Incubate the reaction mixture overnight at room temperature and evaporate the chloroform with a stream of nitrogen gas.

3. Redissolve the reaction mixture in 0.145 M NaCl to hydrolyse non-reacted PEG-OSu.

4. Apply the solution in saline onto a Bio-Gel A-15m column, pre-equilibrated with saline.

5. Pool peak fractions with PEG-PE micelles that are eluted in the void volume, dialyse against water (alternatively, a dialysis bag with large pores, such as Spectra-Por CE, 300 000 MWCO can be used to avoid step 4), and lyophilize.

6. To prepare PEGylated liposomes, add the required quantity of PEG-PE (usually, from 2-8 %mol of total lipids) to a lipid mixture in chloroform or chloroform/ethanol and prepare liposomes by any desirable procedure.

Protocol 2

Preparation of PEG-PE using PEG-succinate (24)

Equipment and reagents

- Membrane filters
- PEG with a molecular weight of 1–10 kDa
- Succinic anhydride, chloroform
- DPPE, DCC
- Ethanol, diethyl ether

Method

1 To prepare PEG-succinate, mix 0.75 mmol of PEG with 0.75 mmol of succinic anhydride in 20 ml distilled chloroform and react overnight.

2 Dissolve 0.75 mmol of DPPE and 0.85 mmol of DCC in 20 ml chloroform containing 0.75 mmol of PEG-succinate.

3 React overnight at 50 °C.

4 Evaporate the chloroform, redissolve the residue in 30 ml of ethanol, and filter.

5 Re-precipitate the product with diethyl ether and dry in vacuum.

6 Disperse the product in 30 ml of distilled water and filter through a 0.2 μm membrane filter.

7 Freeze-dry the filtrate to obtain white powder of PEG-PE.

Protocol 3

Preparation of PEG-PE using carbonyldiimidazole (14)

Equipment and reagents

- Silica gel column chromatography equipment
- PEG
- Carbonyldiimidazole
- Benzene
- DPPE
- Triethylamine

Method

1 Mix 0.5 mmol of PEG with 0.55 mmol of carbonyldiimidazole in benzene and incubate with stirring at 75 °C for 16 h in an N_2 atmosphere.

2 Evaporate the solution. Mix the resulting PEG-imidazolyl carbonyl with 0.5 mmol of DPPE and 0.5 mmol triethylamine in benzene and incubate the reaction mixture for 6 h at 95 °C.

3 Purify the resulting PEG-carbonyl-DPPE (PEG-PE) by silica gel column chromatography.

2.2 Attachment of PEG to previously prepared liposomes

All the methods described above produce PEG-PE that must to be added to the lipid mixture before liposome formation. Alternatively, it was suggested to synthesize single end-reactive derivatives of PEG that can be coupled with certain reactive groups (such as maleimide) on the surface of already prepared liposomes, so called post-coating method (25). Such an approach allows PEG to be post-attached easily to the surface of immunoliposomes.

Protocol 4

Preparation of PEG-succinylcysteine for attachment to the surface of previously prepared liposomes containing DPPE derivative of *m*-maleimidobenzoyl-*N*-hydroxysuccinimide ester (MBPE) (25)

Equipment and reagents

- Reflux equipment
- Sephadex G-10
- PEG, chloroform, succinic anhydride, pyridine
- N-hydroxysuccinimide (NHS)
- Dioxane, 1-ethyl-3-(3-dimethylaminopropyl)-carbodiimide
- Cystine
- Tris–HCl, DTT

Method

1 Dissolve 1 mmol of PEG in 30 ml chloroform and mix with 5 mmol of succinic anhydride and 6.3 mmol pyridine.

2 Reflux the mixture at 40 °C for 4 h with stirring.

3 Wash away the remaining succinic anhydride once with 5 ml of 0.5 N HCl and then twice with 10 ml of water.

4 Dry chloroform layer with sodium sulfate and then in vacuum.

5 To activate the resulting PEG-succinate with N-hydroxysuccinimide (NHS), dissolve the PEG-succinate pellet in 25 ml of dioxane and add 2 mmol of 1-ethyl-3-(3-dimethylaminopropyl)-carbodiimide and 3 mmol of NHS.

6 Heat the mixture at 50 °C for 8 h with stirring.

7 Evaporate the solvent, redissolve the reaction mixture in chloroform, wash with water, and dry as above.

8 With stirring, add 0.2 mmol of solid PEG-succinyl-NHS ester in small portions into 5 ml of the suspension of 1 mmol of cystine in HBS pH 7.4.

9 Maintain the pH value at 7.4 with 0.5 N NaOH and incubate the resulting mixture at room temperature for 16 h.

Protocol 4 continued

10 Remove the insoluble materials by filtration, and mix the filtrate with 1 ml of 1 M Tris–HCl pH 8.6, and 0.7 mmol of dithiotreitol.

11 Incubate at room temperature for 1 h.

12 Purify the reaction mixture on Sephadex G-10 in HBS pH 6.8.

13 Pool the void volume fractions containing thiol residue (as determined by titration with DTNB) and immediately store at –20 °C until used.

14 To prepare PEGylated liposomes or immunoliposomes, incubate (immuno)liposomes containing approx. 5 %mol of MBPE with the required quantity of PEG-succinil-cysteine for 1 h at 37 °C. Then treat with a trace amount of 2-mercaptoethanol for another 30 min.

Use of alternative polymers, such as polyvinylpyrrolidone, polyacrylamide, polyacryloylmorpholine (20, 21), poly(2-methyl-2-oxazoline) and poly(2-ethyl-2-oxazoline) (22), or phosphatidyl polyglycerols (23) for preparing long-circulating sterically protected liposomes has been described in the literature (see some structures in Figure 2).

2.3 Dependence of biodistribution on the size of long-circulating liposomes

When long-circulating liposomes (either coated with PEG or containing ganglio-side G_{M1} in the membrane) were injected intravenously in the experimental animals, significant size dependence was observed in liposome biodistribution. While smaller liposomes (less than approx. 200 nm) circulated freely, larger liposomes (300–400 nm) successfully evaded uptake in the liver but were rapidly trapped in the spleen (26, 27), mostly in the red pulp and marginal zone (28). These results suggest that the size of liposomes used for drug delivery should be chosen carefully.

In another study, where administration of PEGylated liposomes was performed subcutaneously (29), size again proved important for the outcome. Larger liposomes (approx. 200 nm) were retained at the injection site, unless the tissue was massaged (non-PEGylated liposomes were captured by the macrophages). Smaller particles, e.g. PEGylated micelles (30), could migrate into the bloodstream via lymph nodes. Attempts to design a ^{99m}Tc-based liposome sentinel lymph node imaging agent (31) showed that control of liposome size as well as surface charge and PEG content may be necessary to achieve successful sentinel lymph node imaging. Therefore, with either intravenous and subcutaneous administration, liposome size plays an important role in the resulting biodistribution and tissue accumulation patterns. This is an important limitation, because for the optimal drug load into the liposome internal space, higher volume-to-surface ratio and, respectively, a larger particle size, are necessary to achieve a high drug-to-lipid loading ratio.

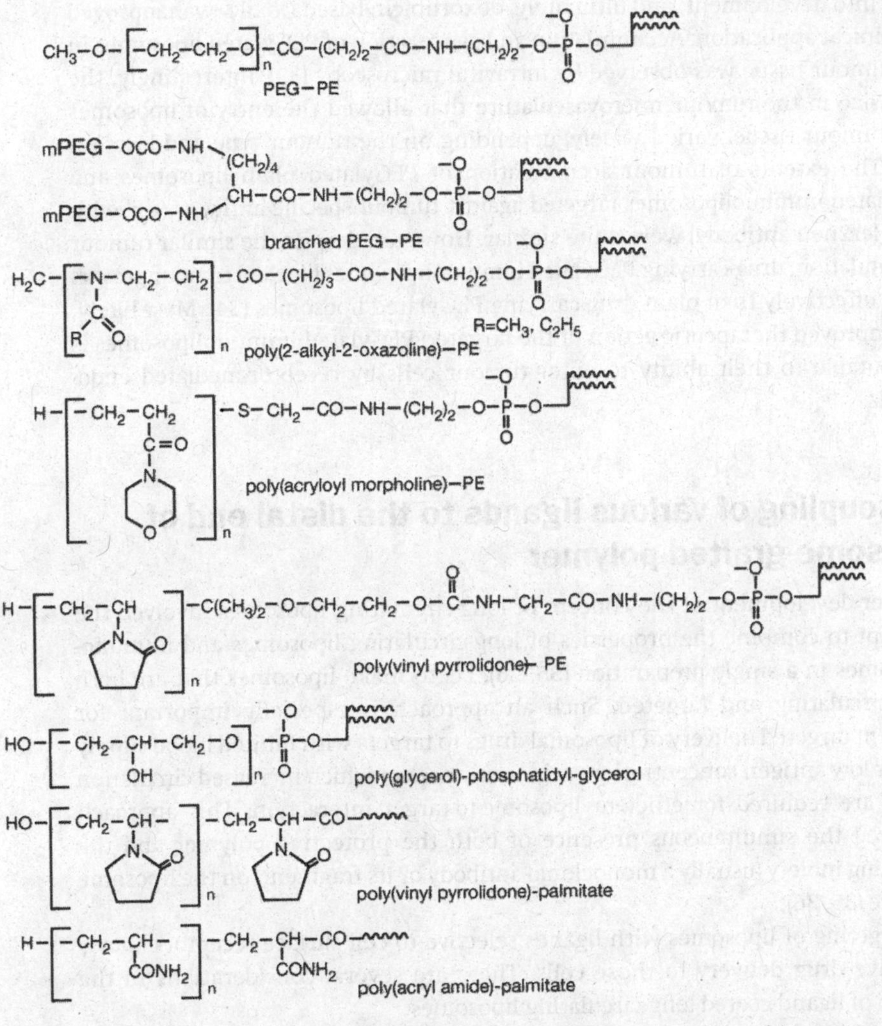

CH$_3$-O-[CH$_2$-CH$_2$-O]$_n$-CO-(CH$_2$)$_2$-CO-NH-(CH$_2$)$_2$-O-P-O

PEG-PE

mPEG-OCO-NH

branched PEG-PE

poly(2-alkyl-2-oxazoline)-PE   R=CH$_3$, C$_2$H$_5$

poly(acryloyl morpholine)-PE

poly(vinyl pyrrolidone)-PE

poly(glycerol)-phosphatidyl-glycerol

poly(vinyl pyrrolidone)-palmitate

poly(acryl amide)-palmitate

Figure 2 The structures of some polymers successfully used for steric protection of liposomes.

2.4 Tumour accumulation of long-circulating liposomes

The fact that tumour endothelium may be 'leaky' and that the porous tumour microvasculature may allow the entrance into the tissue of the particles that would be normally excluded from interstitial space, gave rise to the efforts to deliver therapeutic agents with the aid of long-circulating particles. It would not be possible to pursue this route of tumour drug delivery with the liposome formulations that rapidly leave bloodstream and are captured by RES. Long-circulating liposomes are a reasonable candidate for this approach. It was found that PEGylated liposomes, including those loaded with doxorubicin, can extravasate and enter the tumour interstitium (see relevant data in ref. 9). This finding attracted considerable attention; PEGylated liposome-based anticancer agents went into development; and ultimately, doxorubicin-based Doxil® was approved for clinical application. Accumulation and aggregation of PEGylated liposomes in the tumour tissue was observed by intravital microscopy (32). Interestingly, the pore size in the tumour microvasculature that allowed the entry of liposomes into tumour tissue, varied widely, depending on the tumour type and location (33). The extents of tumour accumulation of PEGylated plain liposomes and PEGylated immunoliposomes targeted against tumour-specific antigens (e.g. with anti-Her2neu antibody) were quite similar. However, despite the similar tumour accumulation, drug-carrying PEGylated immunoliposomes blocked tumour growth more effectively than plain drug-carrying PEGylated liposomes (34). Most likely, the improved therapeutic action of the targeted PEGylated immunoliposomes is attributable to their ability to enter tumour cells by receptor-mediated endo-cytosis.

3 Coupling of various ligands to the distal end of liposome-grafted polymer

Further development of the concept of long-circulating liposomes involved the attempt to combine the properties of long-circulating liposomes and immuno-liposomes in a single preparation (35, 36), i.e. to make liposomes that are both long-circulating and targeted. Such an approach is especially important for efficient targeted delivery of liposomal drugs to targets with limited blood supply and/or low antigen concentration—circumstances in which increased circulation times are required for efficient liposome-to-target interaction. This approach required the simultaneous presence of both the protecting polymer and the targeting moiety (usually a monoclonal antibody or its fragment) on the liposome surface (35, 36).

Targeting of liposomes with ligands selective to cell surface receptors allows selective drug delivery to those cells. There are several considerations in the design of ligand-coated long-circulating liposomes:

(a) A ligand (an antibody, another protein, peptide, or carbohydrate) attached to the liposome may increase the rate of liposome uptake in the liver and spleen, despite the presence of a PEG brush or another molecule on the liposome surface that increases its circulation time. (Ref. 37 and Figure 19.6 therein discuss this issue.)

(b) Ligand-coated liposomes might cause an unwanted immune response against the ligand or other liposome components. The extent of anti-liposome anti-body development would depend on liposome composition and the character of the ligand (e.g. a small peptide or Fv fragment should be much less immunogenic than a complete foreign IgG molecule) (38, 39).

(c) The amount of ligand attached to the liposome may be critical in ensuring successful binding with the target while maintaining an extended liposome circulation time. Thus, the use of liposomes with a lower surface density of ligand may extend the liposome circulation time and improve the overall *in vivo* targeting efficacy to smaller targets with limited blood flow. Such liposomes, however, may not be the best to bind to the same target *in vitro*, when compared with the liposomes fully coated with ligand.

(d) The method of ligand attachment to the liposome surface may also be critical in determining the *in vivo* fate of targeted long-circulating liposomes.

To assemble ligand-bearing PEG-grafted liposomes a few approaches have been used. The simplest approach is to co-immobilize a ligand of potential interest (primarily, an antibody or antibody fragments) together with the protective polymer on the surface of the same liposome (35, 36) (see the schematic pattern in Figure 3A). However, a definite drawback of this approach is that the polymer chains might interfere with the interaction of a ligand and its target (26, 40, 41). The highly mobile PEG chains may also inhibit the conjugation reactions between reactive groups on the surface of the liposome and the ligand molecule.

These concerns led to efforts to couple potential ligands to the far (distal) end of liposome-grafted polymeric chain with significant experimental data demonstrating ligand attachment to the distal ends of PEG chains (Figure 3B). Because the PEG-lipid conjugates used for liposome preparation are derived from commercial methoxy-PEG (mPEG) and carry only inert methoxy terminal groups, several approaches have been developed to functionalize PEG-lipid conjugates (two most elaborated synthetic pathways are presented in Figure 4). For this purpose a number of derivatives of end group functionalized lipopolymers have been introduced (see Table 1). They have the general formula X-PEG-DSPE (42, 43), in which X represents a reactive functional group-containing moiety, and PEG-DSPE represents a urethane-linked conjugate of distearoylphosphatidyl-

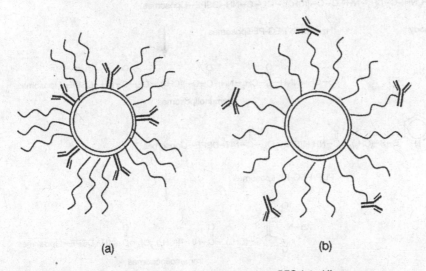

(a) (b)

Figure 3 Two ways to attach specific targeting ligands to PEGylated liposomes. (A) Co-immobilization of a ligand with PEG on the liposome surface. (B) Attachment of a ligand to an activated distal tip of a liposome-grafted PEG chain.

ethanolamine and PEG. Most end group functionalized PEG-lipids were synthesized from a few heterobifunctional PEG derivatives containing hydroxyl and carboxyl or amino groups. Typically the hydroxyl end group of PEG was used to form a urethane attachment with the hydrophobic lipid anchor, DSPE, while the amino or carboxyl groups were used for conjugation or further functionalization reactions. In some instances it was practical to prepare the functionalized lipopolymers by reacting DSPE with a large excess of homobifunctional PEG, followed by purification of the desired product (44, 45). This strategy is successful as long as the formation of DSPE-PEG-DSPE is minimized and/or it is efficiently removed by the purification step.

Three general strategies have been employed to assemble ligand-bearing long-circulating PEGylated liposomes (43, 46). In some instances end group functionalized PEG-lipids (see end groups 1-6 in Table 1) can be incorporated into liposomes and then conjugated to a specific ligand. This approach seems more suitable for macromolecular ligands, such as immunoglobulins. However, this method leads to a ligand-bearing liposome containing some unreacted end groups (though, some protocols involve the use of self-hydrolysable reactive groups, see further). In another method, ligand-PEG-lipids were synthesized first, and then the conjugates were formulated into ligand-bearing vesicles (see the generalized scheme in Figure 5). This second method is more useful for low molecular weight ligands, peptides, oligosaccharides, and vitamins. Both methods have their advantages and drawbacks, which are important to recognize.

The first approach involves conjugation of preformed liposomes and thus does not require complex and labour-intensive preparation of pure ligand-PEG-lipids.

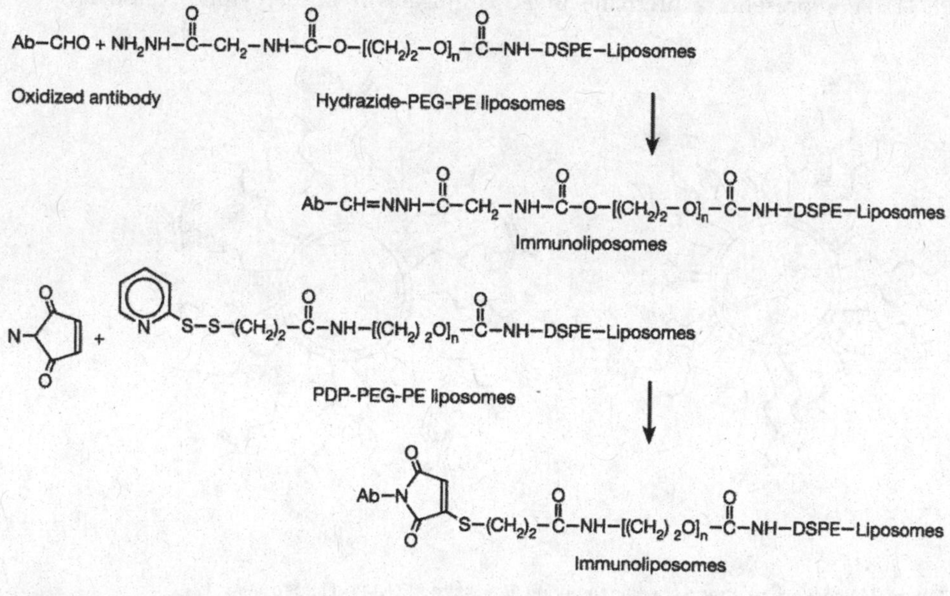

Figure 4 The reaction schemes of two common methods for attaching specific ligands to activated PEG derivatives. (A) Via hydrazide-PEG-PE. (B) Via PDP-PEG-PE.

240

Table 1 Summary of end group functionalized polymer-lipids of general structure X-PEG-DSPE that were used for preparation of ligand-bearing of liposomes [a].

No	X	Comments
1	H₂N–	Used for the preparation of end group functionalized (47, 56) and ligand-PEG-DSPE (48, 49) via the amino group modification. Amino-PEG-PE forms long circulating liposomes, behaving as positively charged particles (53).
2	HO₂C–	Useful for further modification and conjugation reactions via carbodiimide-mediated coupling (45, 57). Was used for immunoliposome preparation.
3	(hydrazide structure)	Hydrazide-PEG-DSPE (52) was introduced for conjugation of antibodies, ozidized on their carbohydrate residues (40, 55), to PEG chains of liposomes and for conjugation of Nterminal Ser or Thr peptides (54)
4	(pyridyl dithio structure)	PDP-PEG-DSPE proved useful for binding thiol-containing ligands through disulfide linkage. Precursor for HS-PEG-DSPE, for attachment of maleimide (56) and bromoacetyl (46) - containing ligands to liposomes.
5	(maleimide structure)	Maleimido-PEG-PE is used for attachment of Fab' fragments and other thiol-containing ligands, e.g. Cysteine-containing peptides (47, 66)
6	R–O–C(=O)–O–	Nitrophenyl carbonates (R= nitrophenyl) are useful derivatives for binding amino-containing ligands and other functional residues forming urethane attachments (44, 58)

[a] The PEG-DSPE residue in most cases was urethane-linked and derived from PEG of average molecular weight 2000.

Because the approach involves conjugation after the formation of liposomes, some of the reactive end groups can remain on the outer surface creating a possibility of crosslinking through the multiple attachments to a single protein (ligand) molecule. Additionally, the reactive groups at the termini of the PEG chains on the inner surface of liposomes remain fully unused. The potential of the unused reactive functionalities on either the inner or outer monolayers for undergoing side reactions with water, drug molecules (if present), or other lipid components is a source of concern. In some instances, it is advisable to quench the unreacted end groups. For example, after conjugation of Fab-thiols to maleimido-PEG-liposomes, an excess of 2-mercaptoethanol has been used to consume the remaining maleimide residues (47).

The above issues are circumvented by the second approach, in which pure ligand-PEG-lipid is mixed with other liposomal matrix-forming components (e.g.

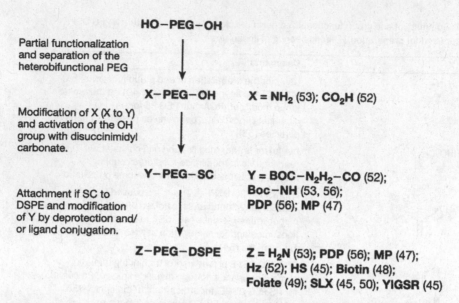

HO–PEG–OH

Partial functionalization
and separation of the
heterobifunctional PEG

X–PEG–OH   X = NH$_2$ (53); CO$_2$H (52)

Modification of X (X to Y)
and activation of the OH
group with disuccinimidyl
carbonate.

Y–PEG–SC   Y = BOC–N$_2$H$_2$–CO (52);
Boc–NH (53, 56);
PDP (56); MP (47)

Attachment if SC to
DSPE and modification
of Y by deprotection and/
or ligand conjugation.

Z–PEG–DSPE   Z = H$_2$N (53); PDP (56); MP (47);
Hz (52); HS (45); Biotin (48);
Folate (49); SLX (45, 50); YIGSR (45)

Figure 5 Possible pathways for transformation of PEG into the ligand-bearing PEG-PE.

lecithin and cholesterol), and then made into unilamellar vesicles (46, 48–50). Three-component conjugates containing various ligands: vitamins (48, 49), peptides, and saccharides (46, 50), were recently synthesized by reacting the appropriate X-PEG-DSPE with suitably functionalized ligands. In some instances, the attachment of the ligand to PEG was performed first, followed by lipid ligation to the other end group of the polymer chain (51). However, this approach is suitable only in special situations, because it generally requires protection/deprotection of the ligand moiety. Ligand-lipopolymer conjugates can be chromatographically purified and characterized by NMR, HPLC, and MALDI. MALDI, in particular, is a powerful technique for characterization of this type of conjugates (46, 48, 49, 51). A straightforward formulation process is one of the main attractive features of the total lipid mixing/extrusion approach to formation of ligand-bearing PEG-liposomes. On the other hand, incorporation of the preformed three-component conjugates into liposomes by this method results in slightly less than half of the ligands facing the inner aqueous compartment, with the remaining 55–60% positioned on the external surface (for 100 nm liposome), where the ligands should exert their biological activity (46), i.e. a substantial portion of the total ligand-PEG-lipid is inner leaflet bound, and is therefore wasted in this approach.

In the third approach to assembling ligand-bearing PEGylated liposomes, it was demonstrated that mPEG-DSPE can be inserted into preformed liposomes achieving similar external surface densities and *in vivo* performance similar to PEGylated liposomes prepared by lipid mixing/extrusion approach (24). A similar insertion strategy was recently applied to several ligand-PEG-DSPE conjugates (46). The incubation of ligand-PEG-DSPE (1.2–1.5 mole%) with preformed liposomes containing mPEG-DSPE (2–3 mole%) at 37 °C resulted in complete insertion of the three-component conjugate. This, aggregation-free, process positioned the PEG-tethered ligands exclusively on the outer leaflet of the liposomal bilayer (oligosaccharide and peptide conjugates were tested). This insertion methodology provides the same external surface densities of both PEG-tethered ligands and mPEG chains as by lipid mixing/extrusion process (46). Perhaps, most important, this insertion approach overcomes the drawbacks of both previously discussed methods. As long as the inserted ligand-lipopolymer is purified and properly characterized, the resulting ligand-bearing liposome is free of any extraneous reactive functional groups, and all ligand moieties are positioned only on the outer leaflet of the liposomal membrane.

3.1 Ligand attachment to hydrazide-activated PEG

Protocol 5

Synthesis of PE-PEG-hydrazide (PEG-PE-Hz) (52) (see Figure 3)

Equipment and reagents

- DEAE-Sephadex A-25 column
- Spectracor CE dialysis tubing (MWCO 300 000)
- 0.2 μm filter
- PEG-diol, toluene, isocyanatoacetate, triethylamine

- NaOH, methylene chloride
- Borate buffer, ammonium bicarbonate
- Pyridine, methylene chloride, acetonitrile, disuccinimidyl carbonate
- Ethyl ether, ethyl acetate
- Chloroform, DSPE

Method

1 Dissolve 42 g of PEG-diol with a molecular weight of 2000 Da in 200 ml of toluene, dry azeotropically, and treat with 2.3 ml (21 mmol) of isocyanatoacetate and 1.5 ml (10 mmol) triethylamine. After overnight reaction at 25 °C evaporate the solution to dryness.

2 Dissolve the residue in 100 ml of 0.2 M NaOH, evaporate the traces of toluene, and maintain pH 12 with periodic dropwise additions of 4 M NaOH. When the pH stops decreasing, acidify the solution to pH 3.0 and extract the product with methylene chloride (100 ml × 2).

3 Dry the solution with MgSO₄, filter, and evaporate to dryness. Dissolve the remaining mixture of unreacted PEG, monocarboxylated PEG, and dicarboxylated PEG in 50 ml water.

4 Load one-third of this solution (approx. 30 ml or 14 g of derivatized PEG) onto the column with 115 ml of DEAE-Sephadex A-25 in borate buffer. Wash underivatized PEG from the column with water (until negative polymethacrylic acid, PMA, test).

Protocol 5 continued

5 Apply a gradient of ammonium bicarbonate (2–20 mM in increments of 1–2 mM every 200 ml) and collect 50 ml fractions. Fractions 1–25 contain only PEG monoacid. Collect these fractions, pool them together, concentrate to approx. 70 ml, acidify to pH 2.0, and extract with methylene chloride (50 ml × 2).

6 Dry methylene chloride solution with $MgSO_4$, concentrate, and pour into cold ether with stirring. Dry the precipitate in vacuum.

7 Dissolve 5 g (2.38 mmol) of the ω-hydroxy acid derivative of PEG from the previous step and 0.91 g (6.9 mmol) of *tert*-butyl carbazate (*t*-Boc-hydrazide) in 7 ml of a methylene chloride/ethyl acetate mixture (1:1).

8 Cool the solution on ice and treat with 0.6 g (2.9 mmol) of dicyclohexylcarbodiimide pre-dissolved in the same solvent mixture. Remove the ice after 30 min and allow the reaction to proceed for an additional 3 h.

9 Filter the precipitated dicyclohexylurea and evaporate. Purify the product by two precipitations from ethyl acetate/ether (1:1) and dry in vacuum.

10 Dissolve 5 g (2.26 mmol) of ω-hydroxy Boc-Hz PEG from the previous step in a mixture of 1.1 ml pyridine, 5 ml methylene chloride, and 2 ml acetonitrile, and treat with 1.4 g (5.5 mmol) of disuccinimidyl carbonate overnight at 25 °C.

11 Filter the solution and gradually add it to 100 ml of cold ethyl ether. Dissolve the precipitate in 45 ml of warm ethyl acetate, chill, and mix with an equal volume of ethyl ether.

12 Collect precipitate by filtration and dry in vacuum over P_2O_5.

13 Dissolve 693 mg (0.29 mmol) of Boc-Hz-PEG-succinimidyl carbonate from the previous step in 4 ml chloroform and treat with 200 mg (0.27 mmol) of solid DSPE and 0.1 ml (0.72 mmol) of triethylamine.

14 Mix the suspension vigorously for 10 min at 45 °C.

15 Add 4.2 ml (0.73 mmol) of acetic acid to the reaction mixture and evaporate it to dryness.

16 Slowly dissolve the solid residue in 5 ml of water and evaporate the remaining traces of chloroform.

17 Transfer the solution into Spectracor CE dialysis tubing (MWCO 300 000) and dialyse against 50 mM saline at 4 °C (3 × 1000 ml, 16 h each period).

18 Dialyse the conjugate solution further against deionized water, filter through 0.2 μm filter, and lyophilize.

19 Deprotect Boc-Hz-PEG-DSPE from the previous step in 4 M HCl in dioxane for 60 min, and vacuum dry.

20 Confirm the identity of the product by NMR, TLC, and derivatization with trinitrobenzene sulfonate or a model aldehyde (17).

The required quantity of PE-PEG-Hz is added to a lipid mixture for the preparation of long-circulating liposomes. Hydrazide group on the distal end of liposome-grafted PEG can be converted into other reactive groups (53) or directly used for the attachment of numerous ligands (54) including glycoproteins, e.g. immunoglobulins (40).

Protocol 6

Coupling of N-terminal Ser or Thr peptides to distal hydrazide groups of PE-PEG-Hz-containing liposomes (54)

The same method should be suitable for conjugation of glycopeptides.

Equipment and reagents

- Biodesign dialysis membrane MWCO 8000
- Liposomes: PE-PEG-Hz, PC, and cholesterol
- Peptide solution
- 25 mM HEPES, 0.9% NaCl pH 7.2
- Sodium periodate
- N-acetylmethionine

Method

1 Prepare liposomes of PE-PEG-Hz, PC, and cholesterol in a weight ratio of 1:3:1 (5:55:38 mol% ratio).

2 Treat 0.2 ml of peptide solution in 25 mM HEPES, 0.9% saline pH 7.2, with 20 μl of a freshly prepared stock solution of sodium periodate for 5 min in the dark at periodate/peptide ratio of 20:1 (100 mM sodium periodate stock solution was used for oxidation of 5 mM peptide solution).

3 Consume the excess of periodate by adding 20 μl of 1 M N-acetylmethionine.

4 Mix 2.2 ml of liposome solution with total phospholipid concentration of about 50 μmol/ml in 0.1 M acetate buffer pH 4.8, with the oxidized peptide solution and incubate overnight at 6 °C.

5 Dialyse the reaction mixture against 25 mM HEPES, 0.9% NaCl pH 7.2, using Biodesign dialysis membrane MWCO 8000.

6 Determine the composition of the peptide-PEG-liposome by amino acid analysis.

A similar protocol can be used for antibody oxidation and subsequent coupling to PE-PEG-Hz-containing liposomes (40, 55).

Protocol 7

Attachment of periodate-oxidized antibody to Hz-PEG-PE-containing liposomes (55)

Equipment and reagents

- Sepharose CL-4B size exclusion column (Pharmacia)
- Antibody, sodium periodate, acetate buffer
- *N*-acetylmethionine
- Hydrazide-PEG-liposomes

Method

1 Incubate a solution of antibody (5.5 ml, at 3 mg/ml) with sodium periodate (2–10 mM, final concentration) in 0.1 M acetate buffer pH 5.5 at 6 °C, for 20 min.

2 Add *N*-acetylmethionine (0.5 ml of 500 mM) to quench the excess periodate.

3 Add hydrazide-PEG-liposomes (5.6 ml at 47 μmole phopholipid/ml) in the same buffer to the solution containing oxidized antibody, and incubate the mixture overnight at 6 °C.

4 Separate the immunoliposomes from the free antibody on a Sepharose CL-4B size exclusion column (Pharmacia).

5 Pool the immunoliposome-containing fractions.

6 Calculate the average number of antibody molecules per liposome from the results of amino acid analysis and phosphate analysis as summarized in ref. 40.

3.2 Ligand attachment to PDP-activated PEG

Alternative chemical pathway for ligand (antibody) attachment to a distal end of liposome-grafted PEG chain involves the use PEG-PE activated at distal terminus with pyridyldithiopropionate (PDP) group (56) (see Figure 3). To be coupled to PDP-activated PEG, the ligand (antibody) must be pre-activated with a maleimide group as described in Protocols 8 and 9.

Protocol 8

Synthesis of PDP-PEG-PE (56)

Equipment and reagents

- Rotary evaporator
- Centrifuge
- SPDP, α-amino-ω-hydroxy-PEG, acetonitrile
- DSC, DSPE
- Ethyl ether, ethyl acetate

Method

1 To prepare PDP-PEG-OH, dissolve 100 mg (0.32 mmol) of SPDP and 0.55 g (0.275 mmol) of α-amino-ω-hydroxy-PEG in 2 ml acetonitrile.

2 React the mixture for 4 h at 25 °C.

3 Evaporate the solvent on a rotary evaporator and add 50 ml of ethyl ether.

4 Store overnight at 4 °C, collect the white solid and dry it in vacuum over P_2O_5.

5 To prepare PDP-PEG-succinimidylcarbonate (PDP-PEG-SC), dissolve 0.4 g (0.18 mmol) of dried PDP-PEG-OH from the previous step in 0.5 ml acetonitrile. React with 81 mg (0.31 mmol) disuccinimidylcarbonate (DSC) and 62 ml (0.79 mmol) pyridine overnight at 25 °C.

6 Precipitate product with 40 ml of ethyl ether at 4 °C, redissolve in 4 ml of ethyl acetate, and precipitate with equal volume of ethyl ether at 4 °C.

7 Collect product by filtration and dry in vacuum over P_2O_5.

8 To obtain PDP-PEG-DSPE, add 36 mg (0.043 mmol) of DSPE to a solution of 100 mg (0.042 mmol) of PDP-PEG-SC from the previous step in 1 ml chloroform, and then add 33 ml (0.237 mmol) triethylamine.

9 Incubate for 10 min at 40 °C until the reaction mixture becomes clear.

10 Evaporate the solvent and replace it with 5 ml acetonitrile.

11 Keep the cloudy solution overnight at 4 °C.

12 To remove traces of insoluble DSPE, centrifuge the solution and separate the clear supernatant.

13 Evaporate the solution in a rotary evaporator under reduced pressure, and dry the residue in vacuum over P_2O_5.

Protocol 9

Preparation of maleimidophenylbutyate-antibody (MPB-Ab) (56)

Equipment and reagents

- Sephadex G-50 column
- 25 mM HEPES, 25 mM MES, 140 mM NaCl pH 6.7

- Antibody
- 25 mM HEPES, 140 mM NaCl pH 7.4
- SMPB, dimethylformamide

Method

1 Dissolve the Ab in 25 mM HEPES, 140 mM NaCl pH 7.4 at a concentration of 10 mg/ml.

2 Slowly add a 25 mM solution of succinimidyl-4-MPB (SMPB) in dimethylformamide to the Ab solution until the molar ratio is 20:1 (SMPB:Ab), and incubate for 30 min at room temperature.

3 Remove the unbound SMPB and lower the pH by passing the solution over a Sephadex G-50 column in 25 mM HEPES, 25 mM MES, 140 mM NaCl pH 6.7 buffer.

Protocol 10

Antibody conjugation with PDP-PEG-PE-containing liposomes (56)

Equipment and reagents

- Sephadex G-50 column
- Sepharose CL-4B column
- 25 mM HEPES, 25 mM MES, 140 mM NaCl pH 6.7
- 25 mM HEPES, 140 mM NaCl pH 7.4

- 100 mM sodium acetate, 70 mM NaCl pH 5.5
- DTT
- Lipid film
- MPB-antibody

Method

1 Hydrate lipid film prepared by any conventional method from PC/Chol/ PDP-PEG-PE at a molar ratio 2:1:0.2 with 100 mM sodium acetate, 70 mM NaCl pH 5.5.

2 Reduce the pyridyldithio groups on the distal ends of the PEG chains by adding dithiothreitol (DTT) to a final concentration of 20 mM and incubating for 30 min at room temperature.

3 Separate DTT and raise the pH by passing the liposomes over a Sephadex G-50 column eluted with 25 mM HEPES, 25 mM MES, 140 mM NaCl pH 6.7.

4 Incubate thiolated liposomes overnight at room temperature with MPB-Ab at Ab/lipid ratio of approx. 1:1000.

5 Remove unbound Ab by passing liposomes over a Sepharose CL-4B column with 25 mM HEPES, 140 mM NaCl pH 7.4.

Protocol 11

Synthesis of maleimido-PEG-PE (47)

Equipment and reagents

- TLC equipment
- Silica gel column
- Amino-PEG-DSPE, dichloromethane, MPS, DMF, triethylamine

- Chloroform, methanol, water
- α-amino-ω-hydroxy-PEG
- DSPE

Method A

1 Dissolve amino-PEG-DSPE (0.5 g, 0.18 mmol) in 3 ml dichloromethane and add N-succinimidyl-3-(N-maleimido)-propionate (MPS, 62.5 mg, 24 mmol) in DMF (75 μl) followed by triethylamine (76 μl, 0.54 mmol).

2 Confirm that the reaction is complete by TLC (chloroform/methanol/ water, 90:18:2, visualized with ninhydrin).

3 Separate the product mixture on silica gel column eluting with a stepwise gradient of methanol (0–15%) in chloroform.

4 Pool the product containing fractions and evaporate the solvent.

5 Dry the pure MP-PEG-DSPE in vacuum over P_2O_5. Yield: 203 mg (44%).

6 Confirm the identity of the product by ^{1}H NMR (CD$_3$OD): δ 0.88 (m, 6H), 1.26 (s, CH$_2$, 56H), 1.58 (br m, CH$_2$CH$_2$C=O, 4H), 2.31 (2 × t, CH$_2$C=O, 4H), 2.48 (t, MP-CH$_2$CH$_2$C=O), 3.53 (t, CH$_2$N, 2H), 3.63 (s, PEG ≈180H), 3.88 & 3.98 (q & t, CH$_2$PO$_4$CH$_2$, 4H), 4.20 (t, CH$_2$O$_2$CN, 2H), 4.17 & 4.39 (2 × dd, OCH$_2$CHCH$_2$OP, 2H), 5.2 (m, PO$_4$CH$_2$CHCH$_2$O, 1H), 6.69 (s, Mal, 4H) ppm.

Method B

1 React MPS with α-amino-ω-hydroxy-PEG as described above for the SPDP reaction.

2 Activate the hydroxyl group using disuccinimidyl carbonate to obtain MP-PEG-SC as described above for the PDP-PEG-SC.

3 Add DSPE (35 mg, 46 μmol) to the solution of MP-PEG-SC (100 mg, 50 μmol) in 2 ml chloroform followed by triethylamine (14 μl, 100 μmol).

4 Allow the reaction to proceed for a few hours at 45 °C.

5 Verify by TLC that the reaction is complete.

6 Purify the product, MP-PEG-DSPE as in Method A. Yield: 118 mg (70%).

3.3 Ligand attachment via COOH-activated PEG

Ligands can be also attached to the distal ends of liposome-grafted PEG via COOH groups (57). In this method, coupling of the PEG carboxylic group with the ligand (antibody) amino group proceeds via activation with a water soluble carbodiimide.

Protocol 12

Synthesis of COOH-PEG-PE (57)

Equipment and reagents

- TLC equipment
- Dialysis equipment
- 5% DSPE in chloroform/methanol
- PEG bis(succinimidyl succinate) (PEG-2OSu) in chloroform
- Triethylamine

Method

1 Add 1 ml of 5% DSPE in chloroform/methanol (3:1, v/v) mixture to ·9.5 ml of PEG bis(succinimidyl succinate) (PEG-2OSu) in chloroform, and then add 20.5 μl triethylamine.

Protocol 12 continued

2 Vigorously stir the reaction mixture overnight at 35 °C in darkness.

3 After separating the products by TLC, confirm by the ninhydrin test full conversion of the amino groups in DSPE.

4 Evaporate the reaction mixture and add a small quantity of water to the residue to form micelles.

5 Dialyse the COOH-PEG-PE micelles for five days against water using a dialysis bag with large pores (Spectrapor CE 300 000 MWCO) and then lyophilize.

Protocol 13

Coupling of antibodies to COOH-PEG-PE-containing liposomes (57)

Equipment and reagents

- Bio-Gel A-15m column
- NaOH, NaCl
- HO₂C-PEG-PE-containing liposomes in MES buffer pH 4–5.5
- 1-ethyl-3-(3-dimethylaminopropyl) carbodiimide
- *N*-hydroxysulfosuccinimide
- Antibody

Method

1 To 300 μl of the suspension of HO₂C-PEG-PE-containing liposomes in MES buffer pH 4–5.5 (total 3 μmol lipids) add 120 μl of a 0.25 M solution of 1-ethyl-3-(3-dimethylaminopropyl)carbodiimide and 120 μl of 0.25 M *N*-hydroxysulfosuccinimide in water.

2 Incubate the mixture for 10 min at room temperature and neutralize it to pH 7.5 with 1 M NaOH.

3 Add the desired quantity of an antibody to the activated liposomes and incubate the reaction mixture for 8 h at 4 °C with gentle stirring.

4 Separate immunoliposomes from unbound antibody on a Bio-Gel A-15m column pre-equilibrated with saline.

5 Collect the peak fractions of immunoliposomes eluted in the void volume, pool them, and when necessary dilute to the required volume with saline.

3.4 Coupling of primary amino group-containing ligands to pNP-PEG-PE-containing liposomes (44, 58)

A new amphiphilic PEG derivative, *p*-nitrophenylcarbonyl-PEG-PE (pNP-PEG-PE), was introduced to further simplify the coupling procedure and to make it suitable for single-step binding of a variety of amino group-containing ligands (including antibodies, proteins, and small molecules) to the distal end of liposome-attached polymeric chains without use of potentially toxic compounds (44, 58). pNP-PEG-PE readily incorporates into liposomes via its phospholipid residue, and easily binds any amino group-containing compound via its water-exposed pNP group forming a stable, non-toxic urethane (carbamate) bond (see the scheme for the synthesis of pNP-PEG-PE and primary amino group-containing ligand to pNP-terminus in Figure 6). The reaction between the pNP group and the ligand amino group proceeds easily and quantitatively at pH around 8.0, and excess free pNP groups are easily eliminated by spontaneous hydrolysis.

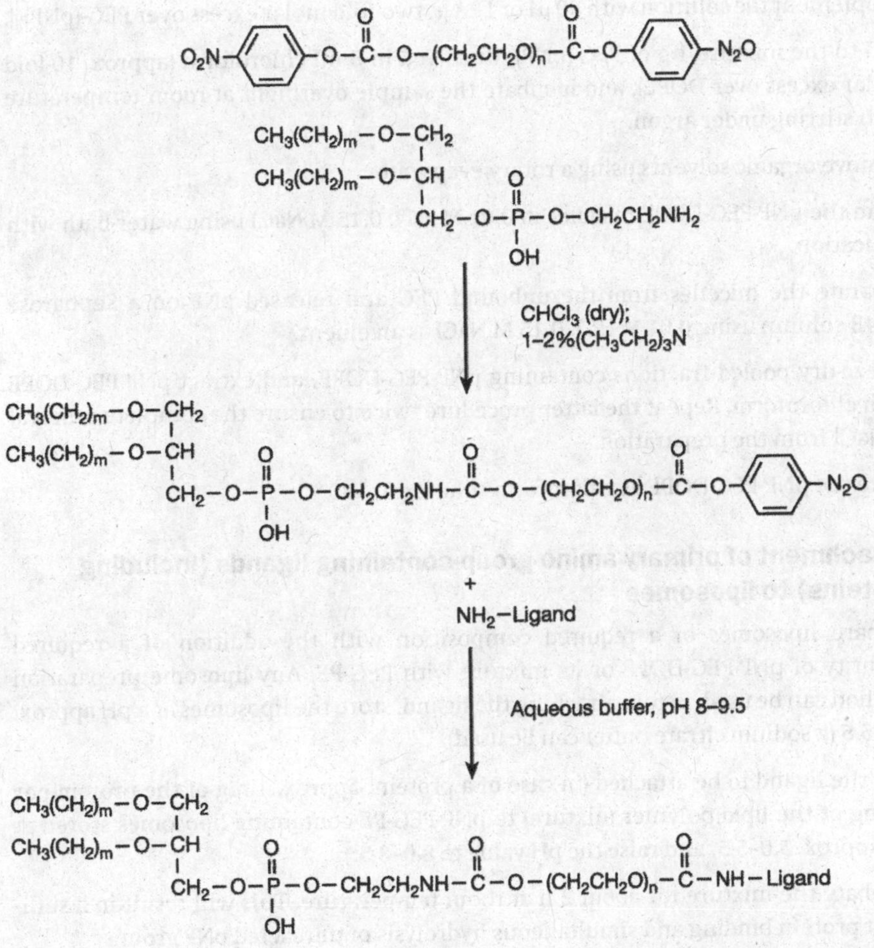

$$O_2N\text{—}\langle\text{—}\rangle\text{—}O\text{—}\overset{\overset{O}{\|}}{C}\text{—}O\text{—}(CH_2CH_2O)_n\text{—}\overset{\overset{O}{\|}}{C}\text{—}O\text{—}\langle\text{—}\rangle\text{—}N_2O$$

$$CH_3(CH_2)_m\text{—}O\text{—}CH_2$$
$$CH_3(CH_2)_m\text{—}O\text{—}CH$$
$$CH_2\text{—}O\text{—}\overset{\overset{O}{\|}}{\underset{\underset{OH}{|}}{P}}\text{—}O\text{—}CH_2CH_2NH_2$$

CHCl$_3$ (dry);
1–2%(CH$_3$CH$_2$)$_3$N

$$CH_3(CH_2)_m\text{—}O\text{—}CH_2$$
$$CH_3(CH_2)_m\text{—}O\text{—}CH$$
$$CH_2\text{—}O\text{—}\overset{\overset{O}{\|}}{\underset{\underset{OH}{|}}{P}}\text{—}O\text{—}CH_2CH_2NH\text{—}\overset{\overset{O}{\|}}{C}\text{—}O\text{—}(CH_2CH_2O)_n\text{—}\overset{\overset{O}{\|}}{C}\text{—}O\text{—}\langle\text{—}\rangle\text{—}N_2O$$

+

NH$_2$–Ligand

Aqueous buffer, pH 8–9.5

$$CH_3(CH_2)_m\text{—}O\text{—}CH_2$$
$$CH_3(CH_2)_m\text{—}O\text{—}CH$$
$$CH_2\text{—}O\text{—}\overset{\overset{O}{\|}}{\underset{\underset{OH}{|}}{P}}\text{—}O\text{—}CH_2CH_2NH\text{—}\overset{\overset{O}{\|}}{C}\text{—}O\text{—}(CH_2CH_2O)_n\text{—}\overset{\overset{O}{\|}}{C}\text{—}NH\text{—}Ligand$$

Figure 6 Synthesis of pNP-PEG-PE and attachment of an amino-containing ligand to pNP-group.

Protocol 14

Coupling of ligands to pNP-PEG-PE

Equipment and reagents

- Rotary evaporator
- Sepharose CL-4B column
- Bio-Gel A-15m column
- DOPE, chloroform
- TEA, PEG-(pNP)$_2$
- HCl, NaCl
- Liposome preparation

A. Synthesis of pNP-PEG-DOPE

1   Dissolve 24 mg (32.2 μmole) of DOPE in chloroform to obtain a 50 mg/ml solution.

2   Supplement the solution with 80 μl of TEA [*c.* two-fold molar excess over PEG-(pNP)$_2$].

3   Add to the mixture 1 g of PEG-(pNP)$_2$ dissolved in 5 ml chloroform (approx. 10-fold molar excess over DOPE), and incubate the sample overnight at room temperature with stirring under argon.

4   Remove organic solvents using a rotary evaporator.

5   Form the pNP-PEG-DOPE micelles in 0.01 M HCl, 0.15 M NaCl using water-bath with sonication.

6   Separate the micelles from the unbound PEG and released pNP on a Sepharose CL-4B column using 0.01 M HCl, 0.15 M NaCl as an eluent.

7   Freeze-dry pooled fractions containing pNP-PEG-DOPE, and extract pNP-PEG-DOPE with chloroform. Repeat the latter procedure twice to ensure the complete removal of NaCl from the preparation.

8   Store the pNP-PEG-DOPE as chloroform solution at –80 °C.

B. Attachment of primary amino group-containing ligands (including proteins) to liposomes

1   Prepare liposomes of a required composition with the addition of a required quantity of pNP-PEG-DOPE or its mixture with PEG-PE. Any liposome preparation method can be used. Before attaching the ligand, store the liposomes at a pH approx. 5.0–5.5 (a sodium citrate buffer can be used).

2   Add the ligand to be attached (in case of a protein, approx. 1 mg of the protein per 10 mg of the lipid/polymer mixture) to pNP-PEG-PE-containing liposomes stored at pH approx. 5.0–5.5, and raise the pH value to 8.0–8.5.

3   Incubate the mixture for about 2 h at room temperature. This will result in a sufficient protein binding and simultaneous hydrolysis of unreacted pNP groups.

4   Purify the ligand-containing liposomes by gel filtration on a Bio-Gel A-15m column.

This method has been successfully used to attach such ligands as monoclonal antibodies, concanavalin A, wheat germ agglutinin, avidin, and TAT peptide to PEG-liposomes at the level of several hundred ligand molecules per single 200 nm liposome (44, 58). This was achieved with complete preservation of the biological activity of the attached ligands.

3.5 Ligand attachment by preparation of ligand-PEG-lipid conjugates and their incorporation into liposomes

Protocol 15

Preparation of oligosaccharide (SLX)-PEG-DSPE (46)

Equipment and reagents

- TLC equipment
- PDP-PEG-DSPE
- Isopropanol
- Tributylphosphine
- $CHCl_3/CH_3OH/H_2O$
- Ether

Method

1. Dissolve PDP-PEG-DSPE (200 mg, 0.064 mmol) in isopropanol/water (1:4.6 ml) containing EDTA (10 mM). Add tributylphosphine (80 μl, 0.32 mmol).

2. After 2 h confirm that the reaction is complete by TLC ($CHCl_3/CH_3OH/ H_2O$, 90:18:2, visualize with iodine). In contrast to the starting material ($R_f = 0.56$) the product— HS-PEG-DSPE ($R_f = 0.58$)—does not absorb UV light. The by-product, 2-thiopyridone, is observed under UV light ($R_f = 0.65$).

3. Lyophilize the reaction mixture.

4. Triturate the yellowish solid residue with ether (3×3 ml), and then dry the resulting white solid in vacuum over P_2O_5.

5. Use the HS-PEG-DSPE from the previous step for coupling with bromoacetylated ligands as described below for SLX and YIGSR-NH$_2$.

Protocol 16

Preparation of Sialyl Lewis^x (SLX)-PEG-DSPE (46)

Equipment and reagents

- TLC equipment
- C8 silica column (8 g, 1 × 40 cm, LC-8 Supelclean, Supelco)
- Bromoacetylated derivative of SLX
- DMF
- HS-PEG-DSPE
- Potassium iodide
- $NaHCO_3$, Na_2EDTA
- $CHCl_3/CH_3OH/H_2O$
- tert-butanol

Protocol 16 continued

Method

1 Add bromoacetylated derivative of SLX (Ref. No. 31, 98 mg, 0.08 mmol) to DMF (2.8 ml) solution of HS-PEG-DSPE (197 mg, 0.07 mmol) followed by potassium iodide (14.3 mg, 0.086 mmol).

2 After 5 min add NaHCO$_3$ (0.4 M) / Na$_2$EDTA (10 mM) solution (pH = 8.0, 328 ml, 0.13 mmol bicarbonate) and let the reaction proceed overnight at room temperature.

3 Confirm by TLC (CHCl$_3$/CH$_3$OH/H$_2$O, 75:36:6) the formation of SLX-PEG-DSPE product (R_f = 0.37, visualized by UV, iodine, and phenol/H$_2$SO$_4$ sprays).

4 Dilute the reaction mixture with water (12 ml) and load it onto a C8 silica column (8 g, 1 × 40 cm, LC-8 Supelclean).

5 Elute the column with a stepwise gradient of methanol (0–70%, v/v) in water (10% increments every 20 ml), and then water/methanol/ chloroform, 15:80:5 (60 ml).

6 Pool the product-containing fractions and evaporate the solvent at ambient temperature to produce a colourless thick liquid.

7 Dissolve the resulting liquid in *tert*-butanol (5 ml), lyophilize it, and further dry in vacuum over P$_2$O$_5$ to obtain white fluffy solid (203 mg, 74%).

8 Confirm the identity of the product by ^{1}H-NMR (CD$_3$OD): δ 0.88 (t, CH$_3$-lipid, 6 H), 1.15 (d, H-6 Fuc, 3H), 1.19 (t, OCH$_2$CH$_3$, 3H), 1.29 (bs, (CH$_2$)$_n$, 56 H), 1.61 (bm, CH$_2$CH$_2$C=O, 4H), 1.73 (t, H-3ax-Sial, 1H), 2.01 (s, NHAc, 3H), 2.32 (2 × t, CH$_2$CO, 4H), 2.58 (t, -SCH$_2$CH$_2$CONH, 2H), 2.87 (dd, H-3eq-Sial, 1H), 2.93 (t, -SCH$_2$CH$_2$CONH, 2H), 3.35 (m, NHCH$_2$, 4H), 3.64 (s, PEG, ≈180H), 3.7–4 (m, overlapping sugar peaks & CH$_2$PO$_4$CH$_2$, 8H), 4–4.31 (m, overlapping, 5H), 4.43 (dd, CHCH$_2$CO, 1H), 4.54 (d, H-1 Gal, 1H), 4.83 (m, H-5 Fuc, 1H), 4.90 (d, H-1 GlcN, 1H), 5.06 (d, H-1 Fuc, 1H), 5.2 (m, POCH$_2$CHCH$_2$, 1H), 7.70 & 7.84 (2 × d, phenyl, 4H) ppm.

9 Confirm the molecular weight of SLX-PEG-DSPE by MALDI-TOFMS producing a bell-shaped distribution of ions spaced at equal 44 Da intervals, and centred at 4056 Da (theoretical value, 4012 Da).

Protocol 17

Preparation of oligopeptide (YIGSR)-PEG-DSPE (46)

Equipment and reagents

- See Protocol 16

- N$^\alpha$-bromoacetyl-YIGSR-NH$_2$

Method

1 Dissolve HS-PEG-DSPE (196 mg, 0.07 mmol) and N$^\alpha$-bromoacetyl-YIGSR-NH$_2$ (54.2 mg, 0.07 mmol, 1.2 equiv.) in DMF (2 ml). Add potassium iodide (14.1 mg, 0.09 mmol, 1.3 equiv.), followed by NaHCO$_3$ (0.4 M)/ Na$_2$EDTA (10 mmol) solution (pH = 8.0, 326 ml).

Protocol 17 continued

2 After stirring for 21 h verify by TLC ($CHCl_3/CH_3OH/H_2O$, 75:36:6) the presence of the expected product ($R_f = 0.55$).

3 Dilute the reaction mixture with 5 ml water, and load it onto a C8 silica column (8 g, 1 × 40 cm, LC-8 Supelclean).

4 Elute the column with 12 ml water, followed by a methanol gradient (0–70%, v/v) in water (10% increments every 25 ml), and then water/ methanol/chloroform, 10:80:10 (60 ml).

5 Pool the product-containing fractions. Evaporate the solvent at ambient temperature producing colourless thick liquid.

6 Dissolve the resulting liquid in *tert*-butanol (5 ml), lyophilize it, and further dry in vacuum over P_2O_5 to obtain a white fluffy solid (174 mg, 69% yield).

7 Confirm the identity of the product by ^{1}H-NMR (CD_3OD): δ 0.9 (3 × t, CH_3 of Ile & lipid, 12H), 1.2 (m, 1H), 1.26 (s, CH_2, 56H), 1.58 (bm, $CH_2CH_2C=O$, 4H), 1.7 (m, 1H), 2.31 (2 × t, $CH_2C=O$, 4H), 2.45 (t, SCH_2CH_2CONH), 2.7 (t, SCH_2CH_2CONH), 2.9 & 3.1 (dd, peptide, 2H), 3.2 (m, 2H), 3.35 (m, $NHCH_2$, 4H), 3.45 (t, 2H), 3.64 (s, PEG, ≈180H), 3.7 (m, 4H), 3.9 (m, CH_2PO_4, 4H), 4.0 (m, 3H), 4.15–4.2 (overlapping peaks, 4H), 4.3–4.45 (overlapping peaks, 3H), 4.6 (m, 2H), 5.2 (m, PO_4CH_2CH, 1H), 6.7 & 7.1 (2 × d, phenyl of Tyr, 4H) ppm.

8 Confirm the molecular weight of the conjugate by MALDI-TOFMS exhibiting a bell-shaped distribution of ions spaced at equal 44 Da intervals, and centred at 3540 Da (theoretical value, 3496 Da).

9 Confirm by amino acid analysis the composition of the YIGSR ligand: Tyr, 0.97; Ile, 1.00; Gly, 0.98; Ser, 0.96; and Arg, 1.08.

Protocol 18

Preparation of amino-PEG-DSPE (53) (see the scheme in Figure 7)

Equipment and reagents

- TLC equipment
- Centrifuge
- *tert*-butyl pyrocarbonate (Boc$_2$O)
- α-amino-ω-hydroxy-PEG2K (Shearwater Polymers)

- Dioxane
- Ethyl ether
- Acetonitrile, DSC, pyridine
- Chloroform, DSPE, triethylamine
- Chloroform/methanol/water

Method

1 Add *tert*-butyl pyrocarbonate (Boc$_2$O, 436 mg, 2 mmol) to a solution of α-amino-ω-hydroxy-PEG2K (2 g, 1 mmol) in 8 ml of dioxane.

Protocol 18 continued

2 Allow the reaction to proceed overnight. Then concentrate the solution and add ethyl ether (40 ml) to precipitate the product Boc-NH-PEG-OH.

3 Filter and dry the product in vacuum, over P_2O_5. Yield: 1.9 g (90%).

4 Confirm the identity of Boc-NH-PEG-OH by ^{1}H-NMR (D6 DMSO): δ 1.37 (s, ^{t}Bu, 9H), 3.06 (m, CH_2NH, 2H), 3.51 (s, PEG, ≈180H), 4.52 (t, HO-PEG, 1H).

5 Dissolve Boc-NH-PEG-OH (1.9 g, 0.9 mmol) in 2 ml acetonitrile and add disuccinimidyl carbonate (DSC, 460 mg, 1.8 mmol) and pyridine (0.36 ml, 4.55 mmol).

6 Allow the reaction to proceed overnight at room temperature.

7 Precipitate the product with ether and then recrystallize it from isopropanol.

8 Filter and dry the product in vacuum, over P_2O_5. Yield: 1.8 g (85%).

9 Confirm the identity of Boc-NH-PEG-SC by ^{1}H-NMR ($CDCl_3$): δ 1.44 (s, ^{t}Bu, 9H), 2.83 (s, SC, 4H), 3.30 (m, CH_2NH, 2H), 3.64 (s, PEG, ≈180H), 4.46 (t, CH_2-SC, 2H), 5.0 (br. S, NH, 1H) ppm.

10 Dissolve Boc-NH-PEG-SC (1 g, 0.47 mmol) in chloroform and add to the solution DSPE (0.33 g, 0.48 mmol) and triethylamine (0.24 ml, 1.6 mmol).

11 Vigorously vortex the resulting suspension while warming it to maintain 40 °C for ≈10 min, until the reaction solution completely clarifies.

12 Evaporate the solution until it dries and extract the residue with acetonitrile (12 ml).

13 After overnight storage at 4 °C, separate the traces of insoluble and unreacted DSPE, by centrifugation.

14 Evaporate the solvent and dry the residue in vacuum, over P_2O_5. Yield: 1.1 g (89%).

15 Confirm the identity of Boc-NH-PEG-DSPE by ^{1}H-NMR ($CDCl_3$): δ 0.88 (t, CH_3, 6H), 1.26 (s, CH_2, 56H), 1.44 (s, ^{t}Bu, 9H), 1.58 (br. CH_2CH_2C=O, 4H), 2.31 (m, CH_2C=O, 4H), 3.31 (br. m, $NHCH_2$, 4H), 3.64 (s, PEG, ≈180H), 4.0–4.3 (overlapping m, CH_2O-P and CH_2OCONH, 6H), 4.39 (dd, glycero-CH_2OCO, 2H), 5.2 (m, CH, 1H), ppm.

16 To remove the amino-protecting group, dissolve Boc-NH-PEG-DSPE in 4 M HCl in dioxane for 2 h.

17 Evaporate the solution until it dries, and then dry the residue carefully in vacuum, over P_2O_5. The recovery is quantitative.

18 Confirm that the deprotection went to completion by TLC (chloroform/methanol/water, 90:18:2, ninhydrin positive spot at R_f = 0.29) and by ^{1}H-NMR ($CDCl_3$): disappearance of the ^{t}Bu peak at 1.44 ppm and appearance of two separate peaks at 3.21 (br. m, CH_2NH, 2H) and 3.46 (m, CH_2NH, 2H), instead of 3.31 (br. m, $NHCH_2$, 4H) in the starting material.

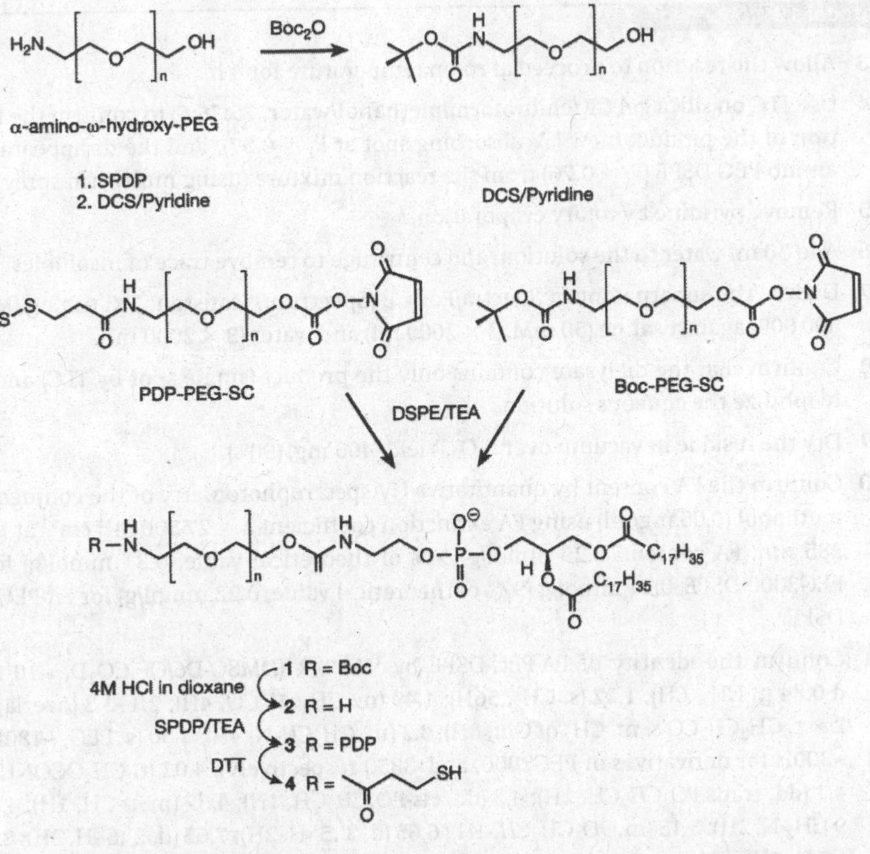

Figure 7 Preparation of amino-PEG-PE.

Protocol 19

Preparation of folate-PEG2000-DSPE (49)

Exactly the same protocol was used to prepare FA-PEG-DSPE from H₂N-PEG3350-DSPE.

Equipment and reagents

- TLC equipment
- Rotary evaporator
- Dialysis equipment
- Folic acid, DMSO

- Amino-PEG2K-DSPE, pyridine, dicyclohexylcarbodiimide
- Chloroform/methanol/water

Method

1 Dissolve folic acid (FA, Fluka, 100 mg, 0.244 mmol) in 4 ml of DMSO.

2 Add amino-PEG2K-DSPE (18) (400 mg, 0.14 mmol), pyridine (2 ml), and dicyclohexyl-carbodiimide (130 mg, 0.63 mmol) to the FA-DMSO solution.

Protocol 19 continued

3 Allow the reaction to proceed at room temperature for 4 h.

4 Use TLC on silica gel GF (chloroform/methanol/water, 75:36:6) to confirm the formation of the product (new UV absorbing spot at $R_f = 0.57$), and the disappearance of amino-PEG-DSPE ($R_f = 0.76$) from the reaction mixture (using ninhydrin spray).

5 Remove pyridine by rotary evaporation.

6 Add 50 ml water to the solution, and centrifuge to remove trace of insolubles.

7 Dialyse the supernatant in Spectra/Por CE (Spectrum, Houston, TX) tubing (MWCO 300 000) against saline (50 mM, 2 × 2000 ml) and water (3 × 2000 ml).

8 Confirm that the dialysate contains only the product (single spot by TLC) and then lyophilize the aqueous solution.

9 Dry the residue in vacuum over P_2O_5. Yield: 400 mg, (90%).

10 Confirm the FA content by quantitative UV spectrophotometry of the conjugates in methanol (0.05 mg/ml) using FA extinction coefficient $\varepsilon = 27\,500$ M^{-1} cm^{-1} at $\lambda_{max} = 285$ nm. FA content: 0.29 mmol/g (94% of theoretical value, 0.31 mmol/g) for FA-PEG2000-DSPE; 0.21 mmol/g (97% of theoretical value, 0.22 mmol/g) for FA-PEG3350-DSPE.

11 Confirm the identity of FA-PEG-DSPE by ^{1}H-NMR (DMSO-D6/CF$_3$CO$_2$D, ~10/1 v/v): d 0.84 (t, CH$_3$, 6H); 1.22 (s, CH$_2$, 56H); 1.49 (m, CH$_2$CH$_2$CO, 4H); 2.1–2.3 (overlapping 2 × t, CH$_2$CH$_2$CO & m, CH$_2$ of Glu, 8H); 3.2 (m, CH$_2$CH$_2$N, 4H); 3.50 (s, PEG, ~180H and ~300H for derivatives of PEG2000, and -3350 respectively); 4.02 (t, CH$_2$OCONH, 2H); 4.1 (dd, trans-PO$_4$CH$_2$CH, 1H); 4.3 (dd, cis-PO$_4$CH$_2$CH, 1H); 4.37 (m, α-CH, 1H); 4.60 (d, 9-CH$_2$-N, 2H); 5.15 (m, PO$_4$CH$_2$CH, 1H); 6.65 (d, 3',5'-H, 2H); 7.65 (d, 2',6'-H, 2H); 8.77 (s, C7-H, 1H) ppm.

12 Confirm the molecular weight of the FA-PEG-DSPE conjugates by MALDI. The spectra should exhibit bell-shaped distribution of 44 Da spaced lines centred at 3284 Da for FA-PEG2000-DSPE (theoretical value 3200 Da), and 4501 Da for FA-PEG3350-DSPE (theoretical value 4540 Da).

Protocol 20

Preparation of biotin-PEG-DSPE (48)

Equipment and reagents

- TLC equipment
- Silica gel column
- Chloroform/methanol/water

- Succinimidyl ester of biotin, DMF
- Amino-PEG$_{2K}$-DSPE
- *tert*-butanol, triethylamine

Method

1 Dissolve succinimidyl ester of biotin (41.31 mg, 0.121 mmol) in 300 ml DMF.

Protocol 20 continued

2 Dissolve amino-PEG$_{2K}$-DSPE (300 mg, 0.11 mmol, Ref. No. 18) in 1.7 ml chloroform.

3 While stirring, add the first solution to the second and then add triethylamine (46 ml, 0.33 mmol).

4 After 20 min confirm the completion of the coupling by TLC (chloroform/methanol/water, 90:18:2, ninhydrin).

5 Filter the reaction mixture and load it onto a silica gel column.

6 Elute the column with a stepwise gradient of methanol (0–14% in chloroform).

7 Pool and evaporate the product-containing fractions ($R_f = 0.51$).

8 Dissolve the residue in *tert*-butanol and lyophilize to obtain white powder (196 mg, 60% yield).

9 Confirm the structure of the product by ^{1}H-NMR (CD$_3$OD): d 0.88 (t, CH$_3$ 6H); 1.26 (s, CH$_2$, 56H); 1.45 (m, CH$_2$ biotin, 2H); 1.58 (broad m, CH$_2$CH$_2$C=O, 4H of each lipid and biotin); 2.22 (t, CH$_2$C=O, biot 2H); 2.31 (2 × t, CH$_2$C=O, 4H); 2.71 & 2.93 (d & dd, SCH$_2$ of biotin, 2H); 3.20 (m, SCH biotin & CH$_2$NH of PEG, 3H); 3.53 (t, CH$_2$NH of PE, 2H); 3.64 (s, PEG, ~180H); 3.88 & 3.98 (q & t, CH$_2$PO$_4$CH$_2$, 4H); 4.17 & 4.39 (2 × dd, OCH$_2$CHCH$_2$OP, 2H); 4.20 (t, CH$_2$O$_2$CN, 2H); 4.3 & 4.5 (2 × dd, CHNHCONHCH, 2H); 5.2 (m, PO$_4$CH$_2$CHCH$_2$OP, 1H) ppm.

10 Confirm the identity of the product by MALDI-TOFMS (bell-shaped distribution of ions spaced at equal 44 Da intervals and centred at 3082 Da; theoretical value, 2986 Da).

Protocol 21

Preparation of ligand-bearing liposomes (PHPC/cholesterol/mPEG-DSPE/ligand-PEG-DSPE, at a molar ratio of 55:40:3:2) by lipid mixing the liganded lipopolymers followed by hydration and extrusion (53)

Equipment and reagents

- 0.2, 0.1, and 0.05 μm pore size polycarbonate membranes
- Reverse-phase HPLC equipped with a UV detector
- Symmetry C-8 column (1 ml, Waters Associates, Milford, MA)
- Prodigy C8 column (Phenomenex, Torrance, CA)
- Lipids, cholesterol
- Chloroform
- Sodium phosphate buffer or HEPES buffer
- Methanol, ammonium phosphate, TFA

Method

1 Dissolve all lipids and cholesterol in chloroform and/or methanol in a round-bottom flask.

Protocol 21 continued

2 Remove the solvent(s) by rotary evaporation to produce a dried lipid film.

3 Hydrate the film with either sodium phosphate buffer (10 mM, 140 mM NaCl pH 7) or HEPES buffer (25 mM, 150 mM NaCl pH 7) to produce large multilamellar vesicles.

4 Pass the resulting vesicles suspension through 0.2, 0.1, and 0.05 μm pore size polycarbonate membranes repeatedly, under pressure, until the average size distribution (monitored by dynamic light scattering) reaches approx. 100 nm in diameter. (The mean particle diameter measured from 12 batches ranged from 92 nm to 111 nm with an average of 98 nm.)

5 Determine the content of ligand-lipopolymers (SLX-PEG-DSPE or DSPE-PEG-YIGSR-NH_2) in liposomes using a reverse-phase HPLC equipped with a UV detector, monitoring $\lambda = 272$ nm. For SLX-PEG-DSPE liposomes, use a Symmetry C-8 column, 1 ml, mobile phase of 92% aqueous methanol containing 20 mM ammonium phosphate, pH 7.0. For DSPE-PEG-YIGSR-NH_2 liposomes, use a Prodigy C8 column with 92% aqueous methanol, containing 0.1% TFA.

6 Determine the peptide content of the YIGSR liposomes by amino acid analysis: Tyr 0.97, Ile 1.00, Gly 0.98, Ser 0.96, Arg 1.08. (The peptide content in 2 mole% formulations calculated from phosphate and amino acid analysis was in the range of 28–32 mmol/mole phospholipid, which was in accord with the ligand contents determined by HPLC.)

Protocol 22

Insertion of ligand-PEG-DSPE into preformed liposomes (46)

Equipment and reagents

- HPLC equipment
- Biogel A50M column
- Sepharose 4B column
- PC/cholesterol unilamellar liposomes

- Ligand-PEG-DSPE
- Sodium phosphate, sodium chloride, NaN_3
- Sucrose, HEPES

Method

1 Prepare unilamellar liposomes (PC/cholesterol) containing 3 mole% mPEG-DSPE and no ligand conjugates.

2 Incubate the liposomes with the ligand-PEG-DSPE conjugate at ambient temperature or 37 °C for up to 48 h with amounts corresponding to 1.2 mole% of SLX-PEG-DSPE or DSPE-PEG-YIGSR-NH_2 (equal to 60% of 2 mole% in the original formulations that had ligands on both sides of lipid bilayer).

3   To confirm the incorporation of ligand-bearing lipopolymers into the liposomes at various time points, separate free ligand conjugates (micelles) from inserted ligands (liposomes) by size exclusion chromatography (SEC). For SLX-liposomes, use Biogel A50M column equilibrated with 10 mM sodium phosphate, 140 mM sodium chloride, 0.02% NaN_3 pH 6.5. For YIGSR-containing liposomes, use Sepharose 4B column with 10% sucrose, 10 mM HEPES pH 7.0 as the eluent. Collect the fractions and analyse them by HPLC to determine the content of the conjugates.

4 Detachable PEG on the liposome surface

The stability of PEGylated liposomes may not always be favourable for drug delivery. In particular, if drug-containing sterically protected liposomes accumulate inside the tumour, they may not necessarily release the drug to kill the tumour cells. Likewise, if the liposome is taken up by a cell via an endocytic pathway, the presence of the PEG coat on the liposome surface may prevent the liposome contents from escaping the endosome and being delivered in the cytoplasm. To solve these problems, chemistry has been devised to detach PEG from the lipid anchor under appropriate conditions. Labile linkages that degrade only in the acidic conditions characteristic of the endocytic vacuole or the acidotic tumour mass are well known from controlled drug release technologies. Such linkages can be based, for example, on the diorto ester acid-labile chemistry (59), or on vinyl ester chemistry (60). The latter reference describes preparation of an acidic medium-cleavable PEG-lipid. Cysteine-cleavable lipopolymers were also described in ref. 61. When the PEG brush is cleaved from the liposome surface, and especially when the liposomal membrane contains phosphatidylethanolamine, the membrane destabilization should occur, and the liposome contents would be delivered to the target (for example, by escaping from the primary endosome into the cell cytoplasm).

Protocol 23

Preparation of pH-sensitive liposomes with a detachable PEG coating (51)

Equipment and reagents

- Silica column
- 0.2 μm Nuclepore filters fitted in a hand-held extruder (Avestin, Canada)
- Sephadex G-75 size exclusion chromatography
- Monomethyl ester of PEG2000

- Distearoyl glycerol
- Molten 3,9-diethylidene-2,4,8,10-tetraoxaspiro[5,5]undecane
- Anhydrous tetrahydrofuran
- p-Toluenesulfonic acid
- Triethylamine, methanol, chloroform

Protocol 23 continued

A. Synthesis and purification of the pH-sensitive lipid-PEG derivative, 3,9-diethyl-3-(2,3-distearoyloxypropyloxy)-9-[methoxypoly(ethylene glycol)2000-1-yl]-2,4,8,10-tetraoxaspiro[5,5]undecane (POD)

1 Dissolve 0.5 mmol monomethyl ester of PEG2000, 0.5 mmol distearoyl glycerol, and 0.5 mmol molten 3,9-diethylidene-2,4,8,10-tetraoxaspiro[5,5]undecane in 5 ml of anhydrous tetrahydrofuran under argon. Avoid contact of the reagents with air.

2 Initiate the reaction by adding *p*-toluenesulfonic acid (0.04 ml, 0.6 mg/ml) and incubate for 2 h at 40 °C.

3 Stop the reaction by adding of 0.2 ml triethylamine (TEA).

4 Place the reaction mixture in 150 ml of 1% triethylamine in methanol, add 4 g of silica gel, and evaporate the solvents under reduced pressure.

5 Pour the dry residue onto a silica column (45 g) pre-equilibrated with 2% TEA in $CHCl_3$, and elute with the same solvent. After the chromatography is completed and pooled product peak has been isolated by solvent evaporation, the yield of the POD product should be around 20%.

B. Preparation and purification of pH-sensitive liposomes by combined reverse-phase evaporation and Nuclepore filtration technique

1 Prepare the liposomes by standard REV technique from a mixture of 9:1 DOPE and POD lipid-PEG using an aqueous buffer solution containing 5 mM HEPES pH 8.5.

2 Filter the prepared liposomes five times through a stack of two 0.2 µm Nuclepore filters fitted in a hand-held extruder to achieve a narrow size distribution (180–200 nm).

3 Remove the non-entrapped solutes by Sephadex G-75 size exclusion chromatography, eluting with 5 mM HEPES-saline pH 8.5. At pH 8.5, the resulting liposomes are stable for two weeks at 4 °C without significant content leakage.

5 Biological factors responsible for the clearance of PEGylated liposomes

It is worth noting that even long-circulating liposomes are eventually eliminated from the blood. The clearance rate of PEGylated liposomes from the bloodstream appears to be dependent on the attachment of serum proteins to the liposome surface, thus marking these particles for removal by phagocytic cells. The barrier properties of the polymer brush were suggested more than a decade ago: avidin attachment to the biotinylated liposome surface was inhibited by increasing concentration of PEG-PE (26). This inhibition of protein penetration to liposomal membrane through PEG brush seems to be kinetic in nature (18). Several proteins, mostly complement components, were implicated in the binding and opsonization of PEGylated liposomes. A recent detailed review of the interaction of polymer brushes with proteins can be found in ref. 62.

Even more complicated events may take place during liposome administration *in vivo*. Apparently, when a second dose of PEGylated liposomes is administered several days after the initial dose, a rapid removal of PEGylated liposomes from the bloodstream takes place (63). This removal is dependent on a heat-labile serum protein factor that may be connected with its release from macrophage-like cells. Further characterization of this opsonization material and its mode of action may be needed to design particulate agents with a truly extended circulation life-span of weeks and months.

When PEGylated liposomes with the targeting antibodies (IgG) attached to the surface (in particular, to the outer tip of the PEG chains) were injected in the experimental animals for extended periods and in multiple doses, the circulation time of liposomes decreased considerably. In this case, it was attributed to the development of an anti-IgG immune response (55). Luckily, the immune response was directed at the constant region of the antibody on the liposome. When smaller targeting ligands were used (e.g. scFv fragments), an immune response did not seem to develop, and scFv-coated liposomes circulated freely after multiple injections (38).

Liposome composition can also affect the liposome clearance rate even after steric protection (PEGylation). For example, the addition of several per cent of phosphatidylserine overcame the protective effect of the PEG brush on the liposome surface, and PS-containing PEG-liposomes rapidly accumulate in the liver and spleen (26). On the other hand, the addition of a hydrophobic prodrug derivatives to the liposome membrane did not seem to reduce the circulation time of liposomes in the bloodstream; in two of three prodrugs, targeting by the liposomes was not affected by prodrug presence (64, 65). However, being long-circulation with a particular prodrug or molecule, liposomes still may manifest rapid clearance from the bloodstream with another molecule or in another animal species. *In vivo* testing should be performed in all the cases, and liposome composition may have to be altered to ensure extended circulation time for liposomes containing additional components.

References

1. Senior, J. H. (1987). *CRC Crit. Rev. Ther. Drug Carrier Syst.*, **3**, 123.

2. Hojo, H., Hoshino, Y., Kurita, T., and Hashimoto, Y. (1985). *Res. Commun. Chem. Pathol. Pharmacol.*, **47**, 373.

3. Patel, K. R., Li, M. P., and Baldeschwieler, J. D. (1983). *Proc. Natl. Acad. Sci. USA*, **80**, 6518.

4. Senior, J., Crawley, J. C., and Gregoriadis, G. (1985). *Biochim. Biophys. Acta*, **839**, 1.

5. Torchilin, V. P., Khaw, B. A., Berdichevskiy, V. R., Klibanov, A. L., Haber, E., and Smirnov, V. N. (1983). *Bull. Exp. Biol. Med. (Russ.)*, **95**, 51.

6. Allen, T. M. and Chonn, A. (1987). *FEBS Lett.*, **223**, 42.

7. Gabizon, A. and Papahadjopoulos, D. (1988). *Proc. Natl. Acad. Sci. USA*, **85**, 6949.

8. Park, Y. S., Maruyama, K., and Huang, L. (1992). *Biochim. Biophys. Acta*, **1108**, 257.

9. Lasic, D. and Martin, F. (ed.) (1995). *Stealth liposomes*. CRC Press, Boca Raton.

10. Mumtaz, S., Ghosh, P. C., and Bachhawat, B. K. (1991). *Glycobiology*, **1**, 505.

11. Illum, L., Davis, S. S., Muller, R. H., Mak, E., and West, P. (1987). *Life Sci.*, **40**, 367.

12. Klibanov, A. L., Maruyama, K., Torchilin, V. P., and Huang, L. (1990). *FEBS Lett.*, **268**, 235.

13. Senior, J., Delgado, C., Fisher, D., Tilcock, C., and Gregoriadis, G. (1991). *Biochim. Biophys. Acta*, **1062**, 77.

14. Allen, T. M., Hansen, C., Martin, F., Redemann, C., and Young, Y. A. (1991). *Biochim. Biophys. Acta*, **1066**, 29.

15. Papahadjopoulos, D., Allen, T. M., Gabizon, A., Mayhew, E., Matthay, K., Huang, S. K., *et al.* (1991). *Proc. Natl. Acad. Sci. USA*, **88**, 11460.

16. Gabizon, A. and Papahadjopoulos, D. (1992). *Biochim. Biophys. Acta*, **1103**, 94.

17. Needham, D., McIntosh, T. J., and Lasic, D. D. (1992). *Biochim. Biophys. Acta*, **1108**, 40.

18. Torchilin, V. P., Omelyanenko, V. G., Papisov, M. A., Bogdanov, Jr. A. A., Trubetskoy, V. S., Herron, J. N., *et al.* (1994). *Biochim. Biophys. Acta*, **1195**, 11.

19. Lasic, D. D., Martin, F. G., Gabizon, A., Huang, S. K., and Papahadjopoulos, D. (1991). *Biochim. Biophys. Acta*, **1070**, 187.

20. Torchilin, V. P., Shtilman, M. I., Trubetskoy, V. S., Whiteman, K., and Milstein, A. (1994). *Biochim. Biophys. Acta*, **1195**, 181.

21. Torchilin, V. P., Trubetskoy, V. S., Whiteman, K. R., Caliceti, P., Ferruti, P., and Veronese, F. M. (1995). *J. Pharm. Sci.*, **84**, 1049.

22. Zalipsky, S., Hansen, C. B., Oaks, J. M., and Allen, T. M. (1996). *J. Pharm. Sci.*, **85**, 137.

23. Maruyama, K., Okuizumi, S., Ishids, O., Yamauchi, H., Kikuchi, H., and Iwatsuru, M. (1994). *Int. J. Pharm.*, **111**, 103.

24. Yoshioka, H. (1991). *Biomaterials*, **12**, 861.

25. Suzuki, S., Watanabe, S., Masuko, T., and Hashimoto, Y. (1995). *Biochim. Biophys. Acta*, **1245**, 9.

26. Klibanov, A. L., Maruyama, K., Beckerleg, A. M., Torchilin, V. P., and Huang, L. (1991). *Biochim. Biophys. Acta*, **1062**, 142.

27. Liu, D., Mori, A., and Huang, L. (1991). *Biochim. Biophys. Acta*, **1066**, 159.

28. Litzinger, D. C., Buiting, A. M. J., Vanrooijen, N., and Huang, L. (1994). *Biochim. Biophys. Acta*, **1190**, 99.

29. Trubetskoy, V. S., Whiteman, K. R., Torchilin, V. P., and Wolf, G. L. (1998). *J. Contr. Rel.*, **50**, 13.

30. Trubetskoy, V. S., Frank-Kamenetsky, M. D., Whiteman, K. R., Wolf, G. L., and Torchilin, V. P. (1996). *Acad. Radiol.*, **3**, 232.

31. Phillips, W. T., Andrews, T., Liu, H., Klipper, R., Landry, A. J., Blumhardt, R., *et al.* (2001). *Nucl. Med. Biol.*, **28**, 435.

32. Wu, N. Z., Da, D., Rudoll, T. L., Needham, D., Whorton, A. R., and Dewhirst, M. W. (1993). *Cancer Res.*, **53**, 3765.

33. Hobbs, S. K., Monsky, W. L., Yuan, F., Roberts, W. G., Griffith, L., Torchilin, V. P., *et al.* (1998). *Proc. Natl. Acad. Sci. USA*, **95**, 4607.

34. Park, J. W., Hong, K., Kirpotin, D. B., Meyer, O., Papahajopoulos, D., and Benz, C. C. (1997). *Cancer Lett.*, **118**, 153.

35. Torchilin, V. P., Klibanov, A. L., Huang, L., O'Donnell, S., Nossiff, N. D., and Khaw, B. A. (1992). *FASEB J.*, **6**, 2716.

36. Torchilin, V. P., Narula, J., Halpern, J., and Khaw, B. A. (1996). *Biochim. Biophys. Acta*, **1279**, 75.

37. Klibanov, A. L. (1998). In *Long-circulating liposomes: long drugs, new therapeutics* (ed. M. C. Woodle and G. Storm), pp. 269–86. Springer–Verlag, Berlin.

38. Park, J. W., Kirpotin, D. B., Hong, K., Shalaby, R., Shao, R., Nielsen, U. B., *et al.* (2001). *J. Contr. Rel.*, **74**, 95.

39. Harding, J. A., Engbers, C. M., Newman, M. S., Goldstein, N. I., and Zalipsky, S. (1997). *Biochim. Biophys. Acta*, **1327**, 181.

40. Hansen, C. B., Kao, G. Y., Moase, E. H., Zalipsky, S., and Allen, T. M. (1995). *Biochim. Biophys. Acta*, **1239**, 133.

41. Zalipsky, S., Hansen, C. B., Lopes de Menezes, D., and Allen, T. M. (1996). *J. Contr. Rel.*, **39**, 153.

42. Zalipsky, S. (1995). *Adv. Drug Deliv. Rev.*, **16**, 157.

43. Zalipsky, S., Gittelman, J., Mullah, N., Qazen, M. M., and Harding, J. (1998). *Targeting of drugs 6: Strategies for stealth therapeutic systems* (ed. G. Gregoriadis), pp. 131–8. Plenum, NY.

44. Torchilin, V. P., Levchenko, T. S., Lukyanov, A. N., Khaw, B. A., Klibanov, A. L., Rammohan, R., *et al.* (2001). *Biochim. Biophys. Acta*, **1511**, 397.

45. Blume, G., Cevc, G., Crommelin, M. D. J. A., Baker-Woundenberg, I. A. J. M., Kluft, C., and Storm, G. (1993). *Biochim. Biophys. Acta*, **1149**, 180.

46. Zalipsky, S., Mullah, N., Harding, J. A., Gittelman, J., Guo, L., and DeFrees, S. A. (1997). *Bioconj. Chem.*, **8**, 111.

47. Kirpotin, D., Park, J. W., Hong, K., Zalipsky, S., Li, W.-L., Carter, P., *et al.* (1997). *Biochemistry*, **36**, 66.

48. Wong, J., Kuhl, T. L., Israelachvili, J. N., Mullah, N., and Zalipsky, S. (1997). *Science*, **275**, 820.

49. Gabizon, A., Horowitz, A. T., Goren, D., Tzemach, D., Mandelbaum-Shavit, F., Qazen, M. M., *et al.* (1999). *Bioconj. Chem.*, **10**, 289.

50. DeFrees, S. A., Phillips, L., Guo, L., and Zalipsky, S. (1996). *J. Am. Chem. Soc.*, **118**, 6104.

51. Zalipsky, S., Mullah, N., Dibble, A., and Flaherty, T. (1999). *Chem. Commun.*, 653.

52. Zalipsky, S. (1993). *Bioconj. Chem.*, **4**, 296.

53. Zalipsky, S., Brandeis, E., Newman, M. S., and Woodle, M. C. (1994). *FEBS Lett.*, **353**, 71.

54. Zalipsky, S., Puntambekar, B., Boulikas, P., Engbers, C., and Woodle, M. C. (1995). *Bioconj. Chem.*, **6**, 705.

55. Harding, J. A., Engbers, C. M., Newman, M. S., Goldstein, N. I., and Zalipsky, S. (1997). *Biochim. Biophys. Acta*, **1327**, 181.

56. Allen, T. M., Brandies, E., Hansen, C. B., Kao, G. Y., and Zalipsky, S. (1995). *Biochim. Biophys. Acta*, **1237**, 99.

57. Maruyama, K., Takizawa, T., Yuda, T., Kennel, S. J., Huang, L., and Iwatsuru, M. (1995). *Biochim. Biophys. Acta*, **1234**, 74.

58. Torchilin, V. P., Rammohan, R., Weissig, V., and Levchenko, T. S. (2001). *Proc. Natl. Acad. Sci. USA*, **98**, 8786.

59. Guo, X. and Szoka, Jr. F. C. (2001). *Bioconj. Chem.*, **12**, 29.

60. Boomer, J. A. and Thompson, D. H. (1999). *Chem. Phys. Lipids*, **99**, 145.

61. Zalipsky, S., Qazen, M., Walker, J. A. 2nd, Mullah, N., Quinn, Y. P., and Huang, S. K. (1999). *Bioconj. Chem.*, **10**, 703.

62. Moghimi, S. M., Hunter, C. M., and Murray, J. C. (2001). *Pharmacol. Rev.*, **53**, 283.

63. Dams, E. T., Laverman, P., Oyen, W. J., Storm, G., Scherphof, G. L., van Der Meer, J. W., *et al.* (2000). *J. Pharmacol. Exp. Ther.*, **292**, 1071.

64. Mori, A., Kennel, S. J., and Huang, L. (1993). *Pharm. Res.*, **10**, 507.

65. Mori, A., Kennel, S. J., van Borssum Waalkes, M., Scherphof, G. L., and Huang, L. (1995). *Cancer Chemother. Pharmacol.*, **35**, 447.

66. Shiahinian, S. and Silvius, J. R. (1995). *Biochim. Biophys. Acta*, **1239**, 157.

Chapter 9
Liposomes in biological systems

Jan A. A. M. Kamps and Gerrit L. Scherphof

Department of Cell Biology, Section Liposome Research, Groningen University Institute for Drug Exploration (GUIDE), Antonius Deusinglaan 1, 9713 AV Groningen, The Netherlands.

1 Introduction

The interaction of liposomes with biological systems is very complex but has bearing on most topics in liposomal drug delivery. In this chapter we will describe the various interactions occurring in biological systems and the factors that determine these interactions. Biological systems in liposome research include relatively simple cell culture set-ups, organ perfusion systems, and the intact organism. Although we will touch on these different systems, emphasis will be on liposome–cell interaction and whole body distribution of liposomes, including the means to determine the interaction processes involved. The first part of this chapter deals with *in vitro* liposome–cell interactions. The different kinds of interaction that can occur at the level of liposome–cell contact will be discussed, including practical methods to distinguish them. The consequences of these interactions for the different liposomal components, i.e. bilayer lipids and the liposomal contents, and various options to analyse these will be reviewed. Most of the above aspects will also be dealt with in the second section of this contribution, which covers biodistribution of liposomes in animal models. Considerable attention will be given to the role of the liver as the main site of uptake from the blood and to the contribution of the different liver cell types to the *in vivo* uptake of liposomes. The experimental protocols given are a selection of protocols available in this research area but they are all practical and generally do not require exceptional laboratory equipment.

2 Interaction of liposomes with cells

2.1 Possible liposome–cell interaction: adsorption, (receptor-mediated) endocytosis, lipid exchange, fusion

We can distinguish four mechanisms of liposome–cell interaction by which liposomes can deliver their contents to cells (1–3) (Figure 1). The occurrence of any one of these interactions largely depends on liposome characteristics such as composition, size, charge, and the presence of homing or targeting devices.

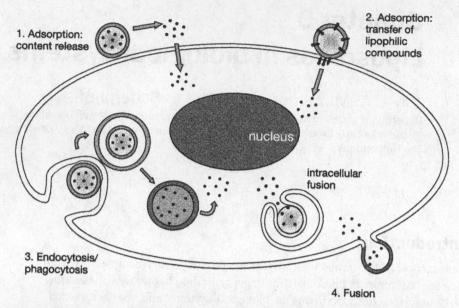

Figure 1 Possible ways by which liposomes can interact with cells and deliver their contents. 1. Adsorption of the liposome followed by extracellular release of the liposome contents and subsequent active or passive transport of these contents into the cell. 2. Adsorption of the liposome followed by selective transfer of lipophilic compounds from the liposomal bilayer to the plasma membrane. 3. Endocytotic internalization of the liposomes followed by intracellular degradation of the liposome via the endolysosomal pathway and subsequent intracellular release of the liposome contents. 4. Fusion of the liposmal membrane with the plasma membrane or, intracellular with the endosomal membrane, thereby releasing the liposomal contents in the cytoplasm.

Other major determinants for the type of mechanism involved in liposome–cell interaction are the type of cell and environmental factors such as the presence of blood or serum.

In vivo, tissue macrophages of liver and spleen but also hepatocytes have been recognized to be heavily involved in the uptake of plain non-targeted liposomes from the blood (4, 5). Interaction of liposomes with these cells, often receptor-mediated, generally leads to endocytosis or phagocytosis of the particles. Upon binding the liposomes are endocytosed by invagination of the cell membrane into endosomal compartments. These endosomes fuse with lysosomes, followed by lysosomal digestion of the endosomal contents and subsequent release of the liposomal contents into the cell. The liposomal phospholipids are hydrolysed to fatty acids in this process, which can be either released from the cell or be recycled and reincorporated into cellular phospholipids. In the endolysosomal system pH varies from 5–5.5 in the endosomes to approximately 4.5 in the lysosomes. These low pH values can be utilized to follow the fate of liposomes and/or liposomal content by means of pH-sensitive fluorescent markers (6). One can also take advantage of the low pH in the endosomes by applying liposomes which in a low pH environment (< pH 6) destabilize possibly followed by mixing of the liposomal lipids with the endosomal membrane, thereby releasing part of the liposomal contents into the cytoplasm of the cells before lysosomal digestion has occurred (7).

Liposome binding or adsorption to cells without uptake of the intact liposome has been described for both targeted and non-targeted liposomes. This type of liposome–cell interaction may lead to two ways of contact-mediated transfer of liposome content. Lipophilic material, e.g. (pro)drugs or certain lipid markers, may be selectively transferred from the liposomal membrane to the cell membrane. Encapsulated water soluble liposome contents can be released under certain circumstances upon adsorption of the liposomes to the cell membrane. Although both these processes are not completely understood, it has become clear that the composition of the liposomal membrane and/or the physico-chemical structure of the exchanged compounds are of major importance (8–10).

Fusion of liposomes with cells involves complete mixing of the liposomal membrane with the cell membrane, thereby releasing the liposomal content into the cytoplasm of the cell. Today it is generally believed that such a process requires specific fusion-inducing agents like fusion proteins or peptides, analogous to viruses. There is no evidence that fusion occurs at the cell membrane with plain liposomes. However, since cytoplasmatic delivery of compounds like DNA or antisense oligonucleotides is highly desired, studies are in progress in which specific fusogenic properties of viruses are combined with liposomes leading to the formation of so called virosomes (11).

2.2 Markers

To investigate liposome–cell interaction a large variety of liposomal markers is available. Since the use of water soluble markers has been extensively dealt with in the contribution of Zuidam *et al.* (Chapter 2), in this section we will give emphasis mainly to lipid markers which allow tracking of the liposome or its components during cell interaction.

When facilities for working with radioactive compounds are available, radio-labels provide a sensitive and a powerful tool to determine liposome–cell inter-action. Most lipids can be purchased in one or more radiolabelled forms. The choice of the radiolabel primarily depends on the aim of the experiment. Radio-active lipid labels can easily be incorporated into the liposomal bilayer when added with the other lipids during liposome preparation, using any method. For determination of the association of liposomes with cells it is important that the marker is stably incorporated in the liposomal bilayer to avoid transfer of the marker from the liposomal membrane to cellular membranes such as the plasma membrane or the endosomal membrane. In addition to stability requirements, the radioactive marker also has to be metabolically inert for the time of the experiment, in order to avoid erroneous interpretations of experimental data. Examples of radioactive markers that fulfil these characteristics are [³H]cholesteryl-hexadecyl ether or [³H]cholesteryloleyl ether, where the ether bond ascertains that the marker is not metabolized by cells. When liposomes are double labelled with a [³H]cholesteryl ether and a radioactive marker such as cholesteryl[¹⁴C]-oleate which is readily hydrolysed in the lysosomes, it is possible to make an estimation of the degradation of liposomes. Due to rapid release from the cells of [¹⁴C]oleate derived from the degraded cholesteryl[¹⁴C]oleate and the complete retention of the metabolically inert [³H]cholesteryl ether the ³H/¹⁴C ratio is a sensitive measure for intracellular degradation (12). It has to be taken in account that the ³H/¹⁴C ratio is also dependent on the presence of a fatty acid acceptor in the extracellular milieu such as albumin and of the nature of the cells used in the experiments. Specialized cells involved in lipid metabolism may not release [¹⁴C]oleate to appreciable extents but, as in the case of hepatocytes, further metabolize it to CO_2 or use it for the production of lipoproteins.

There are also several fluorescent lipid labels on the market, which have been shown to be valuable tools for studying liposome–cell interaction. Fluorescence techniques in liposome research are discussed in Chapter 4.

In addition to labelling of the liposome itself, there are a variety of possibilities to label liposome-associated compounds such as encapsulated material and homing devices. The usefulness of such labels as marker for the fate of liposomes will largely depend on the specifications of the labelled compound and the nature of the label itself. To ensure that a liposomal marker is not processed by the cells differently from other liposomal components or the encapsulated material, double-labelled liposomes may provide an appropriate approach (see also Section 3.3). For morphological studies on the intracellular fate of liposomes and/or their components, fluorescent markers, in combination with conventional fluorescence microscopy or confocal laser scanning microscopy, have been shown to be powerful tools at the light microscopic level (6, 13, 14). For studies at the electron microscopic level liposome encapsulated colloidal gold or the reaction products of liposome encapsulated horseradish peroxidase have been proven to be convenient markers (8, 15–17).

2.3 Cell lines and primary cell cultures

Cell lines form a valuable tool for studying the interaction of liposomes with cells. However interpretation and extrapolation towards more 'natural' and complex systems should be handled with much care, since cell lines often have a life cycle and a cellular make-up different from those of target cells *in situ*. A major advantage of cell lines is their continuous availability and the possibility to control the conditions within an experiment. The latter also applies to primary cells in culture but here availability and/or complicated isolation and culture procedures may form a drawback. Cultured cells allow detailed studies of factors influencing liposome–cell interaction such as the effect of blood or blood components (serum, plasma, and proteins) or the cellular characteristics such as specific receptors. Another important feature of experimentation with cultured cells is that all subsequent events, from binding and uptake to processing of the liposome and its encapsulated material, can be followed without interference by other biological systems (e.g. other cells or organs) in these processes. In the next section the events occurring in liposome–cell interaction will be discussed in more detail, while also some attention will be paid to the isolation and culturing of liver cells involved in liposome uptake. Extrapolation of data obtained in *in vitro* experiments to the *in vivo* situation will be discussed.

2.3.1 Binding, uptake, and processing of liposome components and liposome contents

The first event in liposome–cell interaction *in vitro* is adsorption or binding to the cell membrane. The nature of this interaction will depend on the liposome composition, the experimental conditions, and the cell type (4). Although not many interaction sites for plain liposomes on cells have been identified or characterized thoroughly it seems clear that these interaction sites have a proteinaceous character (18, 19). Studies with uncharged, neutral liposomes and with negatively charged, phosphatidylserine- or phosphatidylglycerol-containing liposomes have shown that different cell lines have different mechanisms by which they interact with liposomes, and that the binding sites for neutral and negatively charged liposomes are not identical (20–22). Experimental conditions will influence binding dramatically; the presence of serum during liposome–cell interaction may lead, depending on the origin of the serum and the cell type, to a substantial decrease in liposome binding (21, 23) (see also Section 3.2). Also effects of divalent cations have been described for liposome–cell interactions (19).

Protocol 1

Liposome binding and uptake by cultured cells

Reagents

- [³H]cholesteryloleyl ether labelled liposomes
- Appropriate serum-free culture medium (depending on cell type and aim of experiment)

- Phosphate-buffered saline (PBS): 10 mM phosphate buffer pH 7.4, 150 mM NaCl
- 0.1 M NaOH

Method

1 Replace the culture medium by serum-free medium and incubate the cells for 1 h at 37 °C in a humidified 5% CO_2/95% air atmosphere.

2 Remove the serum-free medium and add new medium containing appropriate amounts of [³H]cholesteryloleyl ether labelled liposomes and if necessary other additions.

3 Incubate cells for 3 h at 37 °C in a humidified 5% CO_2/95% air atmosphere to determine cell association (binding and uptake) or for 3 h at 4 °C to determine exclusively cell binding.

Protocol 1 continued

4　After the incubation the culture plates are placed on ice and washed six times with ice-cold PBS.

5　The cells are lysed in 0.1 M NaOH for 1 h at 37 °C or overnight at –20 °C and subsequent thawing.

6　The cell-associated radioactivity is determined by liquid scintillation counting of aliquots of the lysed cell suspension and is normalized to the amount of cellular protein as determined according to Lowry (77) using bovine serum albumin as a standard.

The general procedure to determine binding and uptake as presented in Protocol 1, distinguishes between binding plus uptake and exclusive binding of liposomes by incubating the cells either at 37 °C or 4 °C. The difference between liposome association at 37 °C and association at 4 °C is a measure for internalization. However, one has to proceed here with caution since binding at 4 °C may not be representative of binding at 37 °C because of dynamic processes such as receptor recycling which do not occur at 4 °C. Differences between the association of liposomes to cells at 37 °C and 4 °C can also be accounted for by temperature effects on bilayer mobility which may, as was shown for immunoliposomes, affect the amount of liposomes bound to the cells, even in cases that there is no uptake of liposomes (8).

2.3.2 Transfection

Liposome-based or lipid-based gene delivery systems are among the most rapidly progressing fields in liposome research. Although *in vivo* applications of liposomal gene therapeutics are still hampered by relatively low transfection efficiencies, *in vitro* models to study development and efficacy of gene or oligodeoxynucleotide carriers are numerous (24–27). In addition to the methods to determine the interaction of the gene carriers and their contents, as described in Section 2.3.1, the use of plasmids or antisense oligodeoxynucleotides allow and/or require some additional techniques. Especially determination of efficacy of the liposome encapsulated gene material is of importance. For liposome-based gene carrier development, plasmids containing reporter genes for proteins such as (enhanced) green fluorescent protein (GFP), luciferase, or β-galactosidase, are very suitable. The gene products can be determined 6–72 h after incubation of cells with the liposomal gene carriers, either directly using fluorescence microscopy (GFP) or by reporter assays applying relatively simple enzymatic reactions (28).

Another application in which lipid-based gene delivery systems are widely used, are studies on specific gene function. For that purpose model cell lines are transfected with a certain gene followed by determining expression of the protein and its regulation. Especially for these applications several lipid-based transfectants are commercially available (Lipofectin®, Lipofectamine®, FuGENE™, Gene PORTER™, etc.).

2.4 Isolation and culturing of liver cells

A major prerequisite for cells, *in vivo*, to be involved in the elimination of liposomes from the blood is accessibility (see also Section 3.1). It is widely acknowledged that macrophages in liver and spleen and liver parenchymal cells (hepatocytes) are cells that fulfil this requirement, and that, as a matter of fact, these are the most important cell populations responsible for liposome uptake from the blood. Although (vascular) endothelial are also readily accessible for liposomes, so far substantial uptake of liposomes by endothelial cells has only been described for sinusoidal endothelial cells in the liver (29). These considerations imply that understanding the interaction of liposomes with the different cell populations in the liver is important for understanding the mechanisms of liposome elimination *in vivo*. This section focuses on the isolation and culturing of liver cells known to be involved in liposome uptake; the Kupffer cells or liver macrophages, the hepatocytes, and the liver endothelial cells (30–32). These cell types occupy 2.1%, 77.8%, and 2.8% of the liver volume, respectively.

Various methods have been described over the past decades for the isolation of the main liver cell types. It is beyond the scope of this chapter to discuss all these methods and their specific characteristics. We will confine ourselves to the isolation method and culturing method, which in our hands have been proven suitable for liposome research. The liver cell isolation in Protocol 2 describes the separation of the three major liver cell types from one liver using collagenase for digestion of the extracellular matrix. Liver cell isolation starts with digestion, mostly enzymatic, of the extracellular matrix of the liver. After digestion of the liver, cells are isolated based on their density and size by centrifugation, density centrifugation, and centrifugal elutriation. When only non-parenchymal liver cells such as endothelial and Kupffer cells are needed, digestion of the liver by pronase has also been shown to be a convenient isolation method (33). Enzymatic digestion by pronase is harsher on the cells than collagenase digestion and easily leads to non-viable parenchymal cells. This also makes the pronase method less suitable for liposome uptake experiments *in vitro*, since membrane proteins may be removed by the action of the pronase. In Figure 2 the isolation of liver cells after collagenase perfusion and after pronase perfusion are schematically depicted.

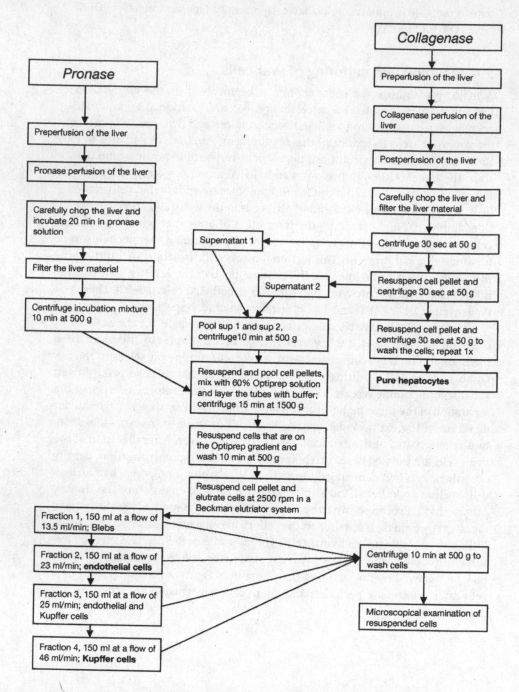

Figure 2 Schematic overview of liver cell isolation and purification. (*Left*) The main steps to isolate and purify liver endothelial cells and Kupffer cells after a pronase perfusion. (*Right*) Isolation and purification of hepatocytes, liver endothelial cells, and Kupffer cells after collagenase perfusion. For further details the reader is referred to Protocol 2.

Protocol 2

Isolation and purification of hepatocytes, Kupffer cells, and endothelial cells by collagenase perfusion

Equipment and reagents

- Peristaltic pump
- Temperature controlled water-bath
- Low speed temperature controlled centrifuge
- Elutriation system (Beckman, type JE-6 elutriation rotor)
- Rats (Wistar or Wag/Rij) (Harlan, The Netherlands)
- Collagenase type A (Boehringer Mannheim)
- Optiprep™ (60% iodixanol, w/v) (Axis-Shield PoC AS)

- Preperfusion buffer: 142 mM NaCl, 6.7 mM KCl, 10 mM N-2-hydroxyethylpiperazine-N'-2-ethanesulfonic acid (HEPES), pH 7.6
- Collagenase buffer: 66.7 mM NaCl, 6.7 mM KCl, 4.8 mM $CaCl_2 \cdot 2H_2O$, 10 mM HEPES pH 7.4
- Hanks' solution: 137 mM NaCl, 5.4 mM KCl, 0.8 mM $MgSO_4 \cdot 7H_2O$, 0.33 mM $Na_2HPO_4 \cdot 2H_2O$, 0.44 mM KH_2PO_4, 10 mM HEPES, 5 mM glucose pH 7.4

A. Buffer preparation

1. Preperfusion buffer. Oxygenate preperfusion buffer by carbogen bubbling for at least 20 min at 37 °C, adjust to pH 7.6 directly before use of the buffer.

2. Collagenase buffer. Oxygenate collagenase buffer by carbogen bubbling for at least 20 min at 37 °C, dissolve bovine serum albumin (BSA) in 10 ml of this buffer (2% BSA in final solution), add collagenase (0.05% collagenase in final solution), mix gently with rest of buffer to avoid air bubbles, and adjust to pH 7.4.

3. Postperfusion buffer. Oxygenate 0.1 litre of the Hanks' solution by carbogen bubbling for at least 20 min at 37 °C, dissolve BSA in 10 ml of this buffer (2% BSA in final solution), adjust to pH 7.4.

4. Dissolve BSA (0.3% BSA in final solution) in remainder of Hanks' solution and adjust to pH 7.4, keep at 4 °C.

B. Preparation of the animal for perfusion

1. Rinse perfusion system with 70% ethanol.

2. Rinse out the pump and tubing with H_2O. Fill the tubing with preperfusion buffer and set the peristaltic pump to deliver 20 ml/min.

3. Anaesthetize the animals with nembutal (50 mg/kg body weight) intraperitoneally 20 min before start of the surgery.

4. Shave the abdominal area. Place the anaesthetized animal on a heated operating surface (if available) or on a cork board.

Protocol 2 continued

5   Open the abdomen with a V-shaped cut out of the skin in the middle of the abdomen. Fold the abdominal flap up onto the chest wall. Scoop the gut to the right side of the animal and, if necessary, displace the lobes of the liver very gently upward to permit the identification of the portal vein. Never use forceps to handle the liver, and, in general, keep handling of the liver to a minimum. Make sure that undue pressure is not placed on the diaphragm as this will hinder breathing.

6   Using a 1 inch, 20 gauge hypodermic braunule, cannulate the portal vein by gently introducing the needle (needle No. 1) into and along the vein (pointing towards the liver). Make sure that the needle does not puncture the far side of the vessel. Tie the needle in place with 4–0 braided silk using two ligatures and again make sure that the ties are not so tight as to cut into the wall of the vein.

7   Ligate (two ties) the posterior vena cava below the liver at the level of the renal vein.

8   Restrain the animal by the limbs so that further movement does not disturb the needle.

9   Open the chest by cutting the rib cage up each side. Leave the diaphragm and the lowest ribs in place.

10 Identify the vena cava where it penetrates the diaphragm. Carefully insert another 16 gauge braunule into the vena cava between the heart and the diaphragm pointing away from the heart. Tie the braunule into place with a ligature of 410 cotton.

11 Ligate the vena cava (two ties) between the needle and the heart.

12 Connect the tubing of the peristaltic pump from the perfusion medium to needle No. 1. Take care not to disturb the needle from its position in the hepatic portal vein.

13 Connect needle No. 2 to the tubing, which in turn is connected to a reservoir for waste perfusate.

C. Liver perfusion

1   Perfuse the liver by allowing the peristaltic pump to pump 400 ml of preperfusion buffer at 20 ml/min. Maintain the temperature of the buffer at 37 °C. As the blood is displaced from the liver by the perfusate, the liver will become progressively paler (tan) in colour. Then increase the pump speed to 28 ml/min.

2   After 300–400 ml of preperfusion medium has passed, change tubing to collagenase buffer reservoir. Do not allow air bubbles into the liver (use bubble trap). Allow the collagenase buffer to recirculate for 10 min at a pump speed of 28 ml/min. Keep the surface of the liver moist with warm buffer. The pH of the perfusate may drop after passage through the liver because of the metabolic activity of the cells. When necessary readjust the pH of the perfusate with 0.1 M NaOH to pH 7.4.

3   Change tubing to postperfusion buffer and allow 100 ml to pass through the liver at a pump speed of 28 ml/min.

4 Remove the liver by cutting round the diaphragm and subsequently cutting the liver free from the remnants of diaphragm. At this stage the liver should have changed into a fragile soft bag of cells indicating a successful perfusion.

D. Preparation of parenchymal cells

1 Wash the perfused liver surface with a small amount of cold Hanks' solution containing 0.3% BSA. Carefully open the liver capsule and release the cell mixture.

2 Carefully filter the cells through a Nylon mesh (100 μm). Transfer the cells which pass through the mesh into 50 ml plastic centrifuge tubes and place them at 4 °C for 5–10 min so that the cells sediment by gravity or centrifuge for 45 sec at 50 g (without centrifuge brake). Cooling the cells too fast (e.g. directly on ice) leads to loss of cell viability in the parenchymal fraction. Note that calcium-free buffer must be used here, since calcium tends to cause macrophages to clump, and would lead to contamination of the sediment with non-parenchymal cells.

3 Remove and save the supernatant from the thick pellet of parenchymal cells. The supernatant should contain only a few parenchymal cells and be rich in non-parenchymal cells.

4 Wash the parenchymal cell pellet five times by centrifugation at 50 g (no brake) with Hanks' solution containing 0.3% BSA. Remove the supernatants and pool the first supernatant from step 4 with the supernatant from step 3 (see part E). Resuspend the cell pellet in 10 ml Hanks' solution or culture medium and count the number of cells. Viability of the cells can be assayed by a trypan blue exclusion test (0.25% trypan blue in phosphate-buffered saline).

5 Cells can now be used for culturing (Protocol 3) or for determination of liposomal components (for calculation see Section 3.4.2).

E. Preparation of liver endothelial and Kupffer cells

1 Centrifuge the supernatants from above (part D, step 4) at 500 g at 4 °C to sediment the non-parenchymal cells. Wash the cells one more time with Hanks' solution containing 0.3% BSA by centrifugation at 500 g, 4 °C. Resuspend the final pellet in two plastic 14 ml tubes with 8.5 ml Hanks' BSA solution each.

2 Mix the non-parenchymal cell suspensions with 3.2 ml Optiprep. Carefully layer the cell mixtures with 1 ml Hanks' solution. Centrifuge for 15 min at 1350 g, 4 °C (no brake).

3 The non-parenchymal cells are now separated from red blood cells and cell debris and can easily be collected as a cell layer in the buffer phase just on top of the Optiprep solution.

4 Resuspend the cells in approx. 10 ml Hanks' BSA solution and centrifuge for 10 min, at 500 g, 4 °C. Resuspend the cell pellet in 5 ml Hanks' BSA solution.

Protocol 2 continued

5. Flush the non-parenchymal cells into the elutriation rotor at 4 °C, at a flow rate of 13 ml/min, and a rotor speed of 2500 r.p.m. (750 g). At this flow rate cell debris is flushed out in 200 ml of Hanks' solution containing 0.3% BSA. Liver endothelial cells are collected in 150 ml at a flow rate of 23 ml/min, an intermediate cell fraction containing large endothelial and small Kupffer cells is collected in 150 ml at a flow rate of 25 ml/min, and Kupffer cells are collected in 150 ml at 46 ml/min.

6. Concentrate the cells by centrifugation for 10 min at 500 g, 4 °C. Resuspend the cell pellets in 10 ml Hanks' solution or culture medium and count the number of cells in the cell fractions. Viability of the cells can be assayed by a trypan blue exclusion test (0.25% trypan blue in phosphate-buffered saline).

7. Liver endothelial and Kupffer cells can now be used for culturing (Protocol 3) or for determination of liposomal components (for calculation see Section 3.4.2).

All three main liver cell types can be cultured (maintenance culture) upon isolation after a collagenase perfusion. In Protocol 3 a general method is given. For parenchymal cells and Kupffer cells most culture plastics can serve as substrate for the cells, although also collagen or fibronectin coating has been used for parenchymal cells. In our hands collagen coating is crucial for culturing liver endothelial cells (7, 32). Ideally, (binding) experiments with liposomes should be performed within three days after isolation. Microscopically the quality of the cells is declining after this period. Kupffer cells and to a lesser extent parenchymal cells show morphological changes, while liver endothelial cells start to detach from the substrate.

Protocol 3

Culturing of hepatocytes, Kupffer cells, and endothelial cells isolated from rat liver

Equipment and reagents

- 24-well cluster plates. For culturing liver endothelial cells these plates should be collagen coated (23, 36). For culturing hepatocytes coating with either fibronectin or collagen is an option, but not a necessity. Kupffer cells can be cultured directly on the plastic substrate.
- Appropriate culture medium (depending on cell type and aim of experiment)
- Culture media for liver endothelial cells: RPMI-1640 supplemented with 20% and 10% heat inactivated fetal calf serum (FCS), 2 mM L-glutamine, 100 IU/ml penicillin, 100 µg/ml streptomycin, and 10 ng/ml endothelial growth factor (Roche)

- Culture media for Kupffer cells: RPMI-1640 supplemented with 20% and 10% heat inactivated FCS, 2 mM L-glutamine, 100 IU/ml penicillin, and 100 µg/ml streptomycin
- Culture media for hepatocytes: Williams' E medium supplemented with 10% heat inactivated FCS, 2 mM L-glutamine, 100 IU/ml penicillin, and 100 µg/ml streptomycin
- PBS
- 0.1 M NaOH

Protocol 3 continued

Method

1 Coated plates can be purchased from various suppliers (Greiner Bio-One, BD Biosciences). If these are not available 24-well plates can be coated with collagen S (type I) (Roche) with 200 μl of a solution containing 100 μg/ml collagen. The solution is allowed to evaporate overnight in a laminar flow cabinet from the wells. Coated plates can be stored for several weeks at 4 °C.

2 Cells, isolated according to Protocol 2, are seeded, after careful resuspension of the cells, at the desired density. Typical cell densities in 24-well plates are 0.5 ml of a suspension of 1×10^6 cells/ml for liver endothelial and Kupffer cells, or 0.5 ml of a suspension of 0.5×10^6 cells/ml for hepatocytes.

3 Cells are allowed to adhere to the substrate for at least 4 h, but preferably overnight, in medium containing 20% FCS.

4 Adhered cells are washed to remove non-attached cells and further cultured in medium containing 10% FCS. Medium is renewed every 24 h.

5 Liposome–cell interaction experiments are performed between the first and third day after culturing of the cells as described in Protocol 1.

3 Biodistribution of liposomes

3.1 Animal models; species differences

Although one might want to extrapolate *in vitro* data directly to the *in vivo* situation, this may be very precarious. Liposomes administered *in vivo* encounter various anatomical barriers and are subject to additional interactions. As far as anatomical barriers are considered, intravenously administered liposomes are able to extravasate only at sites which have a discontinuous or fenestrated endothelium. The liver and spleen fulfil this requirement and in addition these organs also harbour the body's largest resident macrophage populations, explaining the important role of these organs in the *in vivo* handling of liposomes (34–37). So far there are no convincing reports that other readily accessible sites such as the vascular endothelium or blood cells contribute significantly to uptake of liposomes from the blood circulation. In certain pathological conditions such as occurring in solid tumours and at sites of infection or inflammation, leaky vascular endothelium may occur allowing liposomes to extravasate (38, 39).

In vivo studies with liposomes have been performed in most animal models used in laboratories, including guinea pig, dogs, hamster, rabbit, and cats (40–44). Most *in vivo* studies however have been performed in mice and rats. Also with *in vivo* studies interpretation of results deserves attention, especially because of differences between different animal species which may hamper extrapolation of results to other species, e.g. man. Experiments in rats and mice have shown that not only the clearance rate of liposomes is different between these species but also the mechanism by which this clearance rate is regulated (45).

3.2 *In vivo* liposome–cell interactions

It is tempting but not necessarily wise to directly extrapolate the results of *in vitro* studies to the *in vivo* situation. As has become clear from several such *in vitro* studies the addition of serum may have a profound effect. Dijkstra *et al.* noticed at best a slight (maximally two-fold) stimulation of uptake by fetal calf serum but no effect by rat serum (46). Papahadjopoulos and co-workers reported an inhibitory effect of serum (21). Recently, we performed a series of experiments in which we compared the uptake of liposomes with various amounts of PS by Kupffer cells and hepatic endothelial cells both *in vitro* and *in vivo* (23, 47). From these experiments we concluded that various cells *in vitro* quite efficiently internalize liposomes of various compositions and that scavenger receptors are likely to be involved in this uptake. This, however, by no means allows the conclusion that these uptake mechanisms thus play a significant role *in vivo*. As a matter of fact, we found that *in vivo* the liver endothelial cells do not participate at all in uptake of high-PS liposomes from the circulation.

Although it is obvious from a number of studies that macrophages *in vitro* are quite capable of capturing variously composed liposomes in the absence of plasma or individual plasma proteins (46, 48), it is questionable whether such protein-independent uptake is relevant to the *in vivo* situation. Several investigators have shown that liposomes of a wide variety of compositions adsorb substantial amounts of a large collection of individual proteins when incubated with plasma (49, 50). We consider it most likely that, first of all, these proteins effectively mask the phospholipid head groups, preventing specific recognition of any of those head groups by a charge- or head group-specific receptor, if such receptors exist at all. Secondly, among the adsorbed proteins there are likely to be several which can be removed from the blood in a highly specific manner and which will thus also contribute to the removal of the liposomes to which they are adsorbed with the same specificity. It is our view, therefore, that the great majority of liposomes injected into the bloodstream will be cleared by receptor-mediated mechanisms, due to the adsorption of a collection of opsonizing proteins. A limited number of such proteins has been identified to date, e.g. fibronectin (51), complement factors (52, 53), β2-glycoprotein (54), C-reactive protein (55, 56), and α2-macroglobulin (57). In Protocol 4 a method is given for the isolation of adsorbed opsonizing proteins from serum or plasma which is, slightly modified, adapted from the method published by Chonn *et al.* (58). For a more detailed discussion of this topic the reader is referred to other contributions of this issue.

The role of serum and/or proteins in liver uptake can also be studied in liver perfusion systems. Such *in situ* perfusions allow comparison of liposome uptake or clearance of liposomes by the liver under well defined conditions, e.g. serum-free or in serum from different species (45).

Protocol 4

Re-isolation of liposomes from serum

Equipment and reagents

- Tuberculin syringes, 1 ml
- Glass wool
- Bio-Gel A-15m, 200–400 mesh size (Bio-Rad)
- HN buffer: 10 mM HEPES, 135 mM NaCl pH 7.4

Method

1 Plug syringe with glass wool and fill with Bio-Gel.

2 Centrifuge for 2 min, 750 g, at room temperature and repeat this step till the bed volume is 1 ml.

3 Centrifuge for 5 min, 150 g, at room temperature; make sure that the Bio-Gel is uniformly packed and excess buffer is removed.

4 Apply 50 ml samples of liposome/serum incubation mixtures and immediately centrifuge for 1 min, 150 g, at room temperature.

3.3 Markers

In general the remarks on the use of markers in liposome research made in Section 2.2 also hold true for the *in vivo* use of these liposomal compounds. The difference with the *in vitro* system merely lies with the much higher complexity of the biological *in vivo* system. The presence of all these *in vivo* microsystems may have important implications for the stability of the chosen marker but also for its fate in time and thus for the interpretation of the fate of the liposome. In this section some examples will be presented.

Small unilamellar vesicles composed of egg-PC, cholesterol, and PS display, when injected into a rat, a discrepancy between the plasma clearance of the liposome labels N-rhodamine-phosphatidylethanolamine (N-Rh-PE) and phosphatidyl[^{14}C]choline simultaneously present in the liposomes. The N-Rh-PE label was eliminated from the plasma three to four times faster than the radiolabelled PC (59). The fluorescent label was rapidly excreted in the bile, up to 30% of the injected dose within 1 h and 70% after 4 h, indicating efficient processing by hepatocytes of this liposomal label. Since transfer of the different markers to plasma constituents like lipoproteins could be excluded in this study these observations suggest different mechanisms of interaction with hepatocytes for different liposomal compounds. In another study it was found that large (400 nm) PS-containing liposomes labelled with the metabolically inert radioactive label [^{3}H]cholesteryloleyl ether were recovered in substantial amounts in the hepatocytes after intravenous injection into a rat (60). This was a remarkable observation since fenestrations in the liver sinusoidal endothelium are considered to be around 150 nm in diameter. In addition, it was shown that liposomes with a diameter of 400 nm and containing phosphatidylglycerol, did not accumulate in the hepatocytes. In this case selective transfer of the radioactive label across the liver endothelial barrier could be excluded by the use of different labels. The intrahepatic distribution of the [³H]cholesteryloleyl ether was compatible with electron microscopic observations on liver sections following intravenous administration of liposomes of the same size and composition and containing colloidal gold. Also comparison with [¹⁴C]sucrose as an encapsulated marker demonstrated an identical label distribution. In a later study it was concluded that the fluidity of the liposomal PS containing membrane might allow some kind of blood cell mediated forced passage through the fenestrations by a mechanism that does not apply to liposomes containing PG (61).

3.4 Liposome kinetics and tissue distribution

The pharmacokinetics and tissue distribution of liposomes after parenteral administration is determined by a diversity of variables including, liposome size and composition, steric stabilization of the liposome, presence of surface grafted molecules, such as targeting devices, and obviously the organism and the health status of that particular organism. Closely related to this last point is the accessibility of certain tissues or cells for the liposomes. Upon injection liposomes encounter anatomical barriers like the endothelial lining of the vasculature and also of the blood brain barrier which will prevent extravasation of the liposomes. Generally, small liposomes ($\leq$ 100 nm) are eliminated from the blood more slowly than large liposomes, whereas electrostatically charged liposomes disappear faster from the blood than electrostatically neutral liposomes. Under normal conditions intravenously administered liposomes will be taken up from the blood circulation by cells of the mononuclear phagocyte system in the liver and spleen (34–37). In addition, depending on size and composition of the liposomes, in the liver hepatocytes may also play a substantial role in the elimination of liposomes from the blood (5). The ability of liposomes to pass the sinusoidal endothelial lining, allowing uptake by hepatocytes, originates from the presence of fenestrations in these cells. These fenestrations have a size of around 150 nm (62), allowing small liposomes to pass but also larger ones when containing phosphatidylserine (see Section 3.3). As indicated before (Section 3.2), protein adsorption is an important, if not the most important, determinant for cell uptake *in vivo*. In order to diminish protein adsorption and thus prolonging the circulation time of the liposomes, the concept of steric stabilization was developed (63–66). Today lipid-anchored poly(ethylene glycol) (PEG) has proven to be most valuable for *in vivo* applications. Coating of the liposomes with PEG increases the residence time in the blood circulation; in mice and rats the half-life is about 20 hours (65, 67), while in humans half-lives of up to 45 hours have been reported (68). It has been demonstrated that because of their long-circulation properties, PEG liposomes have a relatively high probability to extravasate and accumulate at sites that are characterized by increased vascular permeability (66,

69). This kind of 'leaky' endothelium can be found at various stages of tumour development and at sites of infection or inflammation (70). Under non-pathological conditions a major fraction of the PEG liposomes ultimately ends up, as conventional liposomes, in the cells of the mononuclear phagocyte system in the liver and the spleen. The relative contribution of the spleen to the uptake of PEG liposomes from the blood is somewhat higher than in the case of conventional liposomes (67).

For more than two decades now numerous efforts have been made to specifically target liposomes to specific cells or tissues, in order to improve biodistribution profiles of liposomes and their contents. To enhance the targeting properties of lipsomes a variety of specific ligands have been coupled to the liposome surface, including antibodies (fragments), vitamins, proteins, peptides, and carbohydrates (29, 71–73). Many studies with ligand targeted liposomes show very good *in vitro* target binding properties but the *in vivo* results of targeting to cells other than those present in liver and spleen are scarce and not really impressive (see also Section 3.4.2).

3.4.1 Tissue distribution

A fast way to quantitatively assess the tissue distribution after parenteral administration of liposomes is the use of a stable, metabolically inert marker like [³H]cholesteryloleyl ether. This label has been proven to produce reliable data on tissue distribution both shortly after injection (1–3 h) and also longer times after injection (24 h) (see Protocol 5).

Protocol 5

Determination of tissue distribution of liposomes in rats

Equipment and reagents

- Tuberculin syringe 1 ml, hypodermic needle 25 G
- Rats
- Anaesthetics: halothane and/or nembutal

- Liposomes in an isotonic solution, e.g. phosphate-buffered saline or HEPES-buffered saline
- 10% sodium dodecyl sulfate (SDS) in H_2O

Method

1 Typically 1–2.5 μmol per 100 g of body weight of radiolabelled liposomes is injected into male rats via the penile vein under light halothane anaesthesia.

2 Blood samples can be taken from the tail vein under light anaethesia when a limited number of samples is needed (< six) of relative small volume (< 300 μl). When more extensive blood sampling is required one could consider the introduction of a permanent canule in a vein or artery such as the jugularis or carotis.[a]

Protocol 5 continued

3 Blood samples are allowed to clot for 60 min at 4 °C. The samples are then centrifuged (5 min, 13 000 g). Radioactivity is measured in the serum samples after addition of the appropriate amount of scintillation cocktail. The total amount of radioactivity in the serum can be calculated using the equation:

$$\text{serum volume (ml)} = [0.0219 \times \text{body weight (g)}] + 2.66 \, (74).$$

4 At the last time point of sampling the rat is anaesthetized either with halothane or intraperitoneal injection with nembutal (50 mg/kg body weight). Open the abdomen of the rat as described before, see Protocol 2, steps 5–9 and perfuse the liver with an isotonic buffer to wash out the blood.

5 Gently remove the liver and other tissues of interest.

6 Cautiously remove blood, fat, and/or connective tissue from the surface of the organ and weigh the tissue.

7 Chop the organs using a sharp pair of scissors and homogenize the tissues in a Potter Elvehjem tube in an appropriate volume of isotonic buffer.

8 Radioactivity of the homogenized sample can be determined after solubilization of typically, 400 μl homogenate in 100 μl of 10% SDS and 4 ml scintillation cocktail.

9 For the calculation of the radioactivity per organ, the radioactivity in organs other than the liver has to be corrected for the amount of blood contents (75).

[a] When *in vivo* experiments are performed of a short duration (= 30 min) the whole procedure can be performed in anaesthetized rats. After injection of the liposomes via the penile vein the abdomen can be opened and blood samples can be taken from the vena cava inferior. This procedure also allows liver samples to be taken at given time points by excising liver lobules after ligation of these lobules to prevent blood leakage.

3.4.2 Intra-organ distribution

A variety of methods is available for determination of intra-organ distribution which are generally qualitative or at best semi-quantitative. Labelling of the liposome bilayer with a fluorophore such as 1,1'-dioctadecyl-3,3,3',3'-tetramethyl indocarbocyanine perchlorate (DiI) is in many cases a convenient method to obtain information on intra-organ distribution of the liposomes (see Protocol 6). The importance of carefully looking at the intra-organ distribution is illustrated by a study where immunoliposomes were employed which interacted *in vitro* highly specifically with rat colon adenocarcinoma cells. Upon injection of these immunoliposomes in a rat bearing liver metastases originating from the adenocarcinoma cells, we observed increased uptake of the immunoliposomes in the metastatic tumour nodules in the liver as compared to control liposomes. Visualization of fluorescently or gold labelled immunoliposomes revealed that, although targeting to liver metastases was achieved, the immunoliposomes were not associated with tumour cells but rather localized in other tumour-associated cells, probably macrophages (73).

Intrahepatic distribution in rats can also be determined after i.v. administration of [³H]cholesteryloleyl ether labelled liposomes. The animal is treated as described in Protocol 5, steps 1–4 followed by collagenase perfusion of the liver to isolate parenchymal, Kupffer, and liver endothelial cells, as described in Protocol 2. Subsequently cell numbers in the liver suspension and in the cell fractions are determined microscopically, as is the radioactivity in each cell fraction. To calculate the specific radioactivity in each cell type, total cell numbers in each population can be calculated as follows: parenchymal cells = $(4.50 \times 10^6$ body weight [g]), non-parenchymal cells = $(1.94 \times 10^6$ body weight [g]), liver endothelial cells = $\{0.75 \times (1.94 \times 10^6$ body weight [g])\}, and Kupffer cells = $\{0.25 \times (1.94 \times 10^6$ body weight [g])\}, multiplied by the measured cell-associated radioactivity and expressed as the relative contribution of each cell type to the total liver uptake (76).

Protocol 6

Qualitative determination of intra-organ distribution of liposomes in rats

Equipment and reagents

- Tuberculin syringe 1 ml, hypodermic needle 25 G
- Circular filter paper with a diameter of 2.5 cm
- Cryostat (Leica Microsystems)
- Rats

- Fluorescently labelled liposomes in an isotonic solution, e.g. PBS or HEPES-buffered saline
- Anaesthetics: halothane and/or nembutal
- Isopentane –80 °C

Method

1 Typically 1–2.5 μmol per 100 g of body weight of radiolabelled liposomes is injected into male rats via the penile vein under light halothane anaesthesia.

2 Anaesthetize the rat at a chosen time point either with halothane or intraperitoneal injection with nembutal (50 mg/kg body weight). Open the abdomen of the rat as described before, see Protocol 2, steps 5–9 and perfuse the liver for 2–5 min with an isotonic buffer to rinse out the blood.

3 Gently remove the liver and other tissues of interest and put them immediately on ice.

4 Cautiously remove blood, fat, and/or connective tissue from the surface of the organ and cut tissues in conveniently sized pieces. Place the pieces of, for example, liver, spleen, and kidney together on a buffer-drenched filter paper. This allows direct comparison of the different tissues and will ease the interpretation of the results.

5 Snap-freeze the tissue in isopentane at –80 °C and store frozen tissues at –80 °C until further processing.

6 Cut 4 μm cryostat sections and examine the air dried sections using a fluorescence microscope.[a]

[a] Fixation of the tissue, for example with acetone, may drastically diminish the fluorescent signal on the cryostat sections.

Acknowledgements

We gratefully acknowledge the help of Henriëtte Morselt, Bert Dontje, and Xuedong Yan in the preparation of some of the protocols.

References

1. Pagano, R. E. and Weinstein, J. N. (1978). *Annu. Rev. Biophys. Bioeng.*, **7**, 435.
2. Scherphof, G. L. (1991). In *Handbook of experimental pharmacology* (ed. R. L. Juliano), Vol. 100, p. 285. Springer-Verlag, Berlin Heidelberg.
3. Düzgüneş, N. and Nir, S. (1999). *Adv. Drug Deliv. Rev.*, **40**, 3.
4. Scherphof, G. L. and Kamps, J. A. A. M. (1998). *Adv. Drug Deliv. Rev.*, **32**, 81.
5. Scherphof, G. L. and Kamps, J. A. A. M. (2001). *Prog. Lipid Res.*, **40**, 149.
6. Daleke, D. L., Hong, K., and Papahadjopoulos, D. (1990). *Biochim. Biophys. Acta*, **1024**, 352.
7. Kamps, J. A. A. M., Morselt, H. W. M., Meijer, D. K. F., and Scherphof, G. L. (2001). In *Cells of the hepatic sinusoid* (ed. E. Wisse, D. L. Knook, R. de Zanger, and M. J. P. Arthur), Vol. 8, p. 144. The Kupffer Cell Foundation, Leiden, NL.
8. Koning, G. A., Morselt, H. W. M., Velinova, M. J., Donga, J., Gorter, A., Allen, T. M., et al. (1999). *Biochim. Biophys. Acta*, **1420**, 153.
9. Ho, R. J., Rouse, B. T., and Huang, L. (1986). *Biochemistry*, **25**, 5500.
10. Hoekstra, D., Tomasini, R., and Scherphof, G. L. (1980). *Biochim. Biophys. Acta*, **603**, 336.
11. Daemen, T., De Haan, A., Arkema, A., and Wilschut, J. (1998). In *Medical applications of liposomes* (ed. D. D. Lasic and D. Papahadjopoulos), p. 117. Elsevier Science, Amsterdam.
12. Derksen, J. T. P., Morselt, H. W. M., and Scherphof, G. L. (1988). *Biochim. Biophys. Acta*, **971**, 127.
13. Cerletti, A., Drewe, J., Fricker, G., Eberle, A. N., and Huwyler, J. (2000). *J. Drug Target.*, **8**, 435.
14. Papadimitriou, E. and Antimisiaris, S. G. (2000). *J. Drug Target.*, **8**, 335.
15. Hong, K., Friend, D. S., Glabe, C. G., and Papahadjopoulos, D. (1983). *Biochim. Biophys. Acta*, **732**, 320.
16. Huang, S. K., Hong, K., Papahadjopoulos, D., and Friend, D. S. (1991). *Biochim. Biophys. Acta*, **1069**, 117.
17. Ellens, H., Morselt, H. W., Dontje, B. H., Kalicharan, D., Hulstaert, C. E., and Scherphof, G. L. (1983). *Cancer Res.*, **43**, 2927.
18. Pagano, R. E. and Takeichi, M. (1977). *J. Cell Biol.*, **74**, 531.
19. Dijkstra, J., Van Galen, M., and Scherphof, G. L. (1985). *Biochim. Biophys. Acta*, **813**, 287.
20. Fraley, R., Straubinger, R. M., Rule, G., Springer, L., and Papahadjopoulos, D. (1981). *Biochemistry*, **20**, 6978.
21. Lee, K. D., Hong, K., and Papahadjopoulos, D. (1992). *Biochim. Biophys. Acta*, **1103**, 185.
22. Lee, K. D., Pitas, R. E., and Papahadjopoulos, D. (1992). *Biochim. Biophys. Acta*, **1111**, 1.
23. Kamps, J. A. A. M., Morselt, H. W. M., and Scherphof, G. L. (1999). *Biochem. Biophys. Res. Commun.*, **256**, 57.
24. Lasic, D. D. and Papahadjopoulos, D. (1995). *Science*, **267**, 1275.
25. Zelphati, O. and Szoka, F. C. (1996). *J. Control. Release*, **41**, 99.
26. Wheeler, J. J., Palmer, L., Ossanlou, M., MacLachlan, I., Graham, R. W., Zhang, Y. P., et al. (1999). *Gene Ther.*, **6**, 271.
27. Pagnan, G., Stuart, D. D., Pastorino, F., Raffaghello, L., Montaldo, P. G., Allen, T. M., et al. (2000). *J. Natl. Cancer Inst.*, **92**, 253.
28. Sambrook, J. and Russel, D. W. (ed.) (2001). In *Molecular cloning: a laboratory manual* (3rd edn), p. 17.1. Cold Spring Harbor Laboratory Press, NY.

29. Kamps, J. A. A. M., Morselt, H. W. M., Swart, P. J., Meijer, D. K. F., and Scherphof, G. L. (1997). *Proc. Natl. Acad. Sci. USA*, **94**, 11681.

30. Casteleijn, E., Van Rooij, H., Van Berkel, Th. J. C., and Koster, J. F. (1986). *FEBS Lett.*, **201**, 193.

31. Daemen, T., Veninga, A., Roerdink, F. H., and Scherphof, G. L. (1986). *Cancer Res.*, **46**, 4330.

32. Braet, F., De Zanger, R., Sasaoki, T., Baekeland, M., Janssens, P., Smedsrød, B., *et al.* (1994). *Lab. Invest.*, **70**, 944.

33. Dijkstra, J., Van Galen, W. J. M., Hulstaert, C. E., Kalicharan, D., Roerdink, F. H., and Scherphof, G. L. (1984). *Exp. Cell Res.*, **150**, 161.

34. Poste, G. (1983). *Biol. Cell*, **47**, 19.

35. Senior, J. H. (1987). *Crit. Rev. Ther. Drug Carrier Syst.*, **3**, 123.

36. Allen, T. M. (1988). *Adv. Drug Deliv. Rev.*, **2**, 55.

37. Woodle, M. C. and Lasic, D. D. (1992). *Biochim. Biophys. Acta*, **1113**, 171.

38. Ishida, O., Maaruyama, K., Sasaki, K., and Iwatsuru, M. (1999). *Int. J. Pharm.*, **190**, 49.

39. Maruyama, K. (2000). *Biol. Pharm. Bull.*, **23**, 791.

40. Huong, T. M., Ishida, T., Harashima, H., and Kiwada, H. (2001). *Biol. Pharm. Bull.*, **24**, 439.

41. Bekersky, I., Boswell, G. W., Hiles, R., Fielding, R. M., Buell, D., and Walsh, T. J. (1999). *Pharm. Res.*, **16**, 1694.

42. Devoisselle, J. M., Begu, S., Tourne-Peteilh, C., Desmettre, T., and Mordon, S. (2001). *Luminescence*, **16**, 73.

43. Dams, E. T., Oyen, W. J., Boerman, O. C., Storm, G., Laverman, P., Koenders, E. B., *et al.* (1998). *J. Nucl. Med.*, **39**, 2172.

44. Matteucci, M. L., Anyarambhatla, G., Rosner, G., Azuma, C., Fisher, P. E., Dewhirst, M. W., *et al.* (2000). *Clin. Cancer Res.*, **6**, 3748.

45. Liu, D., Hu, Q., and Song, Y. K. (1995). *Biochim. Biophys. Acta*, **1240**, 277.

46. Dijkstra, J., Van Galen, M., and Scherphof, G. L. (1984). *Biochim. Biophys. Acta*, **804**, 58.

47. Kamps, J. A. A. M., Morselt, H. W. M., and Scherphof, G. L. (1996). *Prog. Drug Deliv. Syst.*, **5**, 89.

48. Dijkstra, J., Van Galen, M., Regts, J., and Scherphof, G. (1985). *Eur. J. Biochem.*, **148**, 391.

49. Maruyama, K., Mori, A., Bhadra, S., Subbiah, M. T., and Huang, L. (1991). *Biochim. Biophys. Acta*, **1070**, 246.

50. Chonn, A., Semple, S. C., and Cullis, P. R. (1992). *J. Biol. Chem.*, **267**, 18759.

51. Rossi, J. D. and Wallace, B. A. (1983). *J. Biol. Chem.*, **258**, 3327.

52. Devine, D. V., Wong, K., Serrano, K., Chonn, A., and Cullis, P. R. (1994). *Biochim. Biophys. Acta*, **1191**, 43.

53. Harashima, H., Sakata, K., Funato, K., and Kiwada, H. (1994). *Pharm. Res.*, **11**, 402.

54. Chonn, A., Semple, S. C., and Cullis, P. R. (1995). *J. Biol. Chem.*, **270**, 25845.

55. Richards, G. L., Gewurz, H., Siegel, J., and Alving, C. R. (1979). *J. Immunol.*, **122**, 1185.

56. Volanakis, J. E. and Narkates, A. J. (1981). *J. Immunol.*, **126**, 1820.

57. Murai, M., Aramaki, Y., and Tsuchiya, S. (1995). *Immunology*, **86**, 64.

58. Chonn, A., Semple, S. C., and Cullis, P. R. (1991). *Biochim. Biophys. Acta*, **1070**, 215.

59. Verkade, H. J., Zaal, K. J. M., Derksen, J. T. P., Vonk, R. J., Hoekstra, D., Kuipers, F., *et al.* (1992). *Biochem. J.*, **284**, 259.

60. Daemen, T., Velinova, M., Regts, J., De Jager, M., Kalicharan, R., Donga, J., *et al.* (1997). *Hepatology*, **26**, 416.

61. Romero, E. L., Morilla, M. J., Regts, J., Koning, G. A., and Scherphof, G. L. (1999). *FEBS Lett.*, **448**, 193.

62. Wisse, E. (1970). *J. Ultrastruct. Res.*, **31**, 125.

63. Allen, T. M. and Choun, A. (1987). *FEBS Lett.*, **223**, 42.

64. Allen, T. M., Hansen, C., and Rutledge, J. (1989). *Biochim. Biophys. Acta*, **981**, 27.

65. Allen, T. M., Hansen, C., Martin, F., Redemann, C., and Yau Yong, A. (1991). *Biochim. Biophys. Acta*, **1066**, 29.

66. Papahadjopoulos, D., Allen, T. M., Gabizon, A., Mayhew, E., Matthay, K., Huang, S. K., *et al.* (1991). *Proc. Natl. Acad. Sci. USA*, **88**, 11460.

67. Scherphof, G. L., Morselt, H. W. M., and Allen, T. M. (1994). *J. Liposome Res.*, **4**, 213.

68. Allen, T. M. (1997). *Drugs*, **54**, 8.

69. Gabizon, A., Catane, R., Uziely, B., Kaufman, B., Safra, T., Cohen, R., *et al.* (1994). *Cancer Res.*, **54**,987.

70. Dvorak, H. F., Nagy, J. A., Dvorak, J. T., and Dvorak, A. M. (1988). *Am. J. Pathol.*, **133**, 95.

71. Mastrobattista, E., Koning, G. A., and Storm, G. (1999). *Adv. Drug Deliv. Rev.*, **40**, 103.

72. Zalipsky, S., Mullah, N., Harding, J. A., Gittelman, J., Guo, L., and DeFrees, S. A. (1997). *Bioconjug. Chem.*, **8**, 111.

73. Kamps, J. A. A. M., Koning, G. A., Velinova, M. J., Morselt, H. W. M., Wilkens, M., Gorter, A., *et al.* (2000). *J. Drug Target.*, **8**, 235.

74. Bijsterbosch, M. K., Ziere, G. J., and Van Berkel, Th. J. C. (1989). *Mol. Pharmacol.*, **36**, 484.

75. Caster, W. O., Simon, A. B., and Armstrong, W. D. (1955). *Am. J. Physiol.*, **183**, 317.

76. Roerdink, F., Dijkstra, J., Hartman, G., Bolscher, B., and Scherphof, G. L. (1981). *Biochim. Biophys. Acta*, **677**, 79.

77. Lowry, O. H., Rosebourgh, N. J., Farr, A. L., and Randall, R. J. (1951). *J. Biol. Chem.*, **193**, 265.

Chapter 10
Cationic liposomes in gene delivery

Sean Sullivan, Yan Gong, and Jeffrey Hughes
University of Florida, Department of Pharmaceutics, Gainesville, FL, USA.

1 Introduction

Gene therapy provides a new paradigm for the treatment of human diseases. Although gene therapy trials have been initiated worldwide for greater than two decades, little has been achieved clinically in curing diseases. A major hurdle is the lack of efficient delivery systems for *in vitro* and *in vivo* studies. An ideal system should have the following characteristics: be targetable, biodegradable, non-toxic, and stable for storage. Gene delivery systems are generally categorized into viral and plasmid-based vectors. Plasmid-based systems are also extremely useful for *in vitro* studies and will be the focus of the chapter.

There are several advantages to using plasmid-based vectors compared to viral vectors including low immunogenicity, no requirement for a specific receptor to transfect cells, simplicity in formulation, and feasibility of production on a large scale. Limitations of non-viral vectors include transient gene expression and a lower transfection efficiency compared to viral vectors. A question that is often asked is 'Why are plasmid-based systems less efficient'? This issue can be addressed by looking at the cellular barriers that face plasmid DNA delivery to the cell. In general, it appears gene delivery systems are similar to other macromolecules in that they enter cells through endocytosis and initially accumulate in an endosomal–lysosomal compartment. A number of potential cell surface receptors for either plasmid DNA or for the liposome/DNA complex have been proposed. Once internalized the accumulated plasmid DNA gradually escapes from endosomes and enters the cytoplasm through a poorly defined mechanism. The majority of the plasmid progresses with the endosome into lysosomes, which ultimately degrade the plasmid. Once in the cytoplasm, the plasmid faces another barrier, the nuclear membrane. Thus plasmid DNA, which initially accumulates in an endosomal–lysosomal compartment, usually represents a pharmacological dead end. Therefore, agents or techniques that enhance transgene expression should:

(a) Promote the initial cellular interaction between plasmid DNA or liposome/DNA complex and the cell membrane.

(b) Promote the transfer from endosomes to the cytosol.

(c) Allow the plasmids to bypass the endosomal compartment.

In most cell culture studies, free plasmid DNA is ineffective as a transfection agent yet becomes active in the presence of an appropriate delivery agent. A number of approaches have been used to enhance the cytoplasmic and nuclear delivery of plasmid DNA. These will be discussed individually in the sections below.

The workhorse of gene delivery systems is known as a plasmid DNA or pDNA. A plasmid is an extrachromosomal, circular segment of DNA, intrinsic to bacteria, yeast, as well as some eukaryotic cells. Features common to plasmid DNA vectors include:

(a) An origin of replication, which codes for the replication of a daughter strand.

(b) A drug-resistance gene, which selects for bacteria transformed with the plasmid.

(c) A multiple cloning region where new DNA fragments can be inserted.

These features give plasmid DNA great value experimentally. Most research laboratories isolate plasmids from *E. coli* via standard protocols or with commercial kits. For cell culture transfections, the purity of the plasmid DNA is not as critical as for *in vivo* experiments, either for local or systemic administration. The contaminants of concern are bacterial chromosomal DNA, RNA, proteins, and endotoxin. A CsCl banding protocol will be provided for plasmid DNA to be used in *in vivo* gene transfer experiments.

Gene expression in transfected eukaryotic or prokaryotic cells is generally studied by linking a promoter sequence to an easily detectable 'reporter' gene within the plasmid. Reporter genes also provide a convenient measure of the expression level of genes mediated by liposome complexes. Standard recombinant methods are used to join the gene of interest to a reporter gene in an expression vector. The resulting recombinant is then introduced into an appropriate cell line, where its expression is detected by measurement of the reporter mRNA or the reporter proteins from cell lysates or growth media using enzymatic or immunological techniques to quantify. The reporter genes should have an easily detected output that can be distinguished from the background of proteins in the host cell. The detection methods should be sensitive, specific, quantitative, reproducible, and rapid to perform.

Commonly used reporter genes include; firefly luciferase, β-galactosidase, alkaline phosphatase, and green fluorescent protein (GFP). These reporter systems use different methods of detection and each has strengths and weaknesses (Table 1).

Firefly luciferase is a monomeric 61 kDa protein found in the gut of the firefly (*Photinus pyralis*) and some marine organisms. However, it does not occur in mammalian cells, thus eliminating any background serves as an excellent reporter for transfection of mammalian cells. The firefly luciferase gene (*Luc*) produces light from luciferin in the presence of ATP and Mg^{2+}:

$$(ATP + luciferin + O_2 \xrightarrow{Mg^{2+}} AMP + oxyluciferin + pp_i + light(560nm)$$

Table 1 Commonly used reporter genes

Reporter gene	Advantages	Disadvantages	Detection[a]
Luciferase (firefly)	High specific activity; no endogenous activity	Requires substrate (luciferin) and O_2, Mg^{2+}, and ATP	BL
β-Galactosidase	Simple colorimetric readouts; sensitive bio- or chemiluminescent assays available	Endogenous activity	CL, CM, FL
Alkaline phosphatase	Colorimetric and luminescent assays available	Endogenous activity in some cells	CL, CM, FL
GFP (jelly fish)	Autofluorescent; no endogenous activity; mutants with improved intensity and spectral qualities available	Low sensitivity (no signal amplification)	FL

[a] BL, bioluminescent; CL, chemiluminescent; CM, colorimetric; FL, fluorescence.

Luminometers or liquid scintillation counters can be used to detect light released by the action of the luciferase enzyme. In the conventional assay for luciferase, a flash of light is generated that decays rapidly after the enzyme and substrates are combined.

The chemiluminescent assay for firefly luciferase activity is an extremely sensitive, rapid, easy-to-handle, and non-isotopic alternative to other reporter gene assay systems. The detectable linear range of firefly luciferase is approximately 10 fg/ml to 1 μg/ml (10^{-16} M to 10^{-8} M).

Different luciferase assays from companies (e.g. Promega, Cat. No. E1500) were developed for reporter quantification in mammalian cells. Luciferase assays can be carried out in 96-well plates to facilitate the analyses of large numbers of transfected cells. The luciferase reporter 1000 Assay System (Cat. No. E4550) is an example of kit designed by Promega to meet this need. This reporter gene can be problematic for *in vivo* gene transfer studies due to the instability of the protein and the rapid turnover of the mRNA.

The *E. coli lacZ* gene codes for the enzyme β-galactosidase, which catalyses the hydrolysis of β-galactosides (e.g. X-Gal and ONPG) to produce colour that is easily detected by colorimetric chemiluminescent assays or histochemical staining. Thus β-galactosidase activity allows for the quick determination of cells expressing the *lacZ* gene as a reporter gene.

ONPG (o-nitrophenyl-β-galactopyranoside) is the most widely used substrate in assays for β-galactosidase in bacterial and eukaryotic cell lysates. ONPG is colourless but the hydrolysis product o-nitrophenol is yellow in alkaline solution and has a maximum absorbance at 420 nm. The reaction can be stopped by adjusting pH to ~11 to inactivate β-galactosidase. More sensitive colorimetric substrates for the detection of β-galactosidase have been developed, such as 4-methylumbelliferyl β-D-galactoside (Sigma, Cat. No. M1600) and chlorophenol red β-D-galactopyranoside (CPRG, Boehringer Mannheim). Assays using chemiluminescent substrates whose hydrolysis products can be detected in a luminometer or scintillation counter are even more sensitive than ONPG-based assays. X-Gal can be used as a substrate for the histochemical staining of β-galactosidase activity in tissues and cells.

The disadvantage of using β-galactosidase as a reporter gene is the endogenous activity of β-galactosidase in mammalian cells. The level of endogenous β-galactosidase activity varies greatly within cells, however, it is possible to distinguish between mammalian and bacterial enzymatic activity by altering the pH. The background staining is particularly problematic for *in vivo* gene transfer experiments due to high background staining in the lungs, liver, and brain.

Alkaline phosphatases are phosphohydrolases that function optimally at alkaline pH. Some alkaline phosphatases can be secreted from cells into culture media, where they can be easily detected and accurately quantified by colorimetric, fluorescent, and chemiluminescent methods according to different characteristics of substrates. Roche Molecular Biochemicals provides a complete range of substrates for human secreted alkaline phosphatase (SEAP). The human placental alkaline phosphatase is a very stable protein. Most endogenous alkaline phosphatase can be heat inactivated by incubating the sample at 65 °C for a half an hour followed by centrifugation. Secondly, the 18 amino acid membrane binding domain can be restored to the protein yielding an extracellular protein. The cell pellet can be assayed for gene expression rather than the supernatant and the cells can be marked for gene expression using either enzyme activity or antibody to the human alkaline phosphatase, such as the one sold by Sigma. *In vivo* gene expression can be quantitated by using a sandwich assay in which a 96-well plate is first coated with goat anti-mouse antibody. The plates are washed and the alkaline phosphatase mouse monoclonal antibody is bound to the plate. Tissue homogenates are first heat activated and then added to the plate. The plate can be incubated overnight at 4 °C. The plates are washed, substrate is added, and real time enzymatic activity can be measured allowing the initial velocity to be determined {Hofland, 1997, No. 52}. This reporter can also be measured using a luminescence assay.

Green fluorescent protein (GFP) from the bioluminescent jellyfish *Aequorea victoria*, absorbs blue light emitted by a Ca^{2+} activated photoprotein aequorin and re-emits the energy as green light. GFP and its engineered variants are the best non-enzymatic reporter systems currently in use. GFP is extremely stable to a wide variety of harsh conditions including heat, extreme pH, and chemical denaturants, and continues to emit fluorescence after fixation in formaldehyde.

GFP is unique among various light-emitting proteins in being autofluorescent, i.e. it does not require substrates or cofactors to emit light. Moreover, GFP is non-lethal when expressed at high levels in variant cells. Most importantly, mutants of GFP can be generated to increase fluorescence intensity and shift wavelengths of excitation and emission. Mutants are also obtainable with shortened intracellular half-lives allowing for observing protein turnover instead of protein stability. However, often because the fluorescent signal is not amplified, detection requires that expression of GFP be driven by very strong promoters or other regulatory elements.

As was discussed above plasmid DNA alone is not active in most *in vitro* evaluations. Liposomes are examples of a vector used in plasmid DNA delivery. Plasmid DNA can be encapsulated within the liposome interior or bound to the surface. Cationic liposomes and plasmids interact via a mixture of electrostatic and hydrophobic interactions. The advantages of the liposome–plasmid interaction are two-fold:

(a) Protect nucleic acids from degradation (e.g. exo- and endonucleases).

(b) Increase the amount of plasmid internalized within cells.

The major problem with liposomes comprised of natural lipids (e.g. neutral and anionic lipids) is that they are associated with low plasmid encapsulation efficiency. The low encapsulation is due in part to the negative charge of the plasmid DNA, which repels the anionic lipids, and the relatively high molecular weight of the plasmid. Huang and others have described methods to overcome these limitations experienced with anionic and neutral lipids (1).

Cationic liposomes employ specific types of lipids as the functional component to transport DNA into the cell. Figure 1 depicts structures of commonly used agents. For the most part there are three distinct regions of cationic lipids.

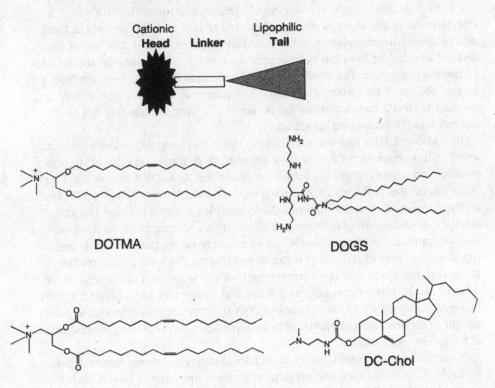

Figure 1 Chemical structure of commonly used cationic lipids.

There is the cationic region (an amine), a linker region (ester, ether, amide, etc.), and a hydrophobic domain. These vesicles do not form the classical bilayer structure of liposomes but may exist as micelles or other forms. This is particularly true after cationic lipids have interacted with nucleic acids (2). Many cationic lipids have been synthesized and have shown activity in delivering genes *in vitro* and *in vivo*. While these compounds are diverse in chemical structure, they do have common features. There is a cationic head group composed of primary, secondary, tertiary, or quaternary amines, which is attached via a connector to a hydrophobic group.

For *in vitro* studies there is a relationship between the net charge of the cationic liposome/DNA complex and its effectiveness. Generally a small net positive charge is required for *in vitro* transfection. Charge ranges from 1:1 to 1:10 (−/+ charge ratio) or greater have been reported in the literature (3). The nitrogen to phosphate ratio can also describe this. The slight positive charge of the complex is hypothesized to enhance the interaction with the net negative charge of cellular membranes from carbohydrates, especially in tissue culture studies.

In a majority of reported studies, the cationic liposomes function most efficiently when the cationic lipid is combined with a second lipid known as a helper. The role of these helper lipids is in stabilization of the liposome/DNA complex or in assisting membrane fusion events within the cell thus leading to escape of DNA from the endosomes. Helper lipids include unsaturated phosphatidylethanolamines, such as dioleoylphosphatidylethanolamine (DOPE). The effectiveness of this agent is generally believed to rest on its propensity to form non-bilayer structures akin to membrane fusion intermediates. The use of cholesterol as a helper lipid has been reported to be effective in animal studies of transgene expression. The reason for the enhancement *in vivo* has been attributed to the ability of cholesterol-containing complexes to maintain the ability to interact with cell membranes in the presence of serum, which may not be the case with DOPE-containing liposomes (4).

In addition to the two component (e.g. lipids and plasmid) delivery system, another important factor is how they are combined. Kinetic instead of thermodynamic processes control the formation of cationic lipid/DNA complexes. This situation creates problems in producing reproducible delivery systems. The key to the formation of stable liposome/DNA complexes appears to be the maintenance of distinguishable intermediate mixtures during complexation in a thermodynamically stable state. When one simply mixes the two components together, a variety of structures result depending on the local concentration of DNA, cationic lipids, and the ionic strength of the solution. Collectively, these differences in physicochemical and structural properties are likely to affect changes in the ability of the complexed DNA to transfect cells. Thus, in a given sample of cationic liposomes/DNA, individual particles may show varying amounts of transgene expression.

A partial list of the variety of commercially obtainable cationic agents is given in Table 2. In most cases, the preformed cationic liposome is mixed with the plasmid DNA and allowed to interact, then the complex is either diluted or

Table 2 Some commercially available cationic agents

Cationic lipid	Commercial source
Lipofect ACE	Life Technologies
Lipofection	Life Technologies
LipofectAMINE	Life Technologies
CellFECTIN	Life Technologies
DMRIE-C	Life Technologies
DDAB	Sigma
DC-Chol	Sigma
DOTAP	Boehringer Mannheim, Avanti Polar Lipids, Biontex
MRX-230 and MRX-220	Avanti Polar Lipids
Transfectam	Promega
TransFast™	Promega
Tfx™-10, Tfx™-20, and Tfx™-50	Promega
ProFection-CaPO$_4$	Promega
ProFection-DEAE-Dextran	Promega
GeneSHUTTLE-40	Quantum Biotechnologies
CLONfectin™	Clontech
METAFECTENE™	Biontex
INSECTOGENE	Biontex
Effectene	Qiagen
FuGENE 6	Roche Molecular Biochemicals
GENESEAL™	MTTI

applied directly onto tissue culture cells. Depending on the lipid either a low serum or serum-containing tissue culture medium is used. Unfortunately, at this time, the best way to select an appropriate cationic liposome is often through trial and error. Each cell line can demonstrate individual responses in terms of both effectiveness and toxicity for the various cationic lipids. Researchers can also produce their own cationic liposome formulations from several readily purchased cationic lipids (this is often more economical than buying pre-made preparations).

Typically, the lipids are dissolved in an organic solvent (e.g. chloroform or methanol). One of the simplest combinations would be DOTAP/DOPE, a combination of the lipids 1,2-dioleoyl-3-trimethylammonium-propane and dioleoyl-phosphatidylethanolamine in a 1:1 molar ratio. The solvent is removed either under vacuum or by blowing an inert gas over the solution followed by rehydration with sterile water or 5% dextrose. A typical concentration would be between 0.5–2 mg of cationic lipid per ml. The heterogeneous population of liposomes is then subject to particle size reduction. The two most common techniques used are sonication and membrane extrusion. Whichever method is used, liposomes or particles close to 100 nm are desired for most studies. Unlike the anionic liposome formulation, sonication can be used in particle size reduction. Sonication does not harm the liposomes but has been shown to degrade plasmid DNA in bulk solution. After production, the cationic particles are stable for several weeks at 4 °C. Cationic liposomes are mixed with the aqueous plasmid DNA solution at a particular weight ratio (ranges from 1–10 to 1), then the lipid/ plasmid DNA complexes are incubated for a period of time (between 15–30 min). For *in vitro* experiments, the complexes are diluted with medium and added to cells. For *in vivo* experiments, the complexes can be used directly. Increased stability can be achieved by lyophilizing the transfection complexes. A cryopreservative, such as lactose, mannitol, dextrose, or sucrose can be added at iso-osmotic concentrations and the complexes can be lyophilized using standard lyophilization cycles.

2 Plasmid DNA isolation

Plasmid DNA is propagated within bacterial cells such as *E. coli*. There exist several methods for the isolation of plasmid DNA from the bacteria. For the majority of these methods the following procedures are observed:

(a) Lysis of the bacterial cell wall.

(b) Separation of plasmid DNA from lipids, proteins, and bacterial genomic DNA.

(c) A concentration of the plasmid.

Researchers can obtain commercial kits for the isolation and purification of plasmids. Since the plasmid is often isolated from Gram negative bacteria, one also needs to be sure to address the chance of having endotoxin in the final plasmid. Plasmid isolation kits designed for endotoxin removal are available. There are also testing kits that can be used to semi-quantify endotoxin amount.

Protocol 1

Plasmid DNA isolation via CsCl centrifugation

Equipment and reagents

- Shaker for 1 and 2 litre bacterial cultures
- Preparative centrifuge
- Preparative centrifuge rotor, 250 ml or 500 ml bottles
- Desktop centrifuge with holder for 15 ml and 50 ml conical centrifuge tubes
- Ultracentrifuge
- Vertical rotor
- Tube sealer
- Isopropanol (Fisher Scientific)
- PhaseLock (Eppendorf Amersham)

- Phenol/chloroform/isoamyl alcohol (Life Technologies, Inc.)
- CsCl
- Miracle cloth
- STE: 0.1 M NaCl, 10 mM Tris, 1 mM EDTA pH 8
- 2 mg/ml lysozyme
- 0.2 N NaOH/1% SDS
- 10 mM Tris, 1 mM EDTA pH 7
- 3 M potassium acetate
- 10 mg/ml ethidium bromide

Method

1. Thaw frozen bacterial pellet from 1 litre culture and resuspend in 10 ml STE.

2. Add 10 ml lysozyme (2 mg/ml) in STE to resuspended pellet and incubate at room temp for 10 min.

3. Add 28 ml of 0.2 N NaOH/1% SDS and incubate at room temp for additional 10 min.

4. Add 60 ml of 3 M potassium acetate. Mix gently by inversion and incubate for 10 min on ice.

5. Centrifuge in 100 ml tubes using a JA18 rotor at 12 000 r.p.m. for 20 min.

6. Filter supernatant through miracle cloth into a 1 litre centrifuge bottle. Precipitate DNA by adding 0.7 vol. of isopropanol and incubate on ice for 10 min.

7. After centrifugation at 13 000 r.p.m. in a JA18 rotor for 20 min at 4 °C, wash pellet once with 70% EtOH.

8. Split solution into two 5 ml aliquots and extracted with 5 ml of phenol/CHCl$_3$/ isoamyl alcohol using 15 ml PhaseLock centrifuge tubes. PhaseLock can be purchased in bulk and used with 50 ml conical centrifuge tubes for larger preparations.

9. Repeat extraction steps until the aqueous phase is clear and no white precipitate is observed underneath or dispersed within the phase lock. Centrifuge tubes at 2000 r.p.m. for 10 min.

10. Extract aqueous phase once with CHCl$_3$ by adding an equal volume of CHCl$_3$ and centrifuging in a desktop centrifuge for 10 min at 2000 r.p.m. The interface should be perfectly clear.

11. Precipitate DNA from the aqueous phase with 0.7 vol. of isopropanol and centrifuging at 2000 r.p.m. for 10 min.

12. Remove isopropanol and briefly dry pellet under a stream of nitrogen for 10 min to evaporate off the residual isopropanol.

13. Dissolve DNA pellet in TE using 0.5 ml step volumes. For example, 0.5 ml TE is added and the pellet is vortexed for a few minutes. If the pellet does not dissolve any further, add an additional 0.5 ml TE. Pellets usually require approx. 2 ml to be completely dissolved.

14. To 4 ml of resuspended DNA add 4.4 g CsCl. The density of the solution should be 1.59. Check density of solution using a balance. Density can be adjusted by adding additional volume of TE. 50 µl of ethidium solution (10 mg/ml) is added to the heat seal centrifuge tube, tube is sealed, and inserted in vertical rotor.

15. Centrifuge gradient either overnight at 65 000 r.p.m. or 4 h at 75 000 r.p.m.

Protocol 1 continued

16 Using a syringe, pierce tube and remove lower band. Band is visible by room light. Avoid use of UV light. Prolonged exposure may result in nicking thus reducing amount of supercoil.

17 Place isolated band in fresh tube and dilute to top with CsCl solution 1.59 g/ml. The sample was rebanded using the previous CsCl density gradient centrifuge conditions.

18 Remove the lower band and extract the ethidium bromide using CsCl saturated butanol. Usually requires five extractions.

19 Dialyse the DNA against 2 × 2 litres of TE over a 24 h period.

20 Check for complete ethidium removal by measuring the fluorescence of the solution at excitation wavelength = 520 nm and the emission wavelength = 590 nm.

3 Quantification of plasmid DNA concentration

Several methods are routinely used to measure the amount of plasmid DNA. If the sample is pure (no protein, phenol, etc.), the simplest method is to use ultraviolet spectrophotometric measurement. If the amount of plasmid is very small or impure, some investigators use a fluorescence method for quantification.'This method uses a chemical that can intercalate within the plasmid thus forming a fluorescent complex. If this method is used, an aliquot of the plasmid is mixed with an identifying compound such as ethidium bromide or Hoechst stain.

Protocol 2

Hoechst fluorescence assay

Equipment and reagents

- 10 × TNE buffer: 100 mM Tris, 10 mM EDTA, 2 M NaCl pH 7.4 (using conc. HCl), filter
- Standard fluorimeter
- 1 mg/ml Hoechst 33258 in water

Method

1 Dilute Hoechst stock 2 µl to 20 ml in TNE for plasmids, and 20 µl/20 ml for genomic DNA.

2 Add 1 ml of diluted Hoechst stock to a 3 ml fluorescent cuvette and zero the instrument.

3 Add 50 ng of plasmid DNA used to prepare complex in a volume of 1–2 µl to 1 ml of diluted Hoechst solution and set scale to 50. Add an additional 50 ng in the same volume four additional times to establish a standard curve.

4   Wash cuvette with ethanol followed by TNE to remove residual ethanol.

5   Add 1 ml of diluted Hoechst, take a reading to ensure that the fluorescence has returned to zero, add 1-2 μl of sample and take reading.

6   Add the same volume of sample one or two times to assure an accurate reading. Fluorescent reading should not exceed 250. This may exceed linearity of the assay because of detection limitations and depletion of Hoechst stain.

Protocol 3

Determination of plasmid DNA concentration by UV spectrophotometry

Equipment and reagents

- Quartz cuvette
- UV spectrophotometer
- TE buffer: 10 mM Tris-HCl, 1 mM EDTA pH 8.0

- Plasmid DNA (for most spectrophotometers the concentration should be >1 mg/ml)

Method

1   Pipette 10 μl of the pure plasmid into 990 μl of TE buffer and mix well.

2   Blank the spectrophotometer at 230 nm, 260 nm, and 280 nm with TE buffer.

3   Measure the absorbency of the plasmid sample at the three wavelengths listed above. If the reading is not between 0.1-1 absorbance unit, prepare a new dilution and repeat the reading.

4   Calculate plasmid concentration in the original solution using the following equation:

$$\text{Plasmid concentration} = 50 \ \mu g/ml \times OD_{260 \ nm} \times DF$$

(a) A solution of 50 mg/ml of an average double-stranded DNA has an $OD_{260 \ nm}$ of 1.

(b) $OD_{260 \ nm}$ is the optical density from the absorbency reading.

(c) DF is the dilution factor (in the above example in would be 100).

In the above example, if the OD was 0.2 and the dilution factor was 100, the plasmid DNA concentration would be 1000 mg/ml.

5   The above calculations assume the plasmid DNA is pure.

Often researchers measure the plasmid at other wavelengths in order to estimate contamination in the purification procedure. Absorption at 230 nm indicates contamination by phenolate ion, thiocynates, etc. Absorption at 280 nm indicates protein contamination. Often a ratio of 1.8 A_{260}/A_{280} is given as means of determining purity. This is a very crude estimate and should not be the only method used to judge protein contamination in the plasmid.

Protocol 4

Lipofection

Equipment and reagents

- Tubes (polystryene or polyproplene)
- Buffers (e.g. 5% dextrose)
- Tissue culture media
- Cell lines
- Cationic lipids (transfection reagent)

A. Preparation of cationic liposomes

For most commercial lipids a detailed protocol is included with the product information. For laboratory produced liposomes the following protocol can be used.

1 Add the appropriate amount of each lipid in chloroform to a round-bottom flask so that you have 10 mg of each final volume. The resultant liposome should contain both lipids in a ratio of 1:1.

2 Evaporate the chloroform on a Rotovap, resulting in a thin lipid film on the surface of the flask (alternately, you can evaporate the chloroform under nitrogen gas).

3 Dry the film under nitrogen gas, then disperse the lipid film in an appropriate volume of distilled water or other solvent.

4 Shake the flask for 10 min to disperse the lipid layer into the liquid, forming liposomes.

5 Allow lipids to hydrate overnight at 4 °C. The liposomes then can be subjected to particle size reduction, by either extrusion or sonication.

B. Cell transfection (lipofection)

1 Use cells which are between 40–70% confluent.

2 Exchange media to serum-free media and add plasmid complex (which has been freshly prepared) and return to incubator for 1–4 h.

3 Remove transfection media and replace with complete media.

4 Incubate cells for 24–48 h.

5 Determine transgene production.

4 Calculation of N/P ratio

(a) Calculation of phosphate. The negative charge in the plasmid DNA backbone arises from the phosphate group from the four deoxyribose nucleotides. Often an average molecular weight of the four bases is assumed to be 330 g/mol.

(b) Calculation of nitrogen. The molecular weight of the cationic lipid is used in this case. For quaternary amines the positive charge is constant and independent of local pH. For other types of lipids there may be a dependence on the local environment.

(c) Example. Complexation of 1 μg plasmid DNA at a DOTAP/DOPE (1 mg/ml DOTAP) to plasmid ratio of 3:1.

Phosphate = 1×10^{-6} g/330 g/mol phosphate = 3 nmol.

DOTAP MW = 698 g/mol.

X (μg) = 698 g/mol $\times$ 3 $\times$ No. moles of phosphate.

X = 6 μg.

References

1. Li, S., Rizzo, M. A., Bhattacharya, S., and Huang, L. (1998). *Gene Ther.*, **5**, 930.
2. Dan, N. (1998). *Biochim. Biophys. Acta*, **1369**, 34.
3. Behr, J.-P., Demeneix, B., Loeffler, J.-P., and Perez-Mutul, J. (1989). *Proc. Natl. Acad. Sci. USA*, **86**, 6982.
4. Crook, K., Stevenson, B. J., Dubouchet, M., and Porteous, D. J. (1998). *Gene Ther.*, **5**, 137.
5. Hofland, H. E., Nagy, D., Liu, J. J., Spratt, K., Lee, Y. L., Danos, O., and Sullivan, S. M. (1997). *Pharm. Res.*, **14**, 742.

II Selected topics and applications

Chapter 11
pH-sensitive liposomes

Regine Peschka-Süss and Rolf Schubert

Albert-Ludwigs-Universität Freiburg, Pharmazeutisches Institut,
Lehrstuhl für Pharmazeutische Technologie, Hermann-Herder-Strasse 9,
D-79104 Freiburg i.Br., Germany.

1 Introduction

In 1980, it was suggested that there might be a possible clinical application of liposomes, which are designed to release their contents in an environment such as tumour tissue with a slightly decreased pH of around 6 (1). An advanced approach of pH-sensitive liposomes is the intracellular pH-triggered release of liposome compounds from the endocytotic pathway to the cytosol.

For this purpose one should understand the cellular mechanisms of uptake and intracellular trafficking (for reviews, see refs 2–5) of colloids and particles such as liposomes. All eukaryotic cells exhibit one or more modes of endocytosis and a significant amount of liposomes is taken up into cells by one of these routes. Early concepts distinguished between phagocytosis ('eating' of particles) or pinocytosis ('drinking' of fluids). However, recent investigations have shown that it is more useful to classify the cellular uptake according to different mechanisms during the first step of the endocytotic pathway (see Figure 1).

After contact with the plasma membrane, liposomes are taken up by a separation of one part of the plasma membrane to form a vesicle, which is then interiorized into the cell (Figure 1, step 1). Three possible endocytotic mechanisms were found and classified as phagocytosis, clathrin-dependent endocytosis, or clathrin-independent endocytosis. The *plasma membrane vesicles* (PMV) have different properties depending on the mode of endocytosis.

(a) *Phagocytosis* occurs in a variety of mammalian immune cells, e.g. in macrophages. Particles opsonized by serum proteins get into contact with receptor proteins and are then caught by pseudopod extensions of the membrane. Then the vesicles are interiorized and rapidly fuse with the early endosome (EE).

(b) *Clathrin-dependent endocytosis* occurs after contact of receptors with specific ligands. After the fusion of the clathrin-coated PMV with the EE, clathrin can be recycled to the plasma membrane.

(c) *Clathrin-independent endocytosis* is found, for example, in endothelial cells. As an alternative uptake mechanism in macrophages, dendritic cells, and

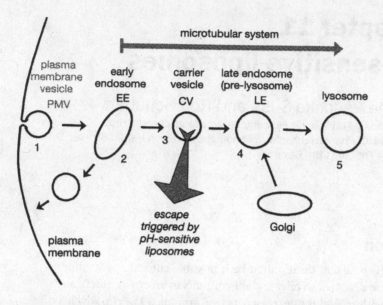

Figure 1 Pathways of endocytosed material. The uptake of particles differs mainly in the first step (1), in which plasma membrane vesicles are formed and internalized. This first step can be phagocytosis, clathrin-dependent endocytosis, or clathrin-independent endocytosis, depending on the cell type. Transport to and fusion with early endosomes is very fast. Content and membrane of EE are rapidly sorted (2) and recycled to the outside or transported in the cell with the help of the microtubular system by carrier vesicles, in which a decreased pH value can induce the release of active material from pH-sensitive liposomes into the cytosol (3). Not released material is transported to perinuclear regions, where it is exposed to even lower pH and lytic enzymes (delivered from Golgi vesicles) in late endosomes (4) and in a further step in lysosomes (5).

fibroblasts, it is defined as *macropinocytosis*, because the size of the formed PMV in these cells can be as large as 1–5 μm.

In general, the first step of the cellular uptake is independent of the microtubular system and is followed by fusion of the interiorized PMV with the *early endosome* (Figure 1, step 2). The EE is a compartment for rapid sorting of compounds such as receptor proteins, which are then recycled to the plasma membrane, and other endocytosed material such as liposomes, which are destined for the transport to the interior of the cell, i.e. to the perinuclear region. Liposomes remain in the EE only for 2–3 min, at a maximum 10 min at a slightly acidic pH of 6.8–6.3. Then they are transported by *carrier vesicles* (Figure 1, CV, step 3), actively mediated by the microtubular system, to the *late endosomes* (LE) and to the *lysosomes*. The contents of the EE are accumulated and concentrated in the LE (Figure 1, step 4). These vesicles already contain hydrolases, which are delivered by fusion with vesicles from the Golgi apparatus. LE are also called pre-lysosomes, because they are likely to initiate the degradative process of their contents, which is finished in the lysosomes (Figure 1, step 5). Before the degradation happens, liposomes, or at least their active compounds, should escape from the endosomal system to the cytosol.

The pH in the CV decreases to a value of about 5.5 within a transportation time of between 20 min and 3 h, depending on the cell type. This drop in pH is used in the concept of pH-sensitive liposomes to trigger the endosomal escape of their compounds.

2 Mechanisms of pH sensitivity

Numerous pH-sensitive liposomes (PSL) with formulations of pH-sensitive lipids or mixtures of lipids with macromolecules were developed (see Table 1) to improve the delivery of active substances to the site of action in the target cell. PSL are formed from components which adopt a lamellar phase at the physiological pH around 7.4. By decreasing the pH to a critical value, or a range around 5.5, the liposomes become fusogenic and favourably fuse with the endosomal membrane. This is the desired mechanism to release the liposomal contents into the cytosol. The predominant reason for fusogenicity is the transition from a lamellar to a hexagonal H_{II} phase, leading to a larger space of the lipophilic part of the lipid structure. Simultaneously—normally an unwanted side-effect—membrane defects occur, which result in the release of entrapped substances into the liposome-surrounding compartment, i.e. the endosome vesicle itself. Therefore, the quantification of both the drug release (see Protocol 3) and the ability to undergo membrane fusion are important in vitro tests for developing PSL. Fusion of liposomes can be monitored by fluorescence resonance energy transfer (FRET) (6, 7).

Compounds which change their molecular shape as a result of a decreased pH are needed for the desired structural changes, as shown for different lipid mixtures in Figure 2.

One possibility is that mixtures of lipids which are shaped conically and inverted conically at neutral pH, adopt an overall lamellar structure (see Figure 2). Cones have a small polar head group and take up a larger space at the hydrophobic tails. Polyunsaturated phosphatidylethanolamine has pronounced properties of this type of membrane lipids. As a single compound, it forms a lamellar phase only at a pH > 9 (8). In the pH range of interest (7.5–4.5) it is zwitterionic. In most cases dioleoylphosphatidylethanolamine (DOPE) is used, which is conically shaped even at temperatures far below 0 °C (9). As the thermal motion influences the dimension of the molecule at the hydrophobic tail, lipid mixtures with DOPE are sensitive to temperature (10).

As a second compound, an inverted conically shaped lipid, normally acidic, and containing a carboxyl group, is needed. Numerous suitable lipids have been studied in the literature (see Table 1). In this chapter only two species are discussed in great detail. One lipid of this type is cholesterolhemisuccinate (CHEMS) (11), which stabilizes the lamellar phase in DOPE/CHEMS mixtures when its amount exceeds 20 mol% (12). CHEMS itself exhibits pH-sensitive

Table 1 pH-sensitive liposomal systems (without coupled targeting molecules)

System	Lipids		Lipid molar ratio	Cationic (c) or anionic (a)	Reference
Lipid mixtures	DOPE/PHC		4:1	a	1, 39
	TPE/CHEMS		Varying	a	11, 12
	DOPE/CHEMS		1:1, 3:2	a	11, 23
			2:1, 7:3		14, 24
	DOPE/OA		7:3	a	6, 40
	DOPE/OA		4:1	a	20, 41
	DOPE/OA/Chol		4:2:4	a	20, 42
			10:5:2	a	43, 44
	ePE/OA/Chol		4:2:4	a	10, 17
	PE + ADA		Varying	a	45
	PE/DPSG		4:1	a	46
	TPE/FA		Varying	a	16
	PE/DASG		Varying	a	47
	DOPE/DOSG		1:1	a	48, 49
	POPE/Chol/THS		8:8:2	a	50
	Acid labile PE or PS derivatives			a	51
	DOPE/sulfatides		≥ 2:1	a	52
	ePC/Chol/N-SCA		9:1	c	53
	DOPE/amphipathic amines		Varying	c	37
	DOPE/DOPC/BHF		3:1:1	a	54
	DOPE/succinyl-PE or glutaryl-PE		7:3	a	55
	DC-Chol/DOPA		(4–1.6):1	a	22
	DODAC/CHEMS		< 0.8:1	a	22
	Lipids	**Additional compound**			
Lipids + biodegrad. surfactants	PC/Chol	DIP	8:2	c	56
	PC/DMPC/Chol	DIP	6:1:8	c	57
Lipids + peptides	ePC/BrPC	GALA	Varying	a	58
	PE/CHEMS	Lysteriolysine	2:1	a	59
	DOPE/DOTAP	GALA	1:1	c	60
Lipids + polymers **(a) Stable**	PC/PS	CAIPEI	4:1	c	61
	PE/FA	Polymeric PE	Varying	a	62
	ePC	PEG-COOH		a	63
	PC/Chol	GALA + polymer-COOH	Varying	a	56
	ePC/Chol	PEG-PE + al-NIPA	3:2	a	64, 65
	DOPE/CHEMS	PEG-PE	6:4	a	15
(b) Biodegradable	DOPE/CHEMS	Cleavable PEG-lipids	4:1	a	66

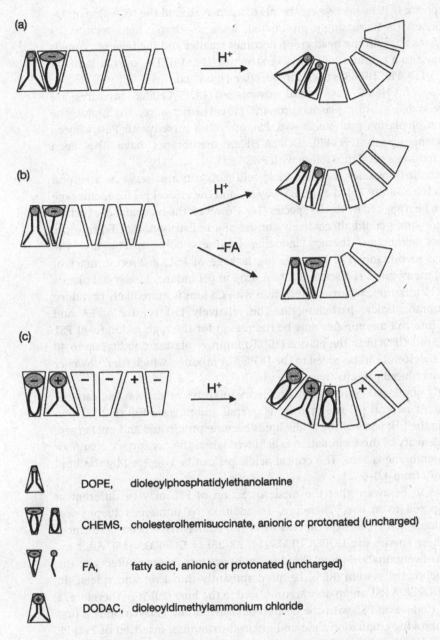

Figure 2 Transition from lamellar to non-lamellar phases in pH-sensitive lipid mixtures. Suitable conically and inverted conically shaped lipids form an overall lamellar structure at neutral pH. Deviation from lamellar membrane structure leads to fusogenicity. This structural reorganization can be induced, when anionic lipids are protonated at lower pH, thereby losing their charge and part of the hydration (a, c, and b, right upper part). In the case of fatty acids, also their release from the membrane can destabilize the lamellar phase (b, right lower part). pH-sensitive lipid mixtures can be prepared by mixtures of neutral and anionic lipids (a and b), as well as by mixtures of cationic and anionic lipids with a surplus of the latter ones (c).

polymorphism (13). By decreasing the pH to a range around the pK_a value of 5.8, the weak acid is increasingly protonated, loses its charge, and reduces its hydration. As a result, the head group becomes smaller and the inverted cone is transformed to a cylinder- or cone-like structure (11, 14). The overall lamellar structure of DOPE/CHEMS is therefore lost (see Figure 2a).

The use of CHEMS has several advantages: DOPE/CHEMS mixtures are relatively stable against plasma proteins (15). Furthermore, to inhibit the adsorption of plasma proteins *in vivo*, PSL are often mixed with PE-anchored poly(ethylene glycol) (PEG-PE). DOPE/CHEMS membranes have also been reported to have a good miscibility with PEG-PE (15).

Long chain fatty acids (FA) like oleic acid (OA) can also serve as a second compound (see Figure 2b) in a similar way (6), and the critical pH for membrane fusion can be triggered by the FA species (16). However, the mechanism of action in the endosomes could alternatively consist of a redistribution of FA into the endosome membrane, thereby inducing leakiness both in PSL and the endosomal membrane (17). For inducing leakage of PSL, a direct contact of liposomal membranes is discussed (18). A drop in pH induces hexagonal phases in DOPE/OA mixtures, whereas interaction with Ca ions is more likely to induce intramembrane lipidic particles (19). The relatively fast release of FA and insertion into cell membranes may be the reason for the high leakiness of PSL composed of DOPE/OA in the plasma (20). To improve plasma stability, up to 40 mol% of cholesterol can be added to the DOPE/OA mixture, which then however possesses a reduced pH sensitivity (21).

Recently developed systems contain binary mixtures of anionic and cationic lipids (22). At neutral pH the mixture is overall anionic (see Figure 2c). Upon decreasing the pH, parts of the acidic lipids become protonated and uncharged. Best fusogenicity of the formulation is achieved when the net surface charge of the PSL membrane is zero. The critical acidic pH can be triggered by the lipid composition from 4.0–6.7.

One has to be aware that the mode of action of PSL may be different *in vitro* compared to *in vivo*. Therefore, in addition to numerous biophysical investigations, many cell experiments or *in vivo* studies have been performed. Most of these studies use DOPE/CHEMS (14, 23–25) or DOPE/OA (15). After i.v. injection conventional pH-insensitive liposomes are rapidly distributed into the reticuloendothelial system (RES), i.e. predominantly into liver and spleen. In contrast, DOPE/OA PSL are mainly accumulated in the lung (20). It is, therefore, a challenge to develop PSL with the desired biodistribution. PEGylation is a first step to improving circulation time and organ distribution. Insertion of PEG-PE into DOPE/CHEMS stabilizes PSL against serum proteins, but it also reduces the pH sensitivity *in vitro*, as measured by the release of a marker. Surprisingly, however, the PEGylated PSL is still capable of inducing the release of compounds from the endosome into the cytosol, which is explained by phase separation of the PSL membrane prior to membrane fusion (15).

The next step in the development of a second generation of PSL is a specific targeting mediated by covalently bound ligands. Conventional coupling procedures require an activated anchor, which is inserted into the membrane during liposome preparation. In most cases the reaction partner is an amino group of the ligand (e.g. peptide or protein). If additional free amino groups on the liposome surface (e.g. lipids such as PE in PSL) are present, the reaction between the activated anchor and the neighbouring amino groups dramatically reduces the coupling efficiency of the ligand. Therefore, in the case of PSL, the ligand has to be pre-coupled to a lipid anchor and inserted into preformed PSL by a suitable measure. This can be done by disturbing the PSL membrane with an organic solvent or a detergent to facilitate the insertion of the anchor–ligand molecule (26–28). Another possibility is the choice of a lipid anchor which by itself has a high tendency to insert into the membrane (29).

In addition to PSL consisting of pH-active lipid mixtures, other formulations have recently been developed, in which surfactants or macromolecules are part of the pH-sensitive principle (see Table 1). Upon a drop in pH, a conformational change of these PSL-attached molecules results in a tendency of the membranes to become leaky or fusogenic. It has to be noted that nucleic acids can also become part of the pH-sensitive system (30).

Most of the pH-sensitive liposome formulations are anionic at physiological pH 7.4. Repulsive forces of negative charges of liposomal and cellular surfaces may reduce their interaction, which limits the cellular uptake of the liposomes. Therefore, alternative PSL with a cationic surface charge at neutral pH are in use (see Table 1).

For other aspects of PSL, see refs 31–35.

3 Methods

3.1 Preparation of pH-sensitive liposomes

In general most of the commonly used liposomal preparation techniques are suitable for the preparation of PSL as long as it is ensured that the pH does not drop to acidic values during the preparation.

As PSL are powerful delivery systems for hydrophilic compounds such as oligonucleotides and proteins, high encapsulation efficiency of the drug of interest is desired. Preparation techniques such as reversed-phase evaporation (Protocol 1) and freeze-thawing (Protocol 2) both followed by extrusion yield high encapsulation values.

Protocol 1

Encapsulation of FITC-dextran in pH-sensitive liposomes (DOPE/CHEMS, 3:2, mol/mol, 50 mM lipid, 2 ml) by reversed-phase evaporation and extrusion

Equipment and reagents

- 50 ml round-bottom flask with elongated neck
- Sonication bath
- LiposoFast® extruder (Avestin) equipped with polycarbonate membranes of 800 nm, 400 nm, and 200 nm pore size (Nuclepore)
- Gel chromatography column (Bio-Rad), 0.7 cm × 20 cm filled with Sepharose CL-4B (Pharmacia) and equilibrated with buffer

- Dioleoylphosphatidylethanolamine (DOPE), cholesterolhemisuccinate (CHEMS), and fluorescein isothiocyanate dextran (FITC-dextran, M_r 4400) (Sigma)
- HEPES buffer: 10 mM HEPES, 150 mM NaCl pH 7.4
- Ether
- FITC-HEPES buffer: 1–10 mM FITC-dextran M_r 4400 in HEPES buffer

Method

1 Prepare buffered ether by mixing 30 ml HEPES buffer with 50 ml ether and shake cautiously.

2 Dissolve 44.6 mg DOPE and 22.9 mg CHEMS in a 50 ml round-bottom flask with an elongated neck in 6 ml buffered ether (see step 1).

3 Add 2 ml FITC-HEPES buffer and sonicate the mixture for 3 min in a sonication bath.

4 Remove organic solvent by evaporation under reduced pressure. During this process a thick gel forms which collapses after some minutes. Continue the evaporation until complete removal of organic solvent.

5 Extrude the preparation with a LiposoFast extruder, first through 800 nm, then 400 nm, and finally 200 nm pore sized membranes (five times for each pore size).

6 Separate non-encapsulated FITC-dextran from liposomes by gel chromatography on a Sepharose CL-4B column.

Instead of FITC-dextran, other suitable hydrophilic drugs such as oligo-nucleotides or proteins may be used in the protocol. When using fluorescent dyes for *in vitro* and *in vivo* studies, certain aspects have to be considered. Most of the fluorescent dyes (such as calcein, FITC, HPTS, etc.) are sensitive to changes in pH. Their fluorescence intensities drop with decreasing pH. FITC-dextrans of different molecular weight can be used to follow the liposomal release and/or cellular uptake in relation to the size of the molecule.

Calcein is often used in high concentrations (> 1 mM) where fluorescence is quenched so that an increase in fluorescence signal corresponds to the release of calcein in compartments of greater volume where fluorescence is no longer quenched.

HTPS (8-hydroxy-1,3,6-pyrenetrisulfonate, synonym: pyranine) is a well known pH-sensitive fluorescent dye for distinguishing between small pH changes (14, 23). This dye has been used to follow the intracellular fate of liposomes after endocytosis. Excitation of HPTS with different wavelengths at a constant emission wavelength (λ_{em} 520 nm) leads to a conclusion about the pH of the environment. The wavelengths of 390 and 450 nm correspond to the maximum in the excitation spectrum of HPTS at acidic and neutral pH, respectively. The ratio of the λ_{exc} 450/390 nm fluorescence measured at λ_{em} 520 nm can be used to determine the pH of the probe, based on a calibration curve of the dye in buffers of differing pH (between pH 3–8). Release experiments can be performed with a combination of HPTS and DPX. Adding DPX (p-xylene-bis-pyridinium bromide) leads to a quench of fluorescence of HPTS and therefore enables the analysis of released HPTS by an increase in fluorescence.

Protocol 2

Encapsulation of HPTS or HPTS/DPX in pH-sensitive liposomes (DOPE/CHEMS, 3:2, mol/mol, 50 mM lipid, 1 ml) by freeze-thawing and extrusion

Equipment and reagents

- LiposoFast® extruder (Avestin) equipped with 200 nm membranes (Nuclepore)
- Gel chromatography columns (0.7 cm × 20 cm) filled with Sepharose CL-4B (Pharmacia) and equilibrated with buffer

- DOPE, CHEMS (Sigma), HTPS and DPX (Molecular Probes)
- HPTS-HEPES buffer: 10 mM HEPES, 150 mM NaCl, 35 mM HPTS pH 7.4
- HPTS-DPX-HEPES buffer: HPTS-HEPES buffer with 50 mM DPX

Method

1 Dissolve 22.3 mg DOPE and 11.5 mg CHEMS in a round-bottom flask in 1 ml chloroform or ethanol.

2 Remove organic solvent by evaporation and vacuum desiccation for 1 h.

3 Suspend the lipid film with 1 ml HPTS-HEPES or HPTS-DPX-HEPES buffer by sonication for 5 min in a sonication bath.

4 Freeze the preparation (transferred into a reaction tube, 1.5 ml) in liquid nitrogen and thaw for 20 min at room temperature. Repeat this procedure three times.

5 Extrude the preparation 11 times with a LiposoFast extruder through filters with 200 nm pore size.

6 Separate non-encapsulated HPTS or HPTS-DPX from liposomes by gel chromatography on a Sepharose CL-4B column.

3.2 Characterization of pH-sensitive liposomes

Characterization of PSL include size, zeta-potential, lipid concentration, degradation products, and others methods as discussed elsewhere (for details see other chapters of this book or ref. 36).

Protocol 3 describes a simple method of investigating pH sensitivity, serum stability, or the influence of any other component of interest to study their interactions with PSL.

As stability of PSL is sensitive to temperature, the experimental conditions have to be carefully considered.

Protocol 3

Stability of pH-sensitive liposomes

Equipment and reagents

- Fluorescence spectrometer and thermostated fluorescence cuvettes
- DOPE, CHEMS, and calcein (Sigma)
- Calcein-HEPES buffer: 10 mM HEPES, 150 mM NaCl, 10 mM calcein pH 7.4
- HPTS-DPX-HEPES buffer (see Protocol 2)
- Release buffers: HEPES buffer (10 mM HEPES, 150 mM NaCl) of different pH (between 5.5–8), HEPES buffer with 10% fetal calf serum or other components of interest

Method

1   Prepare liposomes according to Protocol 1 or 2 using calcein-HEPES buffer or HPTS-DPX-HEPES buffer.

2   Incubate 100 µl purified liposomes (after gel chromatography) with 2900 µl release buffer in a fluorescence cuvette.

3   Thermostat the cuvette (preferable to 37 °C).

4   Measure the fluorescence intensity of the released component at the appropriate wavelengths (calcein: λ_{exc} 494 nm, λ_{em} 524 nm; HPTS: ratio of λ_{exc} 450 nm to λ_{exc} 390 nm at λ_{em} 520 nm). As fluorescence is quenched as long as calcein or HPTS is encapsulated, an on-line analysis can be performed in the cuvette to follow the release kinetics.

3.3 Cellular association of pH-sensitive liposomes

Investigations concerning the cellular uptake and cellular trafficking are of great importance to understand the mechanisms of different delivery systems and to improve the rate of delivery. In the case of PSL, studies on endocytosis are useful to prove that fusion with endosomal membranes triggers PSL to release their contents into the cytosol. The association of liposomes and their contents with cells can be studied according to Protocol 4.

Protocol 4

Cellular association of pH-sensitive liposomes determined by microscopic techniques or FACS analysis

Equipment and reagents

- 6-well plates
- Round glass slides to fit in 6-well plates
- Coverslips
- Fluorescence or confocal microscope
- FACS analyser

- Any cell line or primary cells of interest
- Trypsin/EDTA: 0.02% EDTA containing 0.05% trypsin (w/v)
- Anti-fading media VectaShield®

Method

1   Prepare liposomes according to Protocol 1 or 2.

2   For microscopic analysis add glass slides into some of the wells.

3   Plate cells one to two days prior to incubation studies in 6-well plates (with or without glass slides) so that the cells are 50–80% confluent on the day of experiments (approx. 5×10^6 cells).

4   Change media 2 h prior to beginning incubation. Use 1 ml of the same media as for cultivation of the cells for each well. The effect of serum should be studied by using medium with and without serum.

5   Add 30 μl of purified liposomes after gel chromatography (approx. 200 nmol lipid/well) to each well.

6   Incubate liposomes with cells for the desired incubation time (i.e. 15–120 min) at 37 °C in a humidified atmosphere.

7   Remove media and wash cells twice with PBS (w/o Ca, Mg).

8   For microscopic analysis fix cells with 2% para-formaldehyde (w/v) for 20 min at room temperature. Embed the glass slides in the anti-fading medium and fix the slides on coverslips.

9   For FACS analysis trypsinate the cells with trypsin/EDTA and incubate for 5 min at 37 °C. Centrifuge the cells for 5 min at 1200 g, wash the cell pellet twice with 0.5 ml PBS. Resuspend the pellet with 0.5 ml FACS buffer and store on ice until FACS analysis (preferably count 10 000 cells per experiment).

Microscopic analysis leads to qualitative information by visualizing whether the contents are located in the cytosol, or trapped in vesicular compartments of the cell. FACS analysis offers quantitative data by counting the fluorescent cells in the cell population of the experiment. However, FACS analysis does not give any information on whether the fluorescent contents of liposomes are somehow attached to the cell membrane or internalized into the cell.

To investigate the process of endocytosis, various substances such as NH_4Cl, chloroquine, bafilomycin A1, brefeldin A, and nocodazole, that interfere with this process can be useful (37, 38).

Only small changes in Protocol 4 are required to study some aspects of endocytosis. To demonstrate which role the acidification of the endosome plays in the application of PSL, Protocol 5 uses bafilomycin A1, a specific inhibitor of vacuolar proton ATPases that blocks endosome acidification.

Protocol 5

Study on endocytosis of pH-sensitive liposomes

Equipment and reagents

- See Protocol 4
- Bafilomycin A1 (Sigma): dissolve in DMSO at 20 mM and store at –20 °C

Method

1 Follow Protocol 4, steps 1–5.

2 Prior to step 6 incubate each well for 1 h with 200 nM bafilomycin A1.

3 Add liposomes as described in step 6 and follow the protocol to the end.

Caution: It is important not to remove the substance during the study and to fix the cells immediately after removal because the function of bafilomycin is reversible within 15 min.

References

1. Yatvin, M. B., Kreutz, W., Horowitz, B. A., and Shinitzki, M. (1980). *Science*, **210**, 1253.
2. Silverstein, S. C., Steinmann, R. M., and Cohn, Z. A. (1977). *Annu. Rev. Biochem.*, **46**, 669.
3. Kelly, R. B. (1990). *Cell*, **61**, 5.
4. Mellmann, I. (1996). *Annu. Rev. Cell Dev. Biol.*, **12**, 575.
5. Düzgünes, N. and Nir, S. (1999). *Adv. Drug Deliv. Rev.*, **40**, 3.
6. Düzgünes, N., Straubinger, R. M., Baldwin, P. A., Friend, D. S., and Papahadjopoulos, D. (1985). *Biochemistry*, **24**, 3091.
7. Struck, D. K., Hoekstra, D., and Pagano, R. E. (1981). *Biochemistry*, **20**, 4093.
8. Papahadjopoulos, D. (1968). *Biochim. Biophys. Acta*, **163**, 240.
9. Cullis, P. R. and de Kruijff, B. (1979). *Biochim. Biophys. Acta*, **559**, 399.
10. Torchilin, V. P., Omelyanenko, V. G., and Lukyanov, A. N. (1992). *Anal. Biochem.*, **204**, 109.
11. Ellens, H., Benz, J., and Szoka F. C. (1984). *Biochemistry*, **23**, 1532.
12. Lai, M.-Z., Vail, W. J., and Szoka, F. C. (1985). *Biochemistry*, **24**, 1654.
13. Hafez, I. and Cullis, P. R. (2000). *Biochim. Biophys. Acta*, **1463**, 107.
14. Van Bambeke, F., Kerkhofs, A., Schanck, A., Remacle, C., Sonveaux, E., Tulkens, P. M., *et al.* (2000). *Lipids*, **35**, 213.
15. Slepushkin, A. S., Simões, S., Dazin, P., Newman, M. S., Guo, L. S., Pedroso de Lima, M. C., *et al.* (1997). *J. Biol. Chem.*, **272**, 2382.

16. Hazemoto, N., Harada, M., Komatsubara, N., Haga, M., and Kato, Y. (1990). *Chem. Pharm. Bull.*, **38**, 748.
17. Torchilin, V. P., Lukyanov, A. N., Klibanov, A. L., and Omelyanenko, V. G. (1992). *FEBS Lett.*, **305**, 185.
18. Hazemoto, N., Harada, M., Suzuki, S., Kaiho, F., Haga, M., and Kato, Y. (1993). *Chem. Pharm. Bull.*, **41**, 1003.
19. Collins, D., Connor, J., Ting-Beall, H.-P., and Huang, L. (1990). *Chem. Phys. Lipids*, **55**, 339.
20. Connor, J., Norley, N., and Huang, L. (1986). *Biochim. Biophys. Acta*, **884**, 474.
21. Liu, D. and Huang, L. (1989). *Biochim. Biophys. Acta*, **981**, 254.
22. Hafez, I., Ansell, S., and Cullis, P. R. (2000). *Biophys. J.*, **79**, 1438.
23. Chu, C.-J., Dijkstra, J., Lai, M.-Z., Hong, K., and Szoka, F. C. (1990). *Pharm. Res.*, **7**, 824.
24. Legendre, J.-Y. and Szoka, F. C. (1992). *Pharm. Res.*, **9**, 1235.
25. Lubrich, B., van Calker, D., and Peschka-Süss, R. (2000). *Eur. J. Biochem.*, **267**, 2432.
26. Wang, C.-Y. and Huang, L. (1987). *Proc. Natl. Acad. Sci. USA*, **84**, 7851.
27. Huang, L., Connor, J., and Wang, C. Y. (1987). In *Methods in enzymology*, Vol. 149 (S. Fleischer and L. Packer, eds.), p. 88. Academic Press, London.
28. Spragg, D. D., Alford, D. R., Greferath, R., Larsen, C. E., Lee, K. D., Gurtner, G. C., *et al.* (1997). *Proc. Natl. Acad. Sci. USA*, **94**, 8795.
29. Skalko, N., Peschka, R., Altenschmidt, U., Lung, A., and Schubert, R. (1998). *FEBS Lett.*, **434**, 351.
30. De Oliveira, M. C., Fattal, E., Couvreur, P., Lesieur, P., Bourgaux, C., Ollivon, M., *et al.* (1998). *Biochim. Biophys. Acta*, **1372**, 301.
31. Yatvin, M. B., Tegmo-Larsson, I.-M., and Dennis, W. H. (1987). In *Methods in enzymology*, Vol. 149 (S. Fleischer and L. Packer, eds.), p. 77. Academic Press, London.
32. Nayar, R., Fidler, I. J., and Schroit, A. J. (1988). In *Liposomes as drug carriers* (ed. G. Gregoriadis), p. 771. John Wiley & Sons Ltd.
33. Straubinger, R. M. (1993). In *Methods in enzymology*, Vol. 221 (M. G. Dennis and E. A. Dennis, eds.), p. 361. Academic Press, London.
34. Litzinger, D. C. and Huang, L. (1992). *Biochim. Biophys. Acta*, **1113**, 201.
35. Gerasimov, O. V., Boomer, J. A., Qualls, M. M., and Thompson, D. H. (1999). *Adv. Drug Deliv. Rev.*, **38**, 317.
36. New, R. R. C. (ed.) (1990). *Liposomes: a practical approach.* Oxford University Press, New York.
37. Budker, V., Gurevich, V., Hagstrom, J. E., Bortzov, F., and Wolff, J. A. (1996). *Nature Biotech.*, **14**, 760.
38. Bayer, M., Schober, D., Prchla, E., Murphy, R. F., Blaas, D., and Fuchs, R. (1998). *J. Virol.*, **72**, 9645.
39. Connor, J., Yatvin, M., and Huang, L. (1984). *Proc. Natl. Acad. Sci. USA*, **81**, 1715.
40. Straubinger, R. M., Düzgünes, N., and Papahadjopoulos, D. (1985). *FEBS Lett.*, **179**, 148.
41. Connor, J. and Huang, L. (1986). *Cancer Res.*, **46**, 3431.
42. Wang, C.-Y. and Huang, L. (1989). *Biochemistry*, **28**, 9508.
43. Ropert, C., Lavignon, M., Duberbet, C., Couvreur, P., and Malvy, C. (1992). *Biochem. Biophys. Res. Commun.*, **183**, 879.
44. Ropert, C., Malvy, C., and Couvreur, P. (1993). *Pharm. Res.*, **10**, 1427.
45. Leventis, R., Diacovo, T., and Silvius, R. (1987). *Biochemistry*, **26**, 3267.
46. Liu, D. and Huang, L. (1990). *Biochim. Biophys. Acta*, **1022**, 348.
47. Collins, D., Litzinger, D. C., and Huang, L. (1990). *Biochim. Biophys. Acta*, **1025**, 234.
48. Zhou, F., Rouse, B. T., and Huang, L. (1991). *J. Immunol. Methods*, **145**, 143.
49. Briscoe, P., Caniggia, I., Graves, A., Benson, B., Huang, L., Tanswell, A. K., *et al.* (1995). *Am. J. Physiol.*, **268**, L374.
50. Jizomoto, H., Kanaoka, E., and Hirano, K. (1994). *Biochim. Biophys. Acta*, **1213**, 343.

51. Drummond, D. C. and Daleke, D. L. (1995). *Chem. Phys. Lipids*, **75**, 27.

52. Wu, X., Lee, K. H., and Li, Q.-T. (1996). *Biochim. Biophys. Acta*, **1284**, 13.

53. Cazzola, R., Allevi, P., Cighetti, G., and Cestaro, B. (1997). *Biochim. Biophys. Acta*, **1329**, 291.

54. Jin, J. Y. and Lee, Y.-S. (1998). *Bull. Korean Chem. Soc.*, **19**, 645.

55. Lutwyche, P., Cordeiro, C., Wiseman, D. J., St.-Louis, M., Uh, M., Hope, M. J., *et al.* (1998). *Antimicrob. Agents Chemother.*, **42**, 2511.

56. Hughes, J. A., Aronsohn, A. I., Avrutskaya, A. V., and Juliano, R. L. (1996). *Pharm. Res.*, **13**, 404.

57. Liang, E. and Hughes, J. A. (1998). *J. Membr. Biol.*, **166**, 37.

58. Parente, R. A., Nadasdi, L., Subbarao, N. K., and Szoka, F. C. (1990). *Biochemistry*, **29**, 8713.

59. Lee, K.-D., Oh, Y.-K., Portnoy, D. A., and Swanson, J. A. (1996). *J. Biol. Chem.*, **271**, 7249.

60. Simoes, S., Slepushkin, V., Pires, P., Gaspar, R., Pedroso de Lima, M. C., and Düzgünes, N. (1999). *Gene Ther.*, **6**, 1798.

61. Oku, N., Shibamoto, S., Ito, F., Gondo, H., and Nango, M. (1987). *Biochemistry*, **26**, 8145.

62. Choi, M.-J., Han, H., and Kim, H. (1992). *J. Biochem.*, **112**, 694.

63. Kono, K., Igawa, T., and Takagishi, T. (1997). *Biochim. Biophys. Acta*, **1325**, 143.

64. Meyer, O., Papahadjopoulos, D., and Leroux, J.-C. (1998). *FEBS Lett.*, **421**, 61.

65. Zignani, M., Drummond, D. C., Meyer, O., Hong, K., and Leroux, J. C. (2000). *Biochim. Biophys. Acta*, **1463**, 437.

66. Kirpotin, D., Hong, K., Mullah, N., and Papahadjopoulos, D. (1996). *FEBS Lett.*, **388**, 115.

Chapter 12
Radiolabelled liposomes for imaging and biodistribution studies

Beth A. Goins and William T. Phillips

Department of Radiology, The University of Texas Health Science Center at San Antonio, Mail Code 7800, 7703 Floyd Curl Drive, San Antonio, TX 78229–3900, USA.

1 Introduction

The development of liposome-based agents for diagnostic and therapeutic applications requires an understanding of the blood clearance kinetics and tissue biodistribution of the agents after administration into the body. Non-invasive biodistribution studies of liposomes labelled with gamma (photon)-emitting radionuclides performed with scintigraphic imaging is a powerful approach for studying liposome-based agents *in vivo*. This methodology permits determination of the distribution of liposomes at multiple time points in an individual animal or patient (1, 2). While invasive studies of liposomes labelled with beta-emitting radionuclides such as carbon-14 may be suitable for animal studies, human studies with non-invasive photon imaging is a significantly more efficient approach for liposome-based drug development. Several recent examples clearly illustrate how novel insights can be gained by human scintigraphic imaging of radiolabelled liposomes (3–8). Non-invasive liposome imaging can and should be used more extensively in both liposome drug development and in clinical patient management (optimization versus individualization) (9). For a recent review of the applications of scintigraphic imaging to liposome drug development see ref. 10.

This chapter describes the methodology for conducting scintigraphic experiments by providing a review of both the instrumentation used in carrying out these studies and the techniques for labelling liposomes with radionuclides suitable for scintigraphic studies. Protocols detailing methods for radiolabelling liposomes, image acquisition and analysis, and tissue biodistribution studies are included.

2 Instrumentation for tracking radiolabelled liposomes

2.1 Gamma camera

The instrument used for the scintigraphic imaging of single photon radionuclides such as technetium-99m (^{99m}Tc) (Table 1) is known as a gamma camera (11). A diagram of an imaging procedure using a single photon radionuclide and gamma camera is shown in Figure 1 (*left panel*). Single photons require localization with collimators made of lead to determine the position of the emitted photon within the body. After passing through a lead collimator, the photon strikes a sodium iodide crystal producing a scintillation at a particular location on the crystal. This small scintillation is amplified into an electronic signal by photomultiplier tubes, converted from an analogue signal to a digital signal, and localized in an image matrix that is stored in a computer data bank. The total size of the image matrix can be varied from 64 × 64 to 512 × 512. The time necessary for acquisition of an image ranges from 2 sec to 20 min, depending on the process to be imaged and the amount of radionuclide activity administered. Image acquisition over a fixed time period allows for the summation of counts in the different matrix boxes or pixels, which produces an image of radionuclide activity within the body.

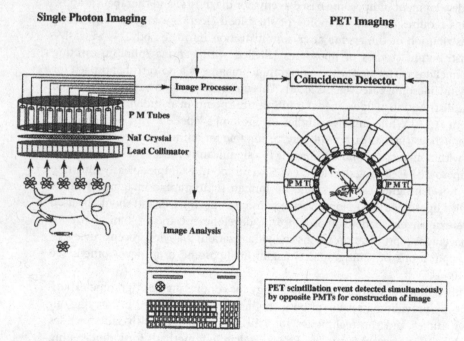

Figure 1 Diagrammatic representation of the processes involved in acquiring an image of an animal after injection of liposomes either radiolabelled with single photon radionuclides using a gamma camera (*left panel*) or positron annihilation photons using a PET camera (*right panel*). PM = photomultiplier, PMT = photomultiplier tube, NaI = sodium iodide, PET = positron emission tomography. Reprinted from ref. 10 with permission from Elsevier Science.

Table 1 Radionuclides used in scintigraphy and their application to liposome labelling

Radionuclide	Abbreviation	Half-life[a]	Photon energy[a] (keV)	Mode of production	Liposome labelling method (ref.)
Single photon radionuclides					
Gallium-67	^{67}Ga	78 h	93 (50%) 185 (30%) 300 (20%)	Cyclotron	After-loading oxine with NTA-liposomes (34); after-loading oxine with DF-liposomes (27)
Indium-111	^{111}In	67 h	173 (50%) 247 (50%)	Cyclotron	Surface chelation DTPA-fatty acid containing liposomes (22, 23); after-loading oxine with NTA-liposomes (35); after-loading ionophore A23187 with NTA-liposomes (25, 36); after- loading oxine with DF-liposomes (5, 30, 37); after-loading oxine with DTPA-liposomes (6)
Iodine-123	^{123}I	13 h	160	Cyclotron	Encapsulation of ^{131}I-sodium iodide or iodinated phospholipid during manufacture (38)
Technetium-99m	^{99m}Tc	6 h	140	Generator	Surface labelling (20, 39); surface chelation DTPA-phospholipid containing liposomes (21); surface chelation HYNIC-phospholipid containing liposomes (24); after-loading HMPAO with GSH-liposomes (26)
Thallium-201	^{201}Tl	72 h	69–81 (90%) 167 (10%)	Cyclotron	
Positron-emitting radionuclides					
Carbon-11	^{11}C	20 min	511	Cyclotron	
Fluorine-18	^{18}F	110 min	511	Cyclotron	Encapsulation of ^{18}F-FDG during manufacture (40)
Nitrogen-13	^{13}N	10 min	511	Cyclotron	
Oxygen-15	^{15}O	2 min	511	Cyclotron	Binding to haemoglobin in preformed liposomes (41, 42)
Gallium-68	^{68}Ga	66 min	511	Generator	
Rubidium-82	^{82}Rb	1.3 min	511	Generator	

[a] Data derived from ref. 43.

Although most clinical single photon images are acquired as two-dimensional planar images, three-dimensional images can be obtained with single photon imaging by rotating the gamma camera around the human or animal while acquiring a set of images at each angle. This set of images is then processed in order to reconstruct a tomographic image slice. These single photon emission computed tomography (SPECT) images provide improved localization of the source of radioactivity in the body. Small animal SPECT imaging is also possible with a special pinhole collimator (12).

2.2 Positron emission tomographic camera

Positron-emitting radionuclides produce imaging photons by emitting a positron which travels a short distance and then collides with an electron in the tissue (13). This collision results in annihilation of the positron and the electron, leading to the release of two annihilation photons that are emitted at 180° angles from each other in a straight line. Positron emission tomographic (PET) cameras, as shown in Figure 1 (*right panel*), take advantage of the two 180° photon emissions by determining a line of activity when photons are detected simultaneously on two different detectors. This simultaneous detection known as coincidence detection allows localization of the radiotracer without the need of lead collimators. The coincidence detection process is much more efficient for localization of the radionuclide activity than single photon imaging so that many more photons are detected per a given amount of radioactivity than with single photon imaging, resulting in a higher quality, higher resolution image compared to a single photon image. This higher efficiency is due to the fact that a filtering lead collimator is not required. Detection of multiple lines of activity at different angles from the same source permits the construction of a three-dimensional PET image. Although the short half-life of positron-emitting radionuclides is a disadvantage associated with PET imaging, particularly for the radiolabelling of liposomes, PET has the advantage of being an efficient imaging process that provides high resolution images while also permitting the study of biologically important molecules (Table 1). The recent development of a commercially available dedicated small animal PET camera promises to accelerate drug research (14). Three-dimensional images provided by the dedicated small animal PET cameras have much higher resolution than is possible with large bore PET cameras currently in use for human imaging. A drawback of PET imaging technology is that it is not as widely available because it is significantly more expensive than single photon technology.

2.3 Gamma well counter

A gamma well counter is the most basic instrument used to determine the amount of radioactivity in a sample. Tubes containing the sample are placed in a scintillation well which is a chamber within a sodium iodide crystal. Scintillations emitted from either single photon agents or positron annihilation photons are detected, and the number of scintillations over a fixed time period are recorded. The system can be automated when large numbers of samples must be counted. To determine the distribution of radioactivity within an animal's body, tissues of interest are collected and placed in separate tubes for counting. Although a tissue biodistribution study is the most quantitatively accurate method for determining the distribution of radionuclides within the body, it requires that an animal be sacrificed and its organs be removed. In general practice, a tissue biodistribution study is usually performed only after prior serial scintigraphic imaging as a method of validating the data derived non-invasively from scintigraphic imaging. Gamma well tissue counting allows for the determination of the percentage of the administered dose per gram of tissue, which can be important for certain drug delivery applications.

The investigator using a particular gamma well counter should be very familiar with its function so that inaccurate counts are not obtained. Ideally, each investigator should perform a study with known standards to determine such factors as the maximum count rate that permits accurate results (saturation), and the maximum amount of tissue that can be counted before the size of the sample is not completely within the counting chamber (geometry). Exceeding the count rate limit or the geometry size limit will result in artefactually reduced counts. An excellent review of the various factors involved in the use of a gamma well counter can be found in ref. 15.

3 Methods for labelling liposomes with gamma-emitting radionuclides

3.1 General overview

The last decade has brought considerable progress in the development of liposome labelling techniques for imaging and biodistribution studies. The most successful of these techniques have many of the following characteristics:

(a) Liposomes are easily labelled independent of their size, surface charge, or lipid composition.

(b) Liposomes can be labelled with radionuclides that are readily available, and have good dosimetric, half-life, and photon energy imaging characteristics.

(c) Previously manufactured liposomes are conveniently labelled in a short time period (< 30 min) and at room temperature with high efficiency.

(d) The label remains with liposomes after injection into the body, and once the labelled liposomes are metabolized, the majority of the label remains at its initial site of retention.

Figure 2 depicts the most common techniques for labelling liposomes with gamma-emitting radionuclides. Liposomes can be radiolabelled either during manufacture or after manufacture and storage (preformed).

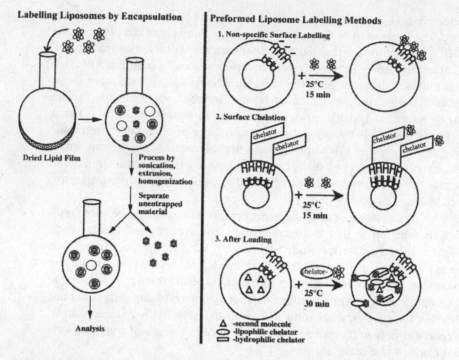

Labelling Liposomes by Encapsulation

Dried Lipid Film

Process by sonication, extrusion, homogenization

Separate unentrapped material

Analysis

Preformed Liposome Labelling Methods

1. Non-specific Surface Labelling

25°C
15 min

2. Surface Chelation

chelator
chelator

25°C
15 min

chelator
chelator

3. After Loading

chelator-

25°C
30 min

△ -second molecule
○ -lipophilic chelator
▭ -hydrophilic chelator

Figure 2 Diagrammatic representation of the methods for radiolabelling liposomes either by encapsulation during manufacture (*left panel*) or after manufacture and storage (*right panel*).

3.2 Radionuclides available for liposome labelling methods

Table 1 lists the most common radionuclides currently used in a clinical setting. Table 1 also summarizes the use of these radionuclides in liposome labelling procedures. The development of new methods for labelling liposomes with both single photon and positron-emitting radionuclides are under investigation.

Single photon radionuclides are the most widely used radionuclides in current clinical nuclear medicine procedures because these radionuclides are readily available and relatively inexpensive. These single photon radionuclides have widely varying half-lives of activity and photon energies (Table 1). The most commonly used clinical radionuclide, ^{99m}Tc, has a half-life of 6 h which permits imaging up to 48 h after injection. ^{99m}Tc is particularly ideal for single photon imaging because its photon energy characteristics and half-life permit generation of the highest quality images currently possible for single photon radionuclides. Also since ^{99m}Tc is produced using a nuclear reactor-derived generator rather than a cyclotron, it is readily available and inexpensive. These attributes of ^{99m}Tc have made it the radionuclide of choice for liposome labelling procedures in the past decade.

Compared to single photon radionuclides, positron-emitting radionuclides tend to have much shorter half-lives (< 2 h) (Table 1), which requires that their site of production must be near their site of usage. While the single photon radionuclides are all heavy elements, most positron-emitting radionuclides are important low molecular weight biological atoms.

3.3 Methods for labelling liposomes using radionuclides

Many methods have been developed for labelling liposomes with gamma-emitting radionuclides for use in scintigraphic imaging (Figure 2) (16, 17). Without the development of these labelling methods, the use of scintigraphy in liposome-based drug research would not be feasible. Only a brief discussion of the methods for the labelling of liposomes will be provided in this chapter since several extensive reviews have been published (16, 17).

3.3.1 Encapsulation

Figure 2 (*left panel*) depicts the typical steps for labelling liposomes by simply encapsulating the radionuclide during manufacture. The encapsulation method, which includes processing, separation, and analysis steps, would take longer than is practical for labelling liposomes with many radionuclides with half-lives under 24 h such as ^{99m}Tc and fluorine-18 (^{18}F). A better approach is the labelling of liposomes after their manufacture and just prior to use. The only method reported to date for labelling liposomes with a positron-emitting radionuclide is the encapsulation of [^{18}F]fluorodeoxyglucose (^{18}F-FDG) within liposomes during liposome manufacture (18).

3.3.2 Non-specific surface labelling

In the non-specific surface labelling method, the liposome membrane is non-specifically labelled with a radionuclide such as reduced ^{99m}Tc (Figure 2, *right panel*). This method proved to produce ^{99m}Tc-labelled liposomes that were not stable when injected *in vivo*, with frequent dissociation of the ^{99m}Tc from the liposome after administration (19, 20).

3.3.3 Surface chelation

In the surface chelation method (Figure 2, *right panel*), a chelator with high affinity for the radionuclide is covalently attached to the head group of a phospholipid such as distearoylphosphatidylethanolamine. This phospholipid chelator is then added to the liposome formulation during manufacture. The radionuclide is then incubated with the chelator–liposomes where it attaches to the chelator on the liposome surface. Various radionuclide-chelator pairs have been used for labelling liposomes, with the most research using either ^{99m}Tc or indium-111 (^{111}In) with diethylenetriamine pentaacetic acid (DTPA) (21–23). The most successful surface chelation method to date has been reported by Laverman *et al.* (24) using the hydrazino nicotinamide (HYNIC) chelator with ^{99m}Tc.

3.3.4 After-loading

The third method of labelling preformed liposomes is known as the after-loading method because the radionuclide is loaded into the liposome interior at some future time following the manufacture and storage of the liposomes (Figure 2, *right panel*). In this method, a radionuclide is incubated with a lipophilic chelator and then mixed with an aliquot of liposomes encapsulating a second molecule. Once the lipophilic chelator carries the radionuclide across the lipid bilayer, the second molecule interacts with the radionuclide-chelator causing the radionuclide to become trapped within the interior of the liposome. This interaction may be due to the second molecule having a higher affinity for the radionuclide than the original lipophilic chelator. An alternative labelling mechanism is that the lipophilic chelator is converted from the lipophilic form to a hydrophilic form after interaction with the second molecule. Since the hydrophilic form cannot cross back through the lipid bilayer, it becomes trapped in the liposome interior. Effective after-loading methods for the post-manufacture labelling of liposomes have been reported with the single photon agents, ^{99m}Tc, ^{111}In, and gallium-67 (^{67}Ga) (25–27). An example of this method is the labelling of liposomes with ^{99m}Tc using the lipophilic chelator, hexamethylpropyleneamine oxime (HMPAO) (Protocol 1) (26). Lipophilic HMPAO enters the liposome where it interacts with reduced glutathione (GSH) and becomes converted to the hydrophilic form, which is trapped in the liposome. All of the materials needed for performing this labelling protocol are commercially available.

Protocol 1

Labelling liposomes with ^{99m}Tc using glutathione-HMPAO after-loading method[a,b]

Equipment and reagents

- Laminar flow hood[c]
- Lead shielding (BIODEX Medical Systems)
- Sephadex G-25 disposable columns (PD-10, Amersham Pharmacia Biotech)[d]
- Dose calibrator (Capintec)
- HMPAO quality control chromatography (BIODEX Medical Systems)
- Paper chromatography strips, 13 cm × 1 cm (Schleicher and Schuell, No. 589)

- Gamma well counter (Canberra, Packard, Perkin Elmer Life Sciences)
- Dulbecco's phosphate-buffered saline (PBS) without Mg^{2+} and Ca^{2+}, pH 6.3, degassed (Sigma)[e]
- Sodium ^{99m}Tc-pertechnetate (Nycomed Amersham, Syncor)[f]
- HMPAO kit, unstabilized (Ceretec™, Nycomed Amersham)[g]
- Liposome preparation[h]

A. Labelling procedure

1 Prepare a lead shielded area in the hood for the sterile radiolabelling and separation procedures.

2 Prepare a Sephadex G-25 column by passing 25 ml of PBS over the column.

3 Pipette 2 ml of the liposome preparation into a tube.

Protocol 1 continued

4 Prepare the HMPAO by adding 5 ml of sodium ^{99m}Tc-pertechnetate in saline to a vial of unstabilized HMPAO. Mix the vial and incubate for 5 min.

5 To label the liposomes, draw the ^{99m}Tc-HMPAO into a syringe and add 2 ml of the ^{99m}Tc-HMPAO to the liposome sample (2 ml). Incubate the ^{99m}Tc-HMPAO/liposome mixture for 15–30 min at room temperature.

6 Immediately after adding the ^{99m}Tc-HMPAO to the liposome preparation, remove a separate aliquot of the ^{99m}Tc-HMPAO and perform the quality control chromatography as described in the HMPAO kit instructions to make certain that the ^{99m}Tc-HMPAO is in the lipophilic form.

B. Column chromatography for separation of free ^{99m}Tc-label from ^{99m}Tc-liposomes and assessment of percentage labelling efficiency

1 Drain any remaining PBS from the Sephadex G-25 column reservoir (part A).

2 Pipette 2.5 ml of the ^{99m}Tc-HMPAO/liposome mixture onto the top of the column (sample loaded on column).

3 Reserve an aliquot (1.5 ml) of the ^{99m}Tc-HMPAO/liposome mixture before passing over the column and accurately measure the volume with a pipette (reserved aliquot).

4 Once the liposomes have completely entered the column packing, add the PBS elution buffer to the column reservoir.

5 The ^{99m}Tc-liposomes will be eluted in the void volume. Collect the ^{99m}Tc-liposomes in a new sterile tube as soon as you see a slight milky eluate coming out of the column and stop when the eluate becomes clear again.[i]

6 Measure the ^{99m}Tc-activity of the post-column ^{99m}Tc-liposome fraction and of the reserved aliquot in a dose calibrator.

7 Calculate the percentage labelling efficiency using the following formula:

$$\frac{\%\text{ labelling}}{\text{efficiency}} = \frac{(\text{mCi in post-column sample})\,(\text{volume of reserved aliquot})}{(\text{mCi in reserved aliquot})\,(\text{volume of sample loaded on column})} \times 100.$$

In our example, the volume of sample loaded onto the column would be 2.5 ml and the volume of the reserved aliquot would be 1.5 ml.

C. Assessment of percentage labelling efficiency using paper chromatography[j]

1 Using a pencil, mark a line 2 cm from the bottom (origin) and 1 cm from the top (solvent front) of a No. 589 paper strip. Also mark a line 7 cm from the bottom of the strip.

2 Prepare a development tank by adding a small amount of 0.9% saline to cover the bottom of the tank.

Protocol 1 continued

3   Apply an aliquot (10 μl) of the ^{99m}Tc-HMPAO-liposome mixture (reserved aliquot) on the origin of the strip.

4   Place strip in the tank containing 0.9% saline, making sure that the saline level is below the origin.

5   Allow the saline to rise up the paper until it reaches the solvent front.

6   Once saline has reached the solvent front, remove the paper from the tube with forceps.

7   Cut the paper at the 7 cm line and place each half in a separate clean tube.

8   Determine the ^{99m}Tc-activity of the top and bottom fractions using a gamma well counter. For most liposome formulations, the ^{99m}Tc-liposomes will remain at the origin.

9   Calculate percentage labelling efficiency using the following equation:

$$\% \text{ labelling efficiency} = \frac{\text{c.p.m. in bottom portion}}{(\text{c.p.m. in top portion} + \text{c.p.m. in bottom portion})} \times 100.$$

[a] Based on the method reported in ref. 26.

[b] The procedure described in this protocol is for labelling 2 ml of liposome preparation. The protocol can be scaled up proportionally according to the amount of liposomes you wish to label. The maximum amount of liposomes that can be loaded per column is 2.5 ml, but multiple columns can be used.

[c] For a sterile radiolabelled liposome product suitable for *in vivo* imaging studies, the labelling procedure is normally performed in a laminar flow hood using aseptic technique and sterile tubes. Disposable syringes, needles, and pipettes are also used.

[d] Alternatively, columns can be prepared in-house by pouring swollen Sephadex G-25 in columns.

[e] Technetium-99m is very sensitive to the presence of oxygen. The buffer used for the labelling procedure should be purged with nitrogen for 15–20 min to remove dissolved oxygen. If possible, liposomes should also be prepared in buffer that has been purged with nitrogen. Liposomes can also be labelled in PBS with higher pH (7.4), 0.9% saline, or other buffer systems.

[f] A local radiopharmacy can supply the ^{99m}Tc-pertechnetate as a single dose by eluting from a technetium generator. If your research facility does not have access to a radiopharmacy, a technetium generator can be purchased and eluted in-house. Irregardless of the source of ^{99m}Tc-pertechnetate, it is very important that the generator has been eluted within the past 24 h before obtaining the ^{99m}Tc-pertechnetate for reconstitution with the HMPAO vial because older ^{99m}Tc-pertechnetate eluate will contain an excessive amount of technetium-99, which is a decay product of ^{99m}Tc that will compete with ^{99m}Tc during the ^{99m}Tc-HMPAO binding reaction (28). For HMPAO labelling, ^{99m}Tc-pertechnetate is normally supplied in a syringe containing a 10–15 mCi (370–555 MBq) dose of sodium ^{99m}Tc-pertechnetate in 5 ml of 0.9% saline. If a higher specific activity is needed, the procedure can be performed with higher doses (30–50 mCi, 1.11–1.85 GBq) of ^{99m}Tc-pertechnetate or by using smaller volumes (1–2 ml) of saline to elute the ^{99m}Tc-pertechnetate from the generator.

g Carefully read the package instructions before attempting the liposome labelling protocol because the HMPAO is only useful for liposome labelling for 30 min after reconstitution. Package instructions for leukocyte labelling using unstabilized product should be followed, not those for brain imaging using the methylene blue stabilized product.

h For successful labelling, liposomes should be prepared in the presence of GSH. It is important that all unentrapped GSH be removed prior to the labelling procedure.

i Occasionally you will see a tailing of the liposomes toward the end of the collection period. When this occurs, stop the collection. The column separation normally increases the volume of the loaded sample by 1.4 times the initial volume.

j Modified from the method given in ref. 29.

4 Characterization of radiolabelled liposomes

4.1 *In vitro* radiolabel stability evaluation

Radiolabel stability should be evaluated *in vitro* by:

(a) Incubating the radiolabelled liposomes in buffer at room temperature to verify a prolonged stable attachment of the radionuclide to the liposomes.

(b) Incubating the radiolabelled liposomes in serum or plasma at 37 °C to mimic body conditions.

In general, radionuclide attachment of most commonly used radiopharmaceuticals remains stable *in vitro* for about 6 h. Radionuclide-liposome attachment should also remain stable for several hours. Prolonged radionuclide attachment is advantageous because the radiolabelled liposomes can be prepared ahead of time so that they are readily available when needed for a study. Another advantage of prolonged radionuclide attachment is that image quality is improved because the presence of dissociated label can degrade the image once the radiolabelled liposomes are injected into the body. Evaluation of radionuclide-liposome attachment is normally carried out by monitoring radionuclide label dissociation using the same chromatography techniques as described in Protocol 1B and 1C. *In vitro* serum stability evaluation is also important because the radionuclide label must remain securely attached to the liposomes after injection in the body. If not, the altered circulation clearance pattern of the dissociated radionuclide can lead to an incorrect assessment of the liposome biodistribution. A good technique for separating the radiolabelled liposome fraction from serum proteins after incubation has been described using a spin column system (21, 30, 31).

4.2 *In vivo* radiolabel evaluation

In vivo radiolabel stability can be assessed by visual review of the early images (0–2 h). One clear indicator of *in vivo* dissociation of the radionuclide label from the liposome is the appearance of radioactivity in the kidneys and bladder, since liposomes do not deposit to any degree in these organs. Whenever possible, serial blood samples should also be collected during the imaging study and counted in a gamma well counter. A more rapid than anticipated decline in the blood activity is also an indicator of *in vivo* radiolabel dissociation.

5 Image acquisition and analysis methods

Protocol 2 describes the general technique for performing a non-invasive bio-distribution study in an animal intravenously injected with radiolabelled liposomes. An intravenous route of administration is the most common for approved liposome drugs, but these methods are very versatile and can be adapted for other administration routes such as intracavitary, intramuscular, subcutaneous, and local administration. This imaging and analysis method without the tissue biodistribution study (Protocol 3) can also be applied to human studies (4–8).

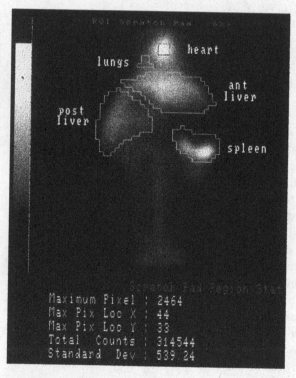

Figure 3 Image of a rabbit acquired 120 min after intravenous injection of ^{99m}Tc-labelled liposome encapsulated haemoglobin demonstrating the methodology used for quantitation of scintigraphic images. Region-of-interest (ROI) boxes are placed on various organs and the total counts in a region displayed. Images acquired at various times are analysed using this methodology to determine the percentage of injected dose that accumulates in the various organs. ant = anterior, post = posterior.

One of most powerful attributes of scintigraphic imaging is that it is inherently quantitative. In addition, scintigraphy is a computer-based system so software has been developed to perform a variety of analysis options. The most common analysis tool is the region-of-interest (ROI) analysis which determines the number of counts in a designated area in an image after being highlighted by the investigator. ROIs can generally be obtained for the liver, spleen, lung, and around a specifically targeted region such as tumour or infection. Figure 3 depicts an image after ROI analysis has been performed. Clearance from the blood can also be estimated by placing a fixed box region over the heart as shown in Figure 3, because the normal heart does not have a significant deposition of radiolabelled liposomes. Generally, counts in the heart ROI correlate with the clearance of the liposomes from the blood.

When the data for each organ has been corrected for decay and for background counts, a time–activity curve can be generated for the organ of interest. Most image analysis systems will automatically generate this curve if the images have been acquired dynamically as shown in Figure 4. This curve provides a fairly accurate estimation of the amount of radioactivity in the organ over time. From this data, an estimation of the percentage of the total injected dose (%ID) in each organ can be made. In human studies, the appropriate volume of the organ or targeted region can be estimated by computed tomography or magnetic resonance imaging so that a %ID/kg of tissue can be estimated (6).

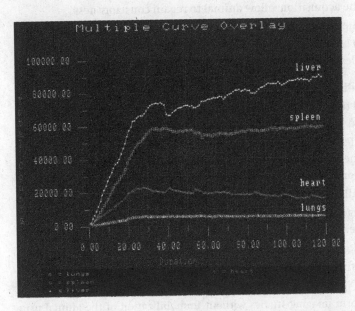

Figure 4 Time–activity curves (total counts in a region versus time) that were generated from region-of-interest (ROI) analysis of various organs drawn in image depicted in Figure 3. The [99mTc]-labelled liposome encapsulated haemoglobin (LEH) was infused over 30 min. After 30 min, the activity in the heart ROI begins to gradually decrease as the [99mTc]-LEH is cleared from the blood, while the activity in the liver increases.

Protocol 2

Imaging study in animals following intravenous injection of radiolabelled liposomes

Equipment and reagents

- Gamma camera with computer workstation (ADAC, Marconi, Siemens)
- Animals
- Anaesthesia[a]
- Radiolabelled liposomes (see Protocol 1)

A. Image acquisition

1. Verify that the gamma camera is calibrated.
2. Set up computer workstation for acquisition and give the study a unique file name so images can be retrieved after acquisition.[b]
3. Anaesthetize animal and insert catheter in a vein for infusion of the radiolabelled liposomes.[c]
4. Position animal under gamma camera so that images of the area of interest will be acquired.[d]
5. Inject radiolabelled liposomes and activate the computer to begin image acquisition.[e]
6. Acquire images for as often and for as long as desired.[f]
7. After completion of the acquisition, allow animal to regain consciousness.
8. Re-administer anaesthesia and perform image acquisition at all time points desired.
9. After the final images have been acquired, a tissue biodistribution study (Protocol 3) can be performed, if desired.[g]

B. ROI analysis of images

1. Draw a region around the organs of interest, typically the liver, spleen, heart, lungs, or specifically targeted location, i.e. tumour or infection, and matching background regions for each time point an image is acquired.[h]
2. Place a box around the whole animal if possible on the first image acquired after liposome infusion is completed.[i]
3. Record the counts in all ROIs.
4. Decay correct the images to the time of the initial image based on the physical half-life of the radionuclide.
5. Correct counts for background and organ blood pool contribution where appropriate.[j]
6. Analyse data by plotting as percentage of total counts after liposome infusion, target-to-background, statistical comparison, etc.[k]

[a] It is very difficult to perform imaging studies without immobilization of the animal using appropriate anaesthesia. The anaesthesia chosen will depend on the length of each image acquisition session. For short imaging sessions, 2–3% isoflurane (Abbott Laboratories) in 100% oxygen is ideal. For longer sessions, rabbits and rats can be intramuscularly injected with ketamine/xylazine (Phoenix Scientific, Inc.) (50 mg/kg:10 mg/kg).

Protocol 2 continued

[b] Images can be acquired either in a static or dynamic mode. A common dynamic image acquisition method is to acquire 1 min images for the first 1–2 h after liposome administration. The camera matrix is set in a matrix size appropriate to the count rate, typically 64×64. Images can also be zoomed.

[c] Typical locations for catheter placement are in the tail vein of rats or ear vein of rabbits. In certain situations, it may be useful to surgically place an indwelling catheter in a large vessel several days prior to the day of the imaging study. A catheter can also be placed in an ear artery of rabbits for blood sampling to determine circulation half-lives.

[d] For small animals such as rats and mice, the camera head is facing up and the animal is laid in the prone position directly on top of the camera head. For larger animals, the camera head is positioned over the animal and the animal is typically in the supine position on an imaging table.

[e] The rate of infusion may be varied depending on the quantity to be infused. Small quantities relative to the weight of the animal are generally infused manually through a syringe while larger quantities may be infused over a slower time period using a syringe pump.

[f] This time can vary depending on the physical half-life of the radionuclide used to label the liposomes and the rate of clearance of the liposomes from the blood. This time period can be determined by visual image assessment to estimate the best time of terminating the study and performing a tissue biodistribution study.

[g] Tissue biodistribution is generally performed at the end of a study to validate the results of the imaging study.

[h] One method is to draw a region around the organs of interest. This permits a global assessment of total organ deposition. A second method is to place fixed size boxes on the organ of interest to observe the changes in counts in the box of that organ over time. The fixed box is less subjective but it only indicates the pattern of uptake of the liposomes over time, while the drawing of regions around the whole organ provides a better estimate of total organ uptake at each time point. Regions can only be drawn around large organs that can be clearly distinguished on the images. For liposome imaging, this is generally the liver, spleen, and heart. Depending on the size of the animal being imaged, it may also be possible to place a region over the lungs to provide an estimate of lung uptake of the liposomes. Regions can also be drawn over the femur to provide an estimation of liposome uptake in the bone marrow.

[i] The standard by which all the regions can be compared is obtained by drawing a large box, if possible, over the whole body image of the animal on the first image acquired immediately after all of the radiolabelled liposomes have been infused. This provides an estimation of the total detectable counts in the injected dose.

[j] If the counts in the images to be analysed are low in comparison to the natural background radiation, a background correction should be performed. This can be performed by determining the background counts per pixel from a ROI placed adjacent to the animal's body and subtracting these counts from each pixel in the ROI. Background correction becomes important on late images (> 12 h after injection) that require a long acquisition time in order to acquire an adequate image. Some organs such as the liver contain a substantial pool of blood. The activity in these organs may need to be corrected for this blood pool activity by subtracting the estimated blood pool activity of each organ region. The activity in the blood can be determined by counting blood samples at each time point in the gamma well counter. The percentage of the blood pool can be determined by performing a study with labelled red blood cells and recording the percentage of labelled red blood cell activity in each organ or by using reported organ blood pool contribution data. This technique is described in detail by Rudolph *et al.* (32).

[k] In many situations it may be useful to compare the liposome accumulation in a targeted site to a control site. For example, target-to-background analysis may be used to compare liposome uptake in a tumour located in the thigh to the normal contralateral thigh.

6 Tissue biodistribution method using gamma well counter

Traditionally, tissue biodistribution studies have used beta-emitting radionuclides, which cannot be detected by scintigraphic imaging. These traditional studies require the use of many more animals because animals must be sacrificed at each desired time point. A better approach using fewer animals is described in Protocol 3. In Protocol 3, the tissue biodistribution is used to validate the imaging results and performed only after images have been acquired at the final time point. All other biodistribution information is determined from the non-invasive imaging study.

Protocol 3

Tissue biodistribution study of animals after intravenous injection of radiolabelled liposomes

Equipment and reagents

- Surgical instruments
- Gamma well counter (Canberra, Packard, Perkin Elmer Life Sciences)
- Animals injected with radiolabelled liposomes (see Protocol 2A)[a]

Method

1 Weigh enough tubes so that each tissue sample can be placed in a separate tube and record the weights.

2 After acquiring images at the last desired time point or at the designated time point if performing no imaging, euthanize the animal.

3 Collect the tissues of interest, rinse with saline, and place each tissue sample in a separate weighed tube. Also remove the entire organ and weigh.

4 Weigh each of the tubes containing the tissue samples and record the weights.

5 Measure the radioactivity of each tissue sample and reserved standard sample in a gamma well counter, and record the results.[b]

6 Enter the weight and radioactive data in a spreadsheet.

7 Calculate the percentage of injected dose in the organ (%ID/organ) as follows:[c]

$$\text{\%ID/organ} = \frac{(\text{c.p.m. in tissue sample/sample weight}) \times \text{total weight of organ}}{(\text{c.p.m. in standard/volume of standard}) \times \text{volume of sample injected}} \times 100.$$

8 Calculate the percentage of injected dose per gram of tissue (%ID/g tissue) as follows:

$$\text{\%ID/g tissue} = \frac{(\text{c.p.m. in tissue sample/sample weight})}{(\text{c.p.m. in standard/volume of standard}) \times \text{volume of sample injected}} \times 100.$$

Protocol 3 continued

[a] A standard of a known percentage of the injected dose should be saved for counting so that total counts injected can be calculated. The standard should be counted in the same approximate volume as the volume of the tissue samples.

[b] It is important that the samples be allowed to decay until the count rates are below the saturation count rate of the gamma well counter. Samples should also be distributed as homogeneously as possible and be distributed so that they do not exceed the geometric size limit of the gamma well counter. These factors are best determined experimentally by the investigator prior to performing tissue biodistribution studies.

[c] For tissues that are not discrete organs such as skin, muscle, and blood, an estimation of the total weight of these tissues in the body can be estimated from the body weight of the animal using previously determined correction factors (33).

References

1. Bhatnagar, A., Hustinex, R., and Alavi, A. (2000). *Adv. Drug Deliv. Rev.*, **41**, 41.
2. Saleem, A., Aboagye, E. O., and Price, P. M. (2000). *Adv. Drug Deliv. Rev.*, **41**, 21.
3. Dams, E. T. and Corstens, F. H. (1999). *Eur. J. Nucl. Med.*, **26**, 311.
4. Dams, E. T. M., Oyen, W. J. G., Boerman, O. C., Storm, G., Laverman, P., Kok, P. J. M., et al. (2000). *J. Nucl. Med.*, **41**, 622.
5. Gabizon, A., Chisin, R., Amselem, S., Druckmann, S., Cohen, R., Goren, D., et al. (1991). *Br. J. Cancer*, **64**, 1125.
6. Harrington, K. J., Mohammadtaghi, S., Uster, P. S., Glass, D., Peters, A. M., Vile, R. G., et al. (2001). *Clin. Cancer Res.*, **7**, 243.
7. Laverman, P., Brouwers, A. H., Dams, E. T. M., Oyen, W. J. G., Storm, G., Rooijen, N. V., et al. (2000). *J. Pharmacol. Exp. Ther.*, **293**, 996.
8. Presant, C. A., Ksionski, G., and Crossley, R. (1990). *J. Liposome Res.*, **1**, 431.
9. Wolf, W. (2000). *Adv. Drug Deliv. Rev.*, **41**, 1.
10. Goins, B. A. and Phillips, W. T. (2001). *Prog. Lipid Res.*, **40**, 95.
11. Graham, L. S. and Muehllehner, G. (1996). In *Diagnostic nuclear medicine* (ed. M. P. Sandler), Vol. 1, p. 81. Williams & Wilkins, Baltimore.
12. Green, M. V., Seidel, J., Vaquero, J. J., Jagoda, E., Lee, I., and Eckelman, W. C. (2001). *Comput. Med. Imaging Graph.*, **25**, 79.
13. Cherry, S. R. and Phelps, M. E. (1996). In *Diagnostic nuclear medicine* (ed. M. P. Sandler), Vol. 1, p. 139. Williams & Wilkins, Baltimore.
14. Phelps, M. E. (2000). *J. Nucl. Med.*, **41**, 661.
15. Early, P. J. and Sodee, D. B. (1995). *Principles and practice of nuclear medicine*, 2nd edn, p. 877. Mosbyl, St. Louis, MO.
16. Phillips, W. and Goins, B. (1995). In *Handbook of targeted delivery of imaging agents* (ed. V. P. Torchilin), p. 149. CRC Press, Boca Raton, FL.
17. Phillips, W. T. (1999). *Adv. Drug Deliv. Rev.*, **37**, 13.
18. Oku, N. (1999). *Adv. Drug Deliv. Rev.*, **37**, 53.
19. Patel, H. M., Boodle, K. M., and Vaughan-Jones, R. (1984). *Biochim. Biophys. Acta*, **801**, 76.
20. Barratt, G. M., Tuzel, N. S., and Ryman, B. E. (1984). In *Liposome technology* (ed. G. Gregoriadis), Vol. 2, p. 94. CRC Press, Boca Raton, FL.
21. Ahkong, Q. F. and Tilcock, C. (1992). *Nucl. Med. Biol.*, **19**, 831.
22. Holmberg, E., Maruyama, K., Litzinger, D. C., Wright, S., Davis, M., Kabalka, G. W., et al. (1989). *Biochem. Biophys. Res. Commun.*, **165**, 1272.

23. Klibanov, A., Maruyama, K., Torchilin, V. P., and Huang, L. (1990). *FEBS Lett.*, **268**, 235.

24. Laverman, P., Dams, E., Oyen, W., Storm, G., Koenders, E., Prevost, R., *et al.* (1999). *J. Nucl. Med.*, **40**, 192.

25. Proffitt, R., Williams, L., Presant, C., Tin, G., Uliana, J., Gamble, R., *et al.* (1983). *J. Nucl. Med.*, **24**, 45.

26. Phillips, W. T., Rudolph, A. S., Goins, B., Timmons, J. H., Klipper, R., and Blumhardt, R. (1992). *Nucl. Med. Biol.*, **19**, 539.

27. Gabizon, A., Huberty, J., Straubinger, R. M., Price, D. C., and Papahadjpulos, D. (1988). *J. Liposome Res.*, **1**, 123.

28. Saha, G. B. (1998). *Fundamentals of nuclear pharmacy*, 4th edn, p. 358. Springer–Verlag, New York.

29. New, R. R. C. (ed.) (1990). In *Liposomes: a practical approach*, 1st edn, p. 265. IRL Oxford University Press, Oxford.

30. Awasthi, V. D., Goins, B., Klipper, R., and Phillips, W. T. (1998). *Nucl. Med. Biol.*, **25**, 155.

31. Chonn, A., Semple, S. C., and Cullis, P. R. (1991). *Biochim. Biophys. Acta*, **1070**, 215.

32. Rudolph, A. S., Klipper, R. W., Goins, B., and Phillips, W. T. (1991). *Proc. Natl. Acad. Sci. USA*, **88**, 10976.

33. Frank, D. W. (1976). In *Handbook of laboratory animal science* (ed. E. C. Melby, Jr.), Vol. 3, p. 23. CRC Press, Boca Raton, FL.

34. Ogihara, I., Kojima, S., and Jay, M. (1986). *J. Nucl. Med.*, **27**, 1300.

35. Hwang, K. J., Merriam, J. E., Beaumier, P. L., and Luk, K. S. (1982). *Biochim. Biophys. Acta*, **716**, 101.

36. Mauk, M. R. and Gamble, R. C. (1979). *Anal. Biochem.*, **94**, 302.

37. Boerman, O. C., Storm, G., Oyen, W. J. G., van Bloois, L., van der Meer, J. W. M., Claessens, R. A. M. J., *et al.* (1995). *J. Nucl. Med.*, **36**, 1639.

38. Hardy, J. G., Kellaway, I. W., Rogers, J., and Wilson, C. G. (1980). *J. Pharm. Pharmacol.*, **32**, 309.

39. Richardson, V. J., Jeyasingh, K., Jewkes, R. F., Ryman, B. E., and Tattersall, M. H. N. (1977). *Biochem. Soc. Trans.*, **5**, 290.

40. Oku, N., Tokudome, Y., Tsukada, H., and Okada, S. (1995). *Biochim. Biophys. Acta*, **1238**, 86.

41. Goins, B., Klipper, R., Martin, C., Jerabek, P. A., Khalvati, S., Fox, P. T., *et al.* (1998). *Adv. Exp. Med. Biol.*, **454**, 643.

42. Phillips, W. T., Lemen, L., Goins, B., Rudolph, A. S., Klipper, R., Fresne, D., *et al.* (1997). *Am. J. Physiol.*, **272**, H2492.

43. Barnes, W. E. (1996). In *Nuclear medicine* (ed. R. E. Henkin, M. A. Boles, G. L. Dillehay, J. R. Halama, S. M. Karesh, R. H. Wagner, and A. M. Zimmer), Vol. 1, p. 43. Mosby, St. Louis, MO.

Chapter 13
Isothermic titration calorimetry (ITC)

J. Lasch
Martin-Luther-University Halle-Wittenberg, Institute for Physiological Chemistry, Halle(Saale), Germany.

1 Introduction

This chapter covers a technique which measures the heats associated with the binding of surfactants to liposomes. It starts with the technique and sample handling and proceeds to the estimation of critical surfactant parameters. The estimation of these parameters is outlined in three main sections comprising the CMC, surfactant partitioning into lipid membranes, and liposome solubilization. Surfactants-induced transitions of lipid bilayers take place in a four-stage process (1). Surfactants added to liposomes are incorporated into the lipid membranes up to a critical (saturating) surfactant/lipid ratio, R_{sat}. Increasing the ratio above R_{sat}, the lipid bilayers are progressively destroyed and mixed vesicles start to coexist with mixed micelles. When the total content of surfactant in the aggregates reaches R_{sol}, all membranes are dissolved leaving only mixed micelles and the solubilization is complete. The micellar intermediate structures are cylindrical mixed micelles (CMM), lipid-rich spherical or ellipsoidal mixed micelles (SMM or EMM), and finally lipid-poor mixed micelles (1) (Figure 1).

2 Instrument and the principle of technique

Calorimetry is a universal technique to measure the heat either generated or absorbed in molecular interactions when substances bind. Isothermal titration calorimetry (ITC) is routinely used to study all types of binding reactions including: protein–protein, DNA–drug, receptor–ligand, and aptamer–ligand, amongst others. ITC has become a standard method for the analysis of solute binding to biological and model membranes (2–7).

This method has been adapted and worked out in detail for the analysis of micellization of amphiphiles and interaction of liposomes with surfactants leading to their solubilization (7–9). ITC measurements provide the characteristic parameters of surfactants in this process: the CMC, the critical concentrations for the onset (R_{sol}) and end (R_{sat}) of membrane solubilization, as well as the partition constant and the reaction enthalpy.

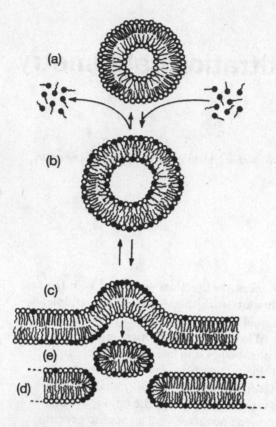

Figure 1 Surfactant-induced transition from lipid vesicles to micelles. (A) Liposomes. (B) Swollen mixed bilayers. (C) Humpbacked vesicles with surfactant at regions of high curvature. (D) Open flat bilayers. (E) Mixed micelles.

In ITC a syringe driven by a computer-controlled stepping motor containing the 'reactant' (in this context a surfactant) is titrated into a cell filled with a 'macromolecule' (in this context lipid vesicles). A schematic representation of a titration calorimeter is shown in Figure 2. It has a reference cell and a measuring cell (both with a volume of about 1.3 ml) filled with the same solution. The tip of the syringe is flat and acts as a very efficient stirrer (the syringe rotates with a speed of about 300 r.p.m.). The injectant is delivered in small aliquots, typically 5–25 μl. As the two materials interact, heat is produced or absorbed in direct proportion to the amount of binding that occurs. As the 'macromolecule' (e.g. lipid vesicles) in the cell become saturated with added ligand (surfactant), the heat signal diminishes until only background heat of dilution is observed. The calorimeter is an adiabatic calorimeter working in a power compensation mode, i.e. all heat effects resulting from the injection are actively balanced by the calorimeter feedback keeping the reference cell and the measuring cell at the same temperature. This is implemented by very precise measurement of the temperature difference between the two cells. The reference cell is heated continuously with a very low power ('RO'), e.g. 20 µW. Thus the increase in temperature is low (30–60 mK/h) and the mixing and reaction process can be regarded as 'isothermal' within the limits of the experiment. The measuring cell, where the mixing occurs, is connected to a second heater ('CFB'), the power of which is controlled by a feedback mechanism eliminating any temperature differences between reference cell and measuring cell. The baseline value of the CFB will be similar to that of the reference cell because size and content of both cells are matched. If heat is generated or absorbed in the measuring cell, a change in the CFB power is required to restore identical temperatures in the two cells. The heat flow is measured and recorded as a function of time. The area underneath each peak is equal to the total heat released for that addition. When this integrated heat is plotted against the molar ratio of ligand added to 'macromolecule' in the cell, a complete binding isotherm for the interaction is obtained. Reference and mixing cell are shielded by an adiabatic jacket equipped with a third heating system ('JFB') keeping the temperature of the shield exactly at that of the reference cell. Thus, no heat exchange can occur with the environment. The instrument measures heats of reaction down to about 1 µcal.

A simple titration sequence with 20 injections is usually finished within 90 minutes. In a simple to perform experiment a complete thermodynamic profile is obtained including binding constant (K), reaction stoichiometry (n), enthalpy (ΔH), and entropy (ΔS).

The cell of the MicroCal system (volume V_o) is completely filled prior to the experiment (see Protocol 1). When the sample in the cell mixes with the inject-

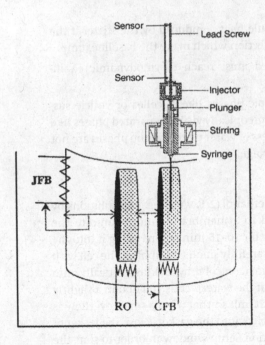

Figure 2 Lollipop-shaped reference and sample cell of the MicroCal MSC ITC.

ant, the injected volume ΔV displaces ΔV of the sample out of the reaction vessel. Thus, the concentration of the compound in V_0 changes a small amount at each injection since the total number of moles in V_0 at the beginning of the experiment is later distributed in the larger volume $V_0 + i\Delta V$. The concentrations of compounds in the cell have to be corrected for these displaced volume effects which occur with each injection. This is done automatically by the software of the instrument (ITC Data Analysis in Origin™) which uses an equation of conservation of mass for this purpose. Only the heat change (ΔH) of the cell is measured; the material change by the volume displacement is isocaloric (10).

3 Computer-assisted measurement with the MCS ITC

The MCS ITC comes with MicroCal Origin which is a general purpose, scientific, and technical data analysis and plotting tool. In addition, Origin can carry add-on routines to solve specific problems, e.g. any non-linear fitting routine based on the Marquardt algorithm.

3.1 Making a calorimetric titration

3.1.1 Prerequisites for ITC samples

(a) Gas-free suspensions. Carefully degas all suspensions before filling them into the measuring cell and the syringe under low vacuum using for instance a membrane pump.

(b) Constant low viscosity. A different Joule heat is induced by the stirrer if the viscosity of the sample varies upon injection which make the baseline jump.

(c) Equilibration. The interaction studied must reach thermodynamic equilibrium between the injections.

(d) Homogeneous suspensions. Microscopic phases like micelles or vesicle suspensions must be homogeneous. Macroscopically visible separated phases like aggregates, inverse micelles in an excess of water or crystalline phases are not to be filled into the cell or even the syringe.

3.1.2 Filling cell and syringe

Clean the sample cell with chloroform/methanol (2:1, v/v). Degas all solutions by stirring while the vessels are connected to a membrane pump. Sonicate the solution to be injected in a bath sonicator for 10–15 min before filling it into the 250 μl syringe avoiding and/or removing carefully small air bubbles. The cell with a volume of 1.3351 ml is filled up to the rim (control it by looking vertically onto it from above—one must see the surface of the water). Thus you obtain a slightly larger volume than that of the cell (1.3351 ml) so that a very small overflow is produced by inserting the syringe with a click into the gasket. Close the jacket of the syringe and click *Run* in the ITC Injection Setup window in order to start the titration.

3.1.3 Instrument settings (MCS ITC) and thermal equilibration

Start Windows and click on the icon *Program Manager*. Choose the *Cell#Status*, then *MCS Observer*: you get the command to switch on the calorimeter. The main switch of the calorimeter is at the back of the instrument. Having this done you click on *Cell 1*. The '*ITC Injection Setup*' window opens. Fill the relevant boxes asking for injection parameters (e.g. volume of the syringe, volume per injection, number of injections, initial injection delay, duration of injection, time between injections for reaching equilibrium), concentrations of injectant in the syringe, and of compound in the cell, both in mM as well as temperature of the experiment.

Especially tricky is the *Reference Offset* setting which has to be done in % full power of the heater. If one expects high exothermic peaks, choose a high Reference Offset (say, 95%); if one expects high endothermic peaks, choose a low Reference Offset (say, 20%). Choose 50% for titrations with both exo- and endothermic peaks. Having done all these settings click on the button *Close*, the Cell1 Plot window appears which shows the plot CFB (μcal/sec) versus time in seconds. An insert window shows the MCS Observer. In its box *temperature* the actual temperature of the calorimeter can be followed. The adjustment of the chosen temperature can take up to 400–600 sec. Reaching the preset temperature exactly, the instrument performs an autostart of the titration.

Along the top of the window you will notice several buttons. Clicking on these buttons gives you access to most of the ITC routines.

3.1.4 Data analysis

Data analysis is carried out by the MicroCal Origin™ software. A number of technical details must be taken into account. First, even for a buffer-into-buffer injection a small heat is measured due to temperature differences between the solution in the syringe and the calorimeter cell. Appropriate control measurements provide the values that must be subtracted. Secondly, changes in the concentration upon successive injections yield heats of dilution which are usually very small. Thirdly, injections into the completely filled cell produce an 'overflow'. The correction for this volume displacement was discussed at the end of Section 2. Finally, the mounting of the syringe might cause a slight inaccuracy of the volume of the first injection. Therefore, at the beginning a small volume (say, 2 μl) is injected and the corresponding heat not included into the calculations.

The data sheets produced by MicroCal Origin™ look like the one in Table 1 from an experiment in this laboratory.

Activating the button 'ITC Final Figure' in the menu 'ITC' at the top of the window you get the corresponding graphical representations (cf. Figure 3). The data in the data sheet (see Table 1) are usually fitted to an appropriate equation with a physicochemical background. The author prefers to copy the data for the purpose of fitting to SigmaPlot. Alternatively, one can get a program listing and instructions for use of the ITC OriginFit function 'PART & RELEASE' from H.

Table 1 Data sheet produced by MicroCal Origin™

ΔH[a]	INJV[b]	Xt[c]	Mt[d]	XMt[e]	NDH[f]
60.77868	10.02094	0.11964	9.92522	0.01205	379.07295
139.74278	10.02094	0.23838	9.85100	0.0242	871.56729
219.25856	10.02094	0.35622	9.77733	0.03643	1367.50244
296.83923	10.02094	0.47316	9.70421	0.04876	1851.36840
336.77268	10.02094	0.58919	9.63162	0.06117	2100.43093
354.75170	10.02094	0.70433	9.55957	0.07368	2212.56499
357.14492	10.02094	0.81856	9.48805	0.08627	2227.49136
361.38386	10.02094	0.93189	9.41704	0.09896	2253.92941
361.97121	10.02094	1.04432	9.34655	0.11173	2257.59264
357.22302	10.02094	1.15585	9.27657	0.12460	2227.97849
364.34563	10.02094	1.26648	9.20710	0.13755	2272.40175
367.35268	10.02094	1.37621	9.13812	0.15060	2291.15658
367.15619	10.02094	1.48503	9.06964	0.16374	2289.93109
360.69703	10.02094	1.59295	9.00165	0.17696	2249.64568
363.35105	10.02094	1.69998	8.93414	0.19028	2266.19863
366.88996	10.02094	1.80610	8.86710	0.20369	2288.27062
364.37087	10.02094	1.91132	8.80054	0.21718	2272.55917
364.83907	10.02094	2.01563	8.73445	0.23077	2275.47934
362.96296	10.02094	2.11905	8.66882	0.24445	2263.77817
362.51835	10.02094	2.22157	8.60365	0.25821	2261.00516

Abbreviations.

[a] Δhi, individual heat change resulting from injection i, in mcal/injection.

[b] µl injected volume.

[c] Concentration of injected solute in the cell before each injection.

[d] Concentration of compound in the cell before each injection after correction of volume displacement.

[e] Molar ratio of injected solute to compound in the cell after injection i.

[f] Normalized heat of injection i, calories per mole of injectant added, kcal/mol.

Heerklotz at the Biozentrum Univ. Basel (Department of Biophysical Chemistry, Biocenter of the University of Basel, Klingelbergstrasse 70, CH-4056 Basel, Switzerland).

4 Estimation of critical micellar concentration

4.1 Thermodynamic background (11)

The heat of micelle formation, ΔH_{mic}, is the molar enthalpy of transfer of surfactant (s) monomers from water (w) into micellar aggregates (m).

The standard free energy of micellization is:

$$\Delta G_s^{0,\,w \to m} = + RT \ln (CMC/55.5)$$

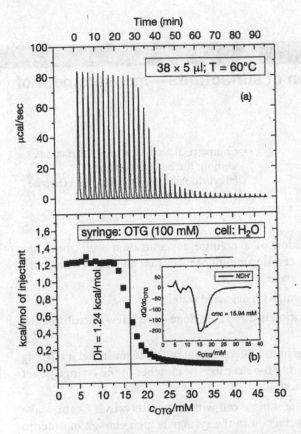

Figure 3 Demicellization experiment with the surfactant octylthioglucoside. (A) Injection of OTG from a solution above its CMC into water leads to demicellization accompanied by the demicellization enthalpy. If the CMC is reached in the sample cell the μcal/sec produced drop to zero. (B) The data of graph (A) are recalculated in kcal/mol as a function of the surfactant concentration in the sample cell.

The factor 55.5 corresponds to the molar concentration of water taking into account the fact that the concentration of surfactant should be given by its molar fraction rather than by the molar concentration mol/l.

The CMC is measured by studying demicellization , i.e. the reverse process of micelle formation (2–8). Thus, if the CMC and the heat of demicellization—both identical to that for micellization, the latter with the opposite sign—are determined, the whole thermodynamic profile of micellization of surfactants can be obtained by the Gibbs–Helmholtz equation:

$$\Delta G_{s,\ demic} = \Delta H_{s,\ demic} - T\ \Delta S_{s,\ demic}$$

4.2 Measurement

Protocol 1

Isothermic microtitration of surfactants—measurement of CMCs

Equipment and reagents

- MCS ITC titration microcalorimeter (MicroCal, Northampton, MA)
- Twice deionized water

- Commercial analytical grade surfactant without further purification (alkyl(thio)glucosides, bile salts, ethylene oxide alkyl ethers, steroids, etc.)

Method

1 Prepare freshly surfactant solution of a definite concentration well above the expected CMC by weighing out a certain amount of surfactant and dilute it up to the required volume with deionized water.

2 Fill the sample cell (volume 1.34 ml) with degassed water.

3 Place the micellar surfactant solution in a 250 μl syringe. Eject a few microlitres and clean the orifice.

4 Insert the syringe in the opening of the filled sample cell. One must feel it clicking into the gasket, so that after starting the titration the clutches in the syringe jacket can correctly take hold of the piston.

5 Inject 25 × 10 μl aliquots into the sample cell with time intervals of 6 min. Make sure that the concentration of surfactant in the syringe is high enough in order to reach the CMC in the sample cell during the run.

The result is shown in Figure 3.

During the run the detergent concentration in the sample cell must vary from well below to above the CMC. How to make sure that during a titration the CMC is covered in the sample cell?

If one has no idea about its value, it is a time-consuming trial and error procedure. On the other hand, making a sound guess from structurally related surfactants, one can calculate the generated concentration series according to the equation given in Figure 4.

Protocol 2

Data analysis

1 Divide the enthalpogram (Figure 3B) into two concentration ranges where the reaction enthalpies are nearly constant.

2 Pin-point the inflection point by calculating the first derivative of the sigmoidal transition curve (Figure 3B) resulting in the curve in the insert.

Protocol 2 continued

3 The minimum of the curve of first derivative is the CMC (15.94 mM for octylthio-glucoside in this example).

4 The enthalpy difference between the two extrapolated lines of constant enthalpy at the inflection point of the transition curve is the heat of demicellization $\Delta H_{s, demic}$, which is the heat of micellization with the opposite sign ($\Delta H_{OTG, demic} = 1.24$ kcal/mol in the example).

$$j := 0 .. 38 \qquad v := 1335.1$$

$$c := 150 \qquad a := 10 \qquad ca := 1500 \qquad c_0 := 0 \qquad v_j := v + j \cdot a$$

$$c_{j+1} := \frac{(c_j \cdot v_j + 1500)}{v_j}$$

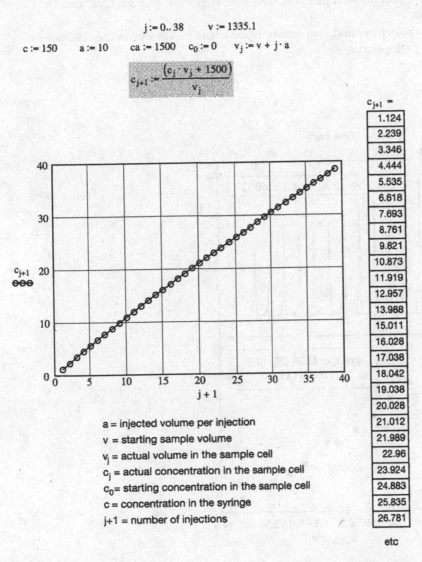

$c_{j+1} =$
1.124
2.239
3.346
4.444
5.535
6.618
7.693
8.761
9.821
10.873
11.919
12.957
13.988
15.011
16.028
17.038
18.042
19.038
20.028
21.012
21.989
22.96
23.924
24.883
25.835
26.781

etc

a = injected volume per injection
v = starting sample volume
v_j = actual volume in the sample cell
c_j = actual concentration in the sample cell
c_0 = starting concentration in the sample cell
c = concentration in the syringe
j+1 = number of injections

Figure 4 Calculation of a concentration series generated by injecting a solution of known concentration into a measuring cell (cuvette).

For a number of surfactants, especially ionic ones, the drop of enthalpy when going from the dissolution of micelles (first range of nearly constant enthalpy) to the simple dilution enthalpy of micelles (second range of nearly constant enthalpy) is not so distinct. However, the CMC can still be found clearly at the minimum of the graph of first derivative. Amphiphiles which do not form micelles but associate with an ever increasing aggregation number or form nanostructures which change with concentration like the bolaamphiphile dequalinium (1,1'-(1,10-decamethylene-bis-[aminoquin- aldinium])-acetate) show no sigmoidal transition between two limiting enthalpies at all. Only slowly decreasing dilution enthalpies are seen (see Figure 5) and no CMC can be determined.

One has to keep in mind, that demicellation enthalpies as well as the CMCs are functions of temperature (9).

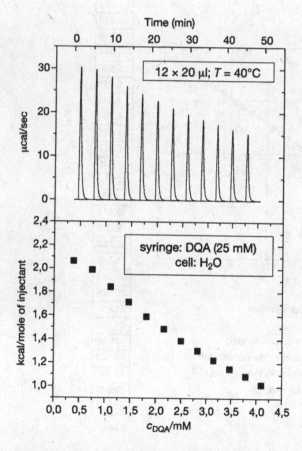

Figure 5 Demicellization experiment with the bolaamphiphile dequalinium. The graphs have the same meaning as in Figure 3, but with DQA as amphiphile instead of OTG.

5 Surfactant–bilayer membrane equilibria

5.1 Surfactant partitioning into lipid membranes

The partition constant K and the heat of transfer, $\Delta H_s^{w \to b}$, of a surfactant from the aqueous phase (w) to the bilayer membrane (b) are determined simultaneously. Figure 5 shows the titration of octylthioglucoside (OTG) with liposomes of 1-palmitoyl-2-oleoyl-sn-glycero-3-phosphocholine (POPC) (see Protocol 3).

Transfer enthalpies $\Delta H_s^{w \to b}$ of the transfer of OTG into POPC liposomes and the partition coefficient K are estimated by fitting the titration data to an appropriate model (see below). From the partition coefficient the Gibbs energy change, $\Delta G_s^{w \to b} = -RT\ln K$, is obtained; the Gibbs–Helmholtz equation:

$$\Delta G_s^{w \to b} = \Delta H_s^{w \to b} - T\,\Delta S_s^{w \to b}$$

then yields the entropy change.

5.1.1 Partitioning models

At surfactant concentrations in the aqueous phase distinctly below its critical micellar concentration ($c_s^o < \text{CMC}$) membrane partitioning upon titration with liposomes will gradually change the physical properties of lipid bilayers (1). Schurtenberger (12) relates the mole ratio of membrane-bound surfactant /total lipid (R) to the surfactant free in solution ($c_{s,\,f}$) by a proportionality constant K which can be viewed as a partition constant with the dimension of a reciprocal concentration:

$$R = K \cdot c_{s,\,f}$$

which can be rewritten as:

$$c_{s,b} / c_L = K\,c_{s,\,f} \tag{1}$$

where c_L is the total lipid concentration in the aqueous phase (cave: the constant lipid concentration in the syringe is denoted by c_L^o). With the law of mass conservation:

$$c_s^o = c_{s,\,b} + c_{s,\,f} \text{ or } c_{s,\,f} = c_s^o - c_{s,\,b}$$

(b for bound and f for free) Equation 1 is transformed into:

$$c_{s,\,b} = c_s^o (K\,c_L) / (1 + K\,c_L) \tag{2}$$

a typical Langmuir-type saturation equation. Derivation with respect to the lipid concentration yields:

$$\delta c_{s,\,b} / \delta c_L^o = c_L K / (1 + K\,c_L)^2 \tag{3}$$

Injecting i-times lipid of concentration c_L^o into the sample cell filled with surfactant solution gives an actual total lipid concentration of $c_L = i\,\delta c_L^o$. The corresponding absolute heat of the ith injection δh_i is:

$$\delta h_i = n_{s,\,b}\,(i)\,\Delta H_s^{w \to b} = \delta c_{s,b}\,V_{cell}\,\Delta H_s^{w \to b}.$$

Substituting $\delta c_{s,b}$ from Equation 3 yields:

$$\delta h_i = V_{cell} \Delta H_s^{w \to b} c_L K / (1 + iK \delta c_L^o)^2 \delta c_L^o \qquad [4]$$

The curvature of δh_i plots is more pronounced than that of the integrated curve (i.e. cumulative heats). Calculating cumulative heats corresponds to a smoothing of curves. Thus, it is better to use as fitting function Equation 4 which is of the type $f = ax / (1 + bx)^2$ (see Figure 6). The right-hand side with the plus sign for endothermic reactions and the minus sign for exothermic ones.

5.1.2 Partitioning measured by ITC

There are two possible partitioning experiments:

(a) A surfactant solution is filled into the sample cell and titrated with a suspension of lipid vesicles.

(b) A monomeric solution of surfactant is titrated to lipid vesicles.

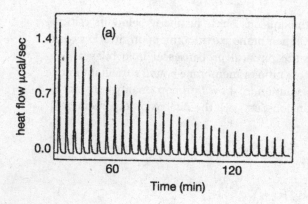

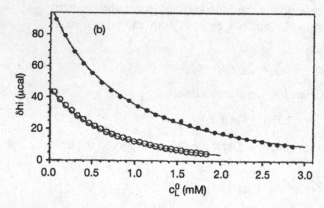

Figure 6 (A) Calorimetric traces (heat flow) observed upon addition of POPC liposomes ($c_L^o = 10$ mM) into 150 µM $C_{10}EO_7$, both in buffer (100 mM NaCl, 10 mM Tris pH 7.4). 10 µl injections of liposome suspension at 6 min intervals. (B) Heats of injection, δh_i, of the data shown in panel A (open circles) and a second experiment, i.e. 250 µM $C_{10}EO_7$ titrated with 14.8 mM POPC (filled circles). Modified from ref. 8 with permission from Elsevier Science.

The signal-to-noise ratio is much lower in the experiment of type (b) because fewer surfactant molecules are transferred from water to the lipid bilayer, but the fitting of experimental data to models assuming ideal mixing behaviour might encounter difficulties (7). The type (a) experiment is described in Protocol 3.

Protocol 3

Surfactant-into-membrane partitioning

Equipment and reagents

- Branson sonifier®, model W-250 (Branson Ultrasonics Corp.)
- MCS ITC titration microcalorimeter (MicroCal)
- Ultra pure water
- Octyl-β-D-thioglucopyranoside (OTG) (Calbiochem-Novabiochem)
- 1-Palmitoyl-2-oleoyl-sn-glycero-3-phosphocholine (Sigma)

Method

1 Prepare OTG solution of a definite concentration below the CMC by weighing out a certain amount of surfactant and dilute it up to the required volume with ultra pure water.

2 Prepare POPC liposomes by sonication (see Chapter 1), corresponding to a high final lipid concentration, e.g. between 15–50 mM.

3 Fill the sample cell (volume 1.34 ml) with OTG solution.

4 Fill the syringe with the liposome suspension free of gas bubbles.

5 Start the titration at a pre-selected temperature, use 10 μl injections or less.

The results are demonstrated in Figure 6A and B. The heats of ith injections, δh_i, are fitted to the fit function of type $f = a\, c_L (1 + b\, c_L)^2$ (see above), $a = V_{cell} \Delta H_s^{w \to b} K$, $b = K$. The solid lines correspond to the theoretical fits. The parameters of the fit yielded $K = 770\ M^{-1}$ and $\Delta H_s^{\ w \to b} = 6.5$ kcal/mol. The partitioning equilibrium model, used here to fit the experimental data, assumes that the mixing of surfactant with the lipid in the vesicles is ideal. The partition coefficient might, however, change with increasing surfactant concentration because of changing physicochemical parameters of the bilayer including clustering of incorporated surfactant molecules (1) (Figure 1C and 1E).

5.2 Solubilization of lipsomes

Micellar surfactant solutions are added to a liposome suspension in such a way that during titration the surfactant/lipid ratios R_{sat} and R_{sol} (see Introduction) are covered. Solubilization of PC bilayers is achieved when the surfactant concentration in the mixture approaches the critical micellar concentration. Three effects

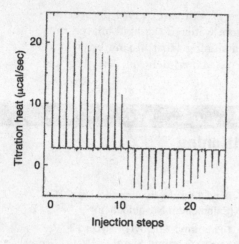

Figure 7 Titration of 33.3 mM micellar solution of $C_{12}EO_6$ to 1.3 ml of 2 mM POPC vesicle suspension in 25 steps of 10 μl each at 25 °C. Modified from ref. 6 with permission from Elsevier Science.

contribute to the reaction enthalpy $\times H$. One is the incorporation of surfactant monomers into the lipid bilayer, $\Delta H_s{}^{w \to b}$, the other the demicellization of injected micelles, $\Delta H_{s, demic}$, and the dilution of the vesicular dispersion, $\times H_{dil}$.

It has been shown (6, 7) that the observed integrated heat, $\times H$ (i.e. enthalpy difference) includes mainly the bilayer transfer enthalpy difference for the added surfactant, $\Delta H_s{}^{w \to b}$.

A solubilizing titration is shown in Figure 7. Depending on surfactant and temperature one finds slowly changing endothermic (upward peaks) (6) or exothermic (downward peaks) (7) heat flows in the beginning (initial injections). Peaks might decrease somewhat with increasing surfactant content of the mixed bilayers. If more surfactant is injected, there is a steep change at R_{sat}. However, the heat flow must not necessarily change from endo- to exothermic. We enter the coexistence region of mixed micelles and mixed bilayers: $R_{sat} < R < R_{sol}$. Now the vesicles start to be dissolved to micelles. Crossing the coexistence region always leads to a sudden and considerable decrease in the heat effect. At surfactant/lipid ratios above R_{sol} ($R > R_{sol}$) no vesicles are left, only mixed micelles. At this point the heat of titration changes again abruptly. Injected surfactant micelles equilibrate with mixed micelles, causing only small heat effects.

Protocol 4

Lipsome solubilization

Equipment and reagents

• See Protocol 3

Protocol 4 continued

Method

1 Prepare OTG solution of a definite concentration well above the CMC, e.g. 50 mM, by weighing out a certain amount of surfactant and dilute it up to the required volume with ultra pure water.

2 Prepare POPC liposomes by sonication (see Chapter 1), corresponding to a concentration of 2 mM.

3 Fill the sample cell (volume 1.34 ml) with POPC liposome suspension.

4 Fill the syringe with the micellar solution of OTC.

5 Start the titration at a pre-selected temperature (choose 25 or 30 °C), use 10 μl injections or less.

References

1. Lasch, J. (1995). *Biochim. Biophys. Acta*, **1241**, 269.
2. Birdi, K. S. (1983). *Colloid. Polym. Sci.*, **261**, 45.
3. Olofsson, G. (1985). *J. Phys. Chem.*, **89**, 1473.
4. Wiseman, T., Williston, S., Brandts, J. F., and Lin, L. N. (1989). *Anal. Biochem.*, **179**, 131.
5. Lehrmann, R. and Seelig, J. (1994). *Biochim. Biophys. Acta*, **1189**, 89.
6. Heerklotz, H., Lantzsch, G., Binder, H., Klose, G., and Blume, A. (1995). *Chem. Phys. Lett.*, **235**, 517.
7. Keller, M., Kerth, A., and Blume, A. (1997). *Biochim. Biophys. Acta*, **1326**, 178.
8. Heerklotz, H. and Seelig, J. (2000). *Biochim. Biophys. Acta*, **1508**, 69.
9. Paula, S., Süs, W., Tuchtenhagen, J., and Blume, A. (1995). *J. Phys. Chem.*, **99**, 11742.
10. Heerklotz, H. and Binder, H. (1997). *Recent Res. Dev. Phys. Chem.*, **1**, 221.
11. Marsh, D. (ed.) (1990). *CRC Handbook of lipid bilayers*, p. 337. CRC Press, Boca Raton.
12. Schurtenberger, P., Mazer, N., and Kanzig, W. (1980). *J. Chem. Phys.*, **89**, 1042.

Chapter 14
Vesicular phospholipid gels

M. Brandl

University in Tromso, Institute for Pharmacy, Department of Pharmaceutics, 9037 Tromso, Norway.

U. Massing

Tumor Biology Center, Breisacher Strasse 117, D-79106 Freiburg, Germany.

1 Background

This chapter discusses some of the common limitations with small liposomes as drug carriers and how vesicular phospholipid gels can be used to circumvent them.

1.1 Biopharmaceutical and technological challenges with liposomes for i.v. application

The purpose of an intravenously injected liposomal drug carrier usually is to circulate in the bloodstream and carry the drug to the desired target organ or tissue. Under ideal circumstances the pharmacokinetics and biodistribution of the carrier-associated drug is merely dependent on the characteristics of the liposomes, not on the drug itself. Size and surface characteristics of the liposomes primarily determine the degree to which they are eliminated from the bloodstream by macrophages and end up in the RES organs spleen and liver (1, 2). Big liposomes (>200 nm) are rapidly eliminated, thus they are inappropriate for i.v. drug delivery. Smaller liposomes are more likely to escape the RES and may thus circulate long enough to reach targets within or nearby the vasculary bed (2). Smaller liposomes furthermore are more likely to extravasate. Under healthy conditions extravasation seems to be restricted to the liver. Within sites of inflammation and certain tumours, however, the lining of the vasculary bed appears to be more leaky. This allows liposomes, which are small enough to extravasate preferentially within such target sites. Together with reduced lymphatic drainage in tumours this may cause a significant accumulation of macromolecular and particulate drug carriers (enhanced permeability and retention effect; EPR-effect) (3–5). In summary, small liposomes (<200 nm) are suited to reach sites of inflammation and solid tumours and accumulate there via passive targeting.

Technologically speaking such small liposomes are unfavourable: the size of a liposome is correlated with the volume of the aqueous core. The volume of the aqueous core in turn determines the capacity of the liposome to carry a drug, at least in the case of hydrophilic drugs. The volume of the aqueous core entrapped at the moment of vesicle formation determines the percentage of a drug being entrapped (encapsulation efficiency). Therefore, loading of small unilamellar vesicles (SUVs) with low molecular weight hydrophilic drugs generally is not a very efficient process. In turn, this usually makes it inevitable to remove non-entrapped drug from the preparation by, for example, gel filtration, dialysis, or others. Such purification processes are difficult to accomplish on a bigger scale and under aseptic conditions. Once the non-entrapped drug is removed, most low molecular weight drugs start to leak out of the interior of liposomes. For most conventional liposomal drug formulations such leakage is shelf-life limiting. Drug leakage is also the main challenge with steam sterilization of conventional SUV dispersions.

1.2 Biopharmaceutical and technological challenges with liposomes for loco-regional administration

The purpose with liposomes for loco-regional administration is to retain and localize the drug within a reservoir at the site of administration. A high drug carrying capacity and good retention is desired. Upon s.c. injection, bigger liposomes escape more easily lymphatic drainage. The retention of the drug within the liposome is primarily governed by the lamellarity, i.e. number of lamellae the drug has to penetrate for release. Multiple lamellae appear advantageous for sustained release (depot-effect). Both size and lamellarity of bigger vesicles have turned out to be difficult to control. Multilamellar vesicle (MLV) preparations usually have a poor reproducibility in terms of liposome size and lamellarity.

1.3 Phospholipid dispersions: swelling and phases

Phospholipids hydrate and swell instantaneously upon contact with aqueous medium forming lamellar structures. For phosphatidylcholine complete hydration of the lipid crystals is first reached at a lipid/water mixing ratio of 55:45 (9). At this mixing ratio the water is fully taken up by the lipid in the form of hydration layers between the bilayer sheets (lamellar phase) and swelling is completed. At higher water contents biphasic preparations are obtained, where hydrated lipid crystal phase and water phase coexist (10).

1.4 Mechanical stress: formation of vesicle dispersions and vesicular phospholipid gels

If swelling of phosphatidylcholine is accomplished under conditions of mechanical stress (stirring, shaking, etc.) or, if pre-swollen lipid crystals are treated mechanically, vesicles are formed. High levels of mechanical stress, e.g. during high pressure homogenization, lead to small and unilamellar vesicles. In excess water, i.e. up to lipid concentrations of about 250 mg/g (325 mM) liposome dispersions (vesicles dispersed in a continuous water phase) are formed. In contrast, above this limit semi-solid, gel-like masses are obtained. We could demonstrate that such masses can be prepared in a way that makes their morphology exclusively vesicular at PC contents far beyond the above limit of 250 mg/g or 325 mM (8). Such preparations do not represent vesicle dispersions rather than three-dimensional gels enclosing aqueous compartments not only within but also in between the vesicular structures. The term 'vesicular phospholipid gels' is thus used for such preparations.

1.5 The vesicular phospholipid gel concept

Vesicular phospholipid gels (VPGs) originally described in refs 6 and 7 are highly concentrated (250–600 mg/g or 325–780 mM lipid) (phospho-) lipid dispersions of semi-solid consistency. They show vesicular morphology (8). This has the following practical implications:

(a) VPGs contain segregated aqueous compartments within the core of the vesicles as well as in between the vesicles.

(b) VPGs can be loaded with hydrophilic, amphiphilic, and lipophilic drugs in different ways.

(c) VPGs retain a constant drug load within the core of the vesicles even during autoclaving or long-term storage because there is no concentration gradient between the vesicles core and surrounding water phase (Figure 1, top).

(d) VPGs appear suited as depots to release drugs in a controlled manner over extended periods of time, e.g. upon implantation or injection.

(e) VPGs can be transferred into 'conventional' small sized liposome (SUV) dispersions by addition of excess aqueous medium and gentle mechanical agitation shortly before use. Under appropriate conditions the preformed vesicles remain intact during this dilution process and retain their drug load (Figure 1, bottom).

  i. Thus, drugs can be entrapped into SUVs with an unusually high efficiency by preparation of VPGs and subsequent dilution.

  ii. Such high ratio of entrapped to unentrapped drug may render removal of free drug unnecessary. In this case diluted VPGs represent dual drug formulations. They contain free and liposomally entrapped drug in a defined ratio.

2 Preparation of vesicular phospholipid gels

2.1 VPGs made of a single phospholipid

For preparing VPGs, which consist of a single phospholipid, Protocol 1 is suitable which is adapted from the one-step liposome preparation technique originally described in ref. 12. A crude mixture of dry crystalline phospholipid is processed

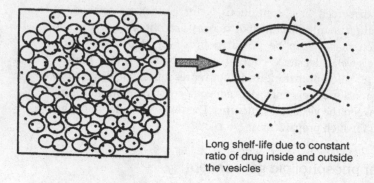

Long shelf-life due to constant
ratio of drug inside and outside
the vesicles

i.v. injection directly after redispersion
(mixture of free drug and liposomally entrapped drug)

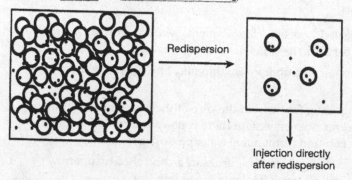

Redispersion

Injection directly
after redispersion

Figure 1 Schematic representation of a drug-containing VPG before and after dilution.

together with buffer (drug solution). APV Micron Lab 40 lab-scale homogenizers are well suited to prepare VPGs. There is also some positive experience with a microfluidizer M110 (not published) in our groups so far. Others have reported problems when preparing conventional liposomes due to insufficient swelling when using a microfluidizer (13).

Protocol 1

Preparation of a VPG from a single lipid

Equipment and materials

- Glass flask with tight screw cap, 100 ml
- Rubber scraper (kitchen type)
- Phosphatidylcholine: natural soy, or egg PC, content 80% or above (e.g. E80, Lipoid GmbH)
- High pressure homogenizer Micron Lab 40 (APV Homogenizer)
- If applicable: hydrophilic drug or marker (calcein), to be dissolved in 40 mM phosphate buffer pH 7.4[a]

Method

1 Disperse the phosphatidylcholine in aqueous medium (e.g. 16 g of E80 in 24 g of phosphate buffer or buffered drug solution, respectively) by manual shaking in a stoppered flask over 1–2 min.

2 Transfer the obtained highly viscous to semi-solid heterogeneous slurry to the educt compartment of the high pressure homogenizer. Use a rubber scraper if necessary. Process it at the chosen pressure. Usually 70 MPa (700 bar) is appropriate.

3 Transfer the mass back from the product to the educt compartment. Repeat the homogenization step until a turbid to opalescent paste is formed, which looks macroscopically homogeneous. Usually five to ten cycles are appropriate.

4 Transfer the VPG to an air-tight container and store it in the fridge at 2–8 °C until used.

[a] With calcein as a model compound, 10 mM EDTA should be included within the buffer in order to complexate cobalt ions which may arise from the stainless steel material of the homogenizer. Otherwise cobalt might affect the fluorometric calcein assay.

2.2 VPGs made of two or more lipids

For preparing VPGs consisting of two or more lipids Protocol 2 is recommended, which first transfers the lipids into a molecular solid solution in order to avoid inhomogeneous distribution of the lipids over the bilayer upon swelling (11, 12). The commonly used thin film hydration technique is not very suited for this due to the relatively big amounts of lipids needed for VPGs. A freeze-drying approach is described instead in Protocol 2.

Protocol 2

Preparation of a VPG from two or more lipids

Equipment and materials

- See Protocol 1
- Freeze-dryer Beta 2–16 (Martin Christ GmbH)[a]
- Phosphatidylcholine: natural or hydrogenated, soy or egg (e.g. E80, Lipoid GmbH)
- Other lipids, e.g. cholesterol (Sigma)
- If applicable: lipophilic or amphiphilic drug
- Methanol, p.a. grade (Merck)
- 40 mM phosphate buffer pH 7.4

Method

1 Dissolve the lipids (and, if applicable drug) in a blend of (organic) solvents[b] under gentle warming (approx. 50 °C). For an equimolar blend of phosphatidylcholine and cholesterol use 10.5 g of E80, 5.5 g of cholesterol, approx. 70 g methanol, and 30 g distilled water.

Protocol 2 continued

2 Transfer the solution into bottles or pans such that the thickness of the fluid layer does not exceed 1 cm.

3 Shock-freeze the solution carefully in liquid nitrogen or, alternatively a freezer at −80 °C until frozen.

4 Transfer the container(s) with the frozen, solid to semi-solid mass without re-thawing to the shelf of the freeze-dryer, which has been pre-cooled to the lowest achievable temperature.

5 Freeze-dry with a cooling trap with liquid nitrogen installed between the freeze-dryer and the vacuum pump.[c] The following initial instrument settings are appropriate for the above example: shelf temperature −55 °C; vacuum 20 Pa; ice condenser temperature below −70 °C. Freeze-dry until the product temperature approximates the shelf temperature. Then increase the shelf temperature to 40 °C and reduce the pressure to its technical lower limit (approx. 2–3 Pa). Continue until the drying is completed.

6 A spongy dry cake should be obtained. Close the container and store it in the fridge at 2–8 °C until used.

7 Disperse the cake in 24 g of aqueous medium and continue as described in Protocol 1.

[a] All parts of the freeze-dryer that come in contact with solvent-vapour must be solvent-resistant.

[b] The solvent must dissolve all components of the formula and the blend have a freezing point above the lowest shelf temperature of the freeze-dryer as well as a high vapour pressure. Methanol/ t-butanol/ water are suitable.

[c] The melting point of pure methanol is −97 °C.

3 Loading of VPGs with drugs

Different approaches have been described to load VPGs with drugs. The choice of the proper technology depends on the physicochemical characteristics of the drug, very much as it is the case with conventional liposomes. According to the drug's ability to interact with phospholipid bilayers or not, the substances may be divided into two main categories:

(a) Water soluble substances which upon loading into VPGs are truly entrapped or encapsulated within the aqueous compartments of the VPG.

(b) Amphiphilic or lipophilic substances which are incorporated into or associated with the bilayers.

Whether a drug belongs to type (a) or type (b) may be judged beforehand by its octanol/water- or oil/water-partition coefficient. Even better predictions allow liposome/water-partition coefficient (14–16). By microcalorimetry drugs can be screened on potential interactions with bilayers (17). For some drugs one even has the choice, depending on pK_a and lipid composition, they may either be entrapped in the aqueous compartment or alternatively associated with the bilayer (18, 19). For hydrophilic drugs one may choose between *direct entrapment* during the formation of the VPG and *passive loading* into preformed VPGs. For amphiphilic or lipophilic drugs the approach described in Section 3.3 may be used.

3.1 Direct entrapment

Direct entrapment is achieved if the formation of VPGs is carried out in drug-containing aqueous medium, e.g. according to Protocols 1 or 2. Together with a distinct volume of aqueous medium a distinct portion of the drug ends up encapsulated within the aqueous core of the vesicles, another part is trapped in the aqueous space between the vesicles. The percentage of drug entrapped in the aqueous core *and* the space between the vesicles is equal to the total amount of drug present (100% entrapment).

3.2 Passive loading

The process of passive loading was originally described by Massing *et al.* (20). In principle it comprises the incubation of 'empty' VPG with drug until the drug is equally distributed throughout the preparation by diffusion. The method takes advantage of the following facts:

(a) With VPGs the ratio of aqueous medium inside as compared to outside the vesicles is high.

(b) Phospholipid bilayers are sufficiently permeable for many drugs.

When added to preformed 'empty' (i.e. drug-free) vesicular phospholipid gels the drug permeates according to the concentration gradient through the bilayers into the vesicles until equilibrium between the interior of the vesicles and the surrounding medium is achieved. Gentle warming can further facilitate the equilibration process. Upon re-cooling and subsequent dilution of the VPG into SUV dispersions (see below) encapsulation efficiencies in the same magnitude as with passive entrapment are reached. For a detailed description of such passive loading process see Protocol 3.

Protocol 3

Passive loading of a VPG with a hydrophilic compound (Gemcitabine)

Equipment and reagents

- Class II biological safety bench for aseptic handling of cytostatics[a] (e.g. Holten Maxisafe)
- Thermostated shaking water-bath (e.g. GFL 1086)
- Containers[b] (e.g. 1.5 ml Eppendorf tubes)
- Drug solution,[b] e.g. Gemcitabine (2',2'-difluoro-2'-deoxycytidine; dFdC) solution: 15 mg dFdC-HCl in 1 ml phosphate buffer, pH 7.3

Protocol 3 continued

Method

1 Prepare a drug-free VPG (empty VPG) as described in Protocols 1 or 2.

2 At the safety bench,[b] transfer approx. 350 mg of the empty VPG into a sterile container. Add the appropriate volume of the drug solution (e.g. 50 μl of the Gemcitabine solution) to the VPG and mix thoroughly using a sterile spatula. Close the container.

3 Incubate the mixture in a water-bath at an appropriate temperature for an appropriate period of time (e.g. for maximum trapping efficiency, incubate the above mixture of Gemcitabine solution and empty VPG for 4 h at 60 °C).

4 Store the drug-loaded VPG in a fridge at 2–8 °C until further use.

[a] Appropriate measures according to local safety regulations are required when handling cytotoxic compounds.

[b] In case the preparation is not subjected to a terminal sterilization step, pre-sterilized media and containers as well as aseptic handling are recommended.

Passive loading has the following advantages: No active ingredient is present during the preparation of the liposomes, which may greatly reduce the extent of safety precautions which have to be taken when toxic drugs are handled. The composition of the medium of the VPG on the one hand and of the drug solution on the other hand may be chosen independently and thus be optimized with respect to increased shelf-life, e.g. pH 6.5 for VPGs and pH 4 for doxorubicin (21) or even freeze-dried state for highly sensitive drugs. Drug and liposomes do not come in contact with each other until shortly before application and possible interactions, which induce degradation, can thus be avoided (22). This approach may allow loading of VPGs in a hospital pharmacy setting.

3.3 Incorporation/association

Drugs that end up incorporated in the liposome membrane are poorly soluble in water but soluble in non-polar solvents (hydrocarbons). For loading into VPGs these lipophilic compounds are treated like lipid compounds, i.e. transferred into a molecular mixture with the lipid components before hydration, e.g. by dissolving drug and lipid(s) in organic solvent and removing the latter to form a cake. Choice of solvent and process conditions during solvent removal should exclude selective recrystallization of one of the components prior to the other(s) in order to ensure homogeneous distribution within the lipid cake and, upon hydration, the bilayer. The amount of hydrophobic drug that can be incorporated in a VPG preparation is dependent on packing restrictions within the bilayer. It is thus vital to choose an appropriate lipid formula. Amphiphilic compounds are usually also treated like lipid compounds. Their association with VPGs, however, is often less stable than that of lipophilic compounds. For preparing a VPG containing a lipophilic drug the binary lipid blends protocol (Protocol 2) can be used with modifications in the composition of the organic solvent, i.e. using a blend of methanol and other organic solvents to dissolve both drug and lipid(s).

4 Sterilization of VPGs

Steam sterilization of the finished product is the method of choice to ensure sterility of parenteral drug products. But, chemical degradation, i.e. hydrolysis of the phospholipid and/or structural rearrangements, vesicle fusion or aggregation, as well as leakage of the drug out of the liposomes have so far mostly ruled out the use of this sterilization technique for production of sterile liposomal drug carriers for parenteral use. Whereas hydrolytic degradation of phospholipids to lyso-phospholipids may be limited by appropriate choice of buffer composition and pH (23, 24), the leakage of encapsulated drug substances during autoclaving has not been overcome with conventional liposomes so far. As with VPGs there is no gradient in drug concentration between the core and the water phase surrounding the vesicles (as long as they are not diluted) no leakage occurs during autoclaving (25). But, structural rearrangements such as fusion to bigger vesicles have been seen with VPGs. This in turn influences their visco-elastic behaviour (see below), sustained release behaviour (see below), and encapsulation efficiency (see below) and requires stringent monitoring (25). Nevertheless the results gained so far do not seem to rule out steam sterilization as an approach to gain sterile VPGs.

5 Characteristics of VPGs

VPGs are primarily characterized by their morphology, visco-elastic behaviour, and sustained release of drugs.

5.1 Morphology

The morphology of VPGs can be analysed by freeze-fracture transmission electron microscopy (FFTEM). The technique used for FFTEM studies of VPGs is described in ref. 8. Here, the influence of mechanical stress on the morphology of highly concentrated phospholipid dispersions was studied. Phospholipid type and concentration are of key importance for the morphology of VPGs (8): with natural egg or soy PC-containing VPGs prepared as described in Protocol 1, one can expect predominantly small unilamellar vesicular structures (diameter around 30 nm) up to lipid contents of 450 mg/g, with occasionally bigger vesicles occurring filled with SUVs (diameters up to several hundred nm). With higher lipid contents, an increasing fraction of such multivesicular vesicles along with multilamellar morphologies is obtained. With VPGs made of synthetic, saturated PC, a higher tendency to form multilamellar structures is observed irrespective of lipid content (27).

5.2 Rheology, viscosity

The rheological behaviour of VPGs can be studied by a rotational viscometer (pate/plate set-up, diameter 20 mm) in the rotational or, preferably, in the oscillating mode as described in ref. 27. VPGs represent visco-elastic bodies with pronounced yield points. The yield point depends on lipid composition, concentration, vesicle size, and vesicle size distribution (27). Yield points in the magnitude 4–40 Pa were observed (27, 29).

5.3 Sustained release behaviour *in vitro*

For assessment of the *in vitro* release of drug from VPG-formulations a test method based on a custom-made flow-through cell, as displayed in Figure 2, has been established. The method is described in Protocol 4. The rationale for the cell design is given in ref. 28. An acceptor medium (buffer) is run through the cell at a rate of 10 ml/h, to mimic the flow of tissue fluid at the site of injection or implantation. As in this model the donor and acceptor compartments are *not* separated by a (semi-permeable) membrane, not only drug release via diffusion through the matrix, but also erosion of the lipid matrix can be followed. Fractions collected over distinct time intervals are analysed for both drug and phospholipid. The drug in the eluate is quantified by HPLC or another appropriate method. Differentiation between drug released in free and liposomal form can be done by (sub-)fractionation of the eluate using size exclusion chromatography on Sepha-

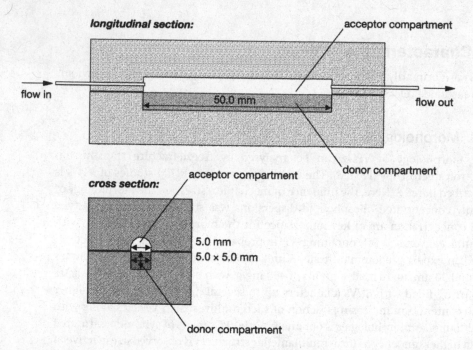

Figure 2 Flow-through cell for analysis of *in vitro* drug release from VPGs. Adapted from ref. 28.

dex G-50 gel. The amount of lipid released can be quantified gravimetrically upon freeze-drying, as described in ref. 28, unless too little. Or, lipids are quantified by techniques such as Bartlett or Stewart assays, as described elsewhere in this book.

Protocol 4

Assessment of *in vitro* drug release behaviour of a VPG

Equipment and reagents

- Custom-made release cell with a rectangular donor compartment (5 × 5 × 50 mm), to take up about 1 g of the VPG and an acceptor compartment of semicircular cross-section (radius 2.5 mm) and 50 mm length (Figure 2)
- Pulse-free pump, providing a constant flow rate of 10 ml/h, e.g. piston pump P-500 (Pharmacia Biotech)
- Water-bath set to 37 °C

- Fraction collector and tubes, suitable to collect 10 ml fractions per hour (or multiples of that), e.g. RediFrac (Pharmacia Biotech)
- Buffer reservoir, e.g. 2 litre flask
- VPG sample to be analysed, approx. 1 g
- Acceptor medium, e.g. the buffer which has been used for VPG preparation[a]

Method

1. Place the buffer reservoir with the acceptor medium in the water-bath for equilibration at 37 °C.

2. Determine the mass of the empty, dry release cell and fill the donor compartment of the cell with the VPG sample bubble-free, using an ointment spatula. Clamp or screw the two halves of the cell tightly together.

3. Weigh the filled release cell to determine the accurate mass of the VPG loaded into the cell.

4. Mount the tubing and place the cell in the water-bath[b] and expel all air from the tubing by pumping acceptor medium through the system.

5. Start the pump and fraction collector and pump the acceptor medium through the system at a flow rate of 10 ml/h and collect fractions (1 fraction/h, or alternative settings).

6. Analyse an aliquot of each fraction for overall drug and for lipid content.

7. Fractionate an aliquot of each fraction on Sephadex G-50 gel and analyse the subfractions for liposomal and free-drug content respectively.

8. At the end of the experiment collect the VPG remaining in the cell (if any) by rinsing it off with excess acceptor medium. Analyse it for its drug and lipid content.

[a] Alternatively plasma can be used to mimic more closely the *in vivo* situation.

[b] If the cell is placed in a plastic bag for submersion in the water-bath eventual leaks are more easily detected.

An example for the sustained release behaviour of calcein from a 450 mg/g egg phosphatidylcholine VPG is given in Figure 3. In general, release of drugs from a VPG matrix is slow with release half-times ranging from a couple of hours up to several weeks. Depending on the lipid type, lipid concentration, and the intrinsic ability of the drug to permeate through phospholipid membranes, one of the following two release mechanisms may be rate limiting:

(a) Diffusion of the drug through the VPG matrix.

(b) Erosion of the VPG matrix resulting in the release of whole liposomes.

A systematic study on the influence of lipid concentration on the matrix erosion and release mechanism and rate of low molecular weight hydrophilic compounds from egg PC VPGs is found in ref. 28. Steam sterilization alters the release behaviour of a VPG (25). Data on the sustained release of various drug compounds from VPGs can be found in the following references: Gemcitabine (29), vincristine (32), carboplatin (33), and the peptide hormone antagonist Cetrorelix® (34). In conclusion, the release of drugs from VPGs can be adapted over a wide range. The results gained so far seem to indicate that VPGs may be suited as depots both for loco-regional as well as systemic therapy.

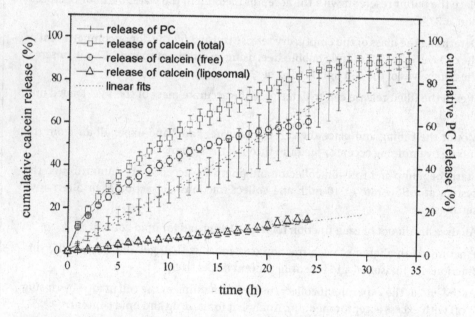

Figure 3 *In vitro* release of PC and calcein from an EPC-gel (450 mg/g). Cumulative release versus time. PC release (mean ± sd, n = 4). Calcein release total (mean ± sd, n = 5), free (mean ± sd, n = 3); liposomal (mean ± sd, n = 3). Linear fits for PC release over the time period 0–30 h, r = 0.9986; for liposomal calcein release over the time period 0–19 h, r = 0.9983. From ref. 28.

6 Preparation of SUV dispersions from VPGs

Upon addition of excess aqueous medium, VPGs can be transferred into dispersions of liposomes by gentle mechanical agitation. Manual shaking as well as treatment by a ball mill have proven appropriate for this. Both intensity and duration of mechanical agitation have an influence on liposome size and loss of entrapped drug, i.e. encapsulation efficiency measured for the overall process (VPG formation and re-dilution, see below) (26). A detailed description of the dilution process is given in Protocol 5.

Protocol 5

Transfer of a VPG into a liposome dispersion

Equipment and reagents

- 2 ml vials with screw cap (Sarstedt)
- Glass beads (diameter 1–2 mm)
- Oscillating ball mill (MM200 Retsch) with adapter for 2 ml vials
- Bench centrifuge (Biofuge Pico, Heraeus Instruments)
- 40 mM phosphate buffer pH 7.4

Method

1 Transfer approx. 1 g of a VPG from Protocols 1 or 2 into a 2 ml vial. Add three to five glass beads and 100 μl of aqueous medium, e.g. 40 mM phosphate buffer pH 7.4. Close the vial tightly and set it on an oscillating ball mill. Agitate at maximum speed for 2–3 min.

2 Add another 100 μl aliquot of aqueous medium and shake again for 2–3 min.

3 Repeat step 2 another three to eight times, or until the desired final dilution is achieved. A slightly turbid to opalescent liposome dispersion should be obtained.

4 Spin the resultant SUV dispersion at 2500 g in a bench centrifuge for 20 min at room temperature to remove eventual bigger particles or aggregates.

---

7 Characterization of SUV dispersions prepared from VPGs

Diluted VPGs are primarily characterized by their liposome size distribution and encapsulation efficiency.

7.1 Vesicle size distribution

The vesicle size of dispersed VPGs may be assessed by any standard technique suitable for SUV dispersions such as photon correlation spectroscopy or electron microscopy. One should be aware, however, that a minor 'contamination' of the SUV dispersions with bigger vesicles might render it difficult to gain proper PCS results of dispersed VPGs. To gain a better quantitative insight in the amount of multivesicular vesicles (MVVs) one can remove them by filtration through 0.2 μm pore membranes and quantify both drug and lipid content before and after filtration as described in ref. 26. In another approach dispersed VPGs are fractionated by size exclusion chromatography prior to PCS analysis (27). Electron microscopic techniques, especially cryo-electron microscopy, have proven useful because they not only measure vesicle sizes but also judge vesicle morphologies (26, 27).

In general, the vast majority of vesicles within dispersed VPGs are small, around 30 nm when determined by cryo-electron microscopy with a minor fraction of multivesicular vesicles in the several hundred nm range. There is only limited data available how lipid composition and concentration as well as the extent of mechanical energy applied during preparation and dilution of VPGs influence the vesicle sizes of dispersed VPGs (22, 26, 27).

7.2 Encapsulation efficiency

During dilution of VPGs in excess aqueous medium the gel matrix is transformed into separate dispersed vesicles and the preparation becomes fluid. Under appropriate conditions the fraction of drug which had been trapped in the core of the vesicles stays entrapped, the fraction of drug which had been trapped in the aqueous space between the vesicles is set free. The encapsulation efficiency for hydrophilic drugs is thus determined by the ratio of vesicle core volume compared to overall aqueous space within the original VPG. This ratio is in general quite high. Encapsulation efficiencies in the magnitude 30–70% are experimentally found for hydrophilic model compounds like calcein and carboxyfluorescein (26). As expected from theory, rising encapsulation efficiencies are obtained with increasing lipid concentrations (Figure 4). Under the assumption that exclusively small uniform (diameter 21 nm) unilamellar vesicles are formed, theoretically the encapsulation efficiency should reach its maximum at a phospholipid concentration of about 550 mg/g. At this lipid concentration, vesicles would adopt maximum density sphere packing with 74% of the total volume of the preparation taken by the vesicles and the aqueous core of these vesicles representing 51% of the total volume of all aqueous compartments. 51% thus represents the theoretical upper limit for encapsulation efficiency with VPGs of this vesicle size. Experimental values may deviate from theory because the above assumptions may not be fully fulfilled. Tighter packing may be achieved due to elastic deformation of the vesicles. In practice, however, it is hard to achieve experimentally the theoretically predicted maximum encapsulation efficiency and small unilamellar vesicles. Preparations which have a lipid content at or close to the maximum density packing tend to be inhomogeneous in terms of vesicle size and lamellarity. Experimentally obtained encapsulation efficiencies of drug substances within redispersed VPGs in the literature are 35% for Gemcitabine (29), 56% for vincristine (32), and 55% for carboplatin (33). In any case these values are significantly higher than those of other small unilamellar

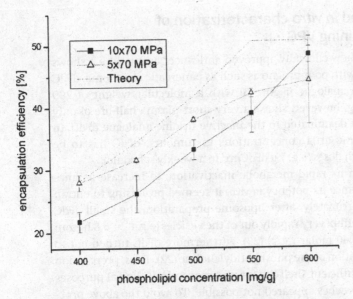

Figure 4 Encapsulation efficiency of carboxyfluorescein in VPGs of different PC content. VPGs prepared from egg phosphatidylcholine (E80, Lipoid GmbH, Ludwigshafen) according to Protocol 1 employing five or ten homogenization cycles at a pressure of 70 Mpa, respectively. Adapted from ref. 26.

vesicle preparations (SUVs), i.e. SUVs prepared by common techniques which typically yield encapsulation efficiencies in the magnitude 2–20% (30). To our knowledge there are only two exceptions found in the literature where encapsulation efficiencies (of hydrophilic compounds) have been achieved in the same magnitude as with VPGs or even higher:

(a) With radiolabelled compounds. Here, however, one should be aware that radiolabelling changes the physicochemical characteristics of a compound often inducing considerable association of the drug with the bilayer, at least in case of iodine (31). This results in falsely too high encapsulation efficiency values.

(b) With SUVs, which were actively loaded by a pH or ammonium sulfate gradient (see respective section in this book for references). The active loading approach, however, is not generally applicable rather than limited to certain weak amphipathic bases or acids.

8 *In vivo* applications

Gemcitabine has been used as an example to demonstrate the entrapment of a low molecular weight, water soluble drug into VPGs and the resulting change of its anticancer properties upon both i.v. and intra-tumoral injection (22, 29).

8.1 Preparation and *in vitro* characterization of Gemcitabine-containing VPG

Gemcitabine (dFdC) is a new clinically approved anticancer agent, which shows efficacy in solid cancers with poor prognosis such as pancreatic carcinoma. dFdC is a fluorinated cytidine analogue (Figure 5) with a molecular weight of 299 (hydrochloride). The drug, however, shows a very short plasma half-life of only 8–12 min, as it is rapidly deaminated to the inactive uridine analogue dFdU. In order to reach therapeutic drug concentrations in tumours, dFdC has to be administrated in very high doses (e.g. 1 g dFdC/m² in a weekly schedule).

To prevent dFdC from its rapid metabolic inactivation, to increase its anti-cancer efficacy, and enhance its potency *in vivo*, it seemed promising to entrap dFdC in liposomes. Unfortunately, after liposome preparation, the small dFdC molecules turned out to efflux very rapidly out of the vesicles (e.g. $t_{\frac{1}{2}}$ = 6.8 h from DSPC/Chol-liposomes, 60:40 molar ratio) (29). Furthermore dFdC turned out to induce hydrolytic degradation of the phosphatidylcholine (22). Thus, preparation of dFdC-liposomes with sufficient shelf-life for pharmaceutical/ clinical purposes by the conventional approaches appeared not possible. To avoid the above problems dFdC was entrapped into VPGs with the aim to achieve preparations with long shelf-life and high trapping efficiency. Anti-tumour activity both after intra-tumoral and i.v. application as well as pharmacokinetics and biodistribution of the redispersed Gemcitabine-containing VPG (GemLip) was evaluated in a human bladder xenograft BXF 1301 (s.c. growing in athymic nude mice) compared to the free drug (GemConv).

dFdC-containing VPG was prepared using the passive loading technique as described in Protocol 3 using a total of 400 mg/g lipid (hydrogenated egg PC and Chol in equimolar ratio); vesicle diameter, 40–60 nm; entrapping efficiency, 35%; shelf-life, > 14 months. Directly prior to use, the VPGs were diluted as described in Protocol 5 in a ratio of 2:1 for intra-tumoral and 1:2 for i.v. injection. Slight dilution of the GemLip intended for intra-tumoral application turned out to be necessary in order to be able to press it through a 27 gauge needle. The resulting GemLip preparations represent dual drug formulations consisting of 35% of liposomally entrapped dFdC and 65% of free drug.

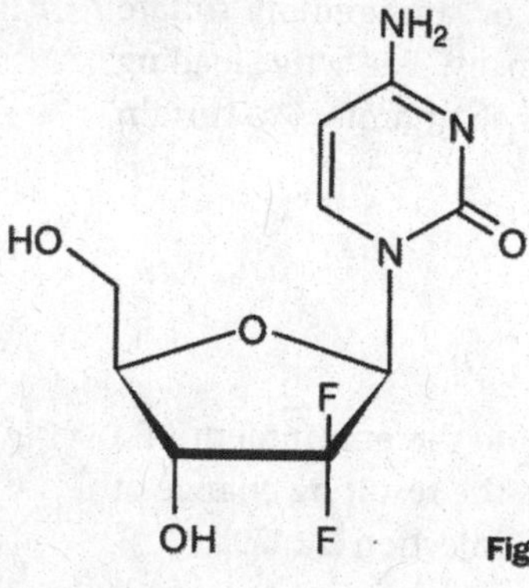

Figure 5 Gemcitabine (2′,2′-difluoro-2′-deoxy-cytidine; dFdC).

8.2 Intra-tumoral application of Gemcitabine-containing VPG

In a pilot study groups of tumour-bearing nude mice who were treated intra-tumorally with 4 and 6 mg/kg GemLip showed an initial tumour regression and subsequent regrowth (29). At the same time necrotic changes of the tumour-surrounding tissue were observed. Astonishingly, control tumours subcutaneously growing on the opposite flank of the mice were significantly reduced as well, which pointed towards a considerable redistribution of the cytotoxic agent. The study on intra-tumoral application was thus terminated in favour of the more promising systemic administration of Gemcitabine-containing VPGs.

8.3 i.v. application of Gemcitabine-containing VPG

GemLip and GemConv were administered i.v. on days 1, 8, and 15 at a dFdC dose of 6 mg/kg and a volume of 10 ml/kg into BXF 1301 bearing nude mice. Growth of the tumours was followed by serial calliper measurements. For pharmacokinetic studies, dFdC in serum were quantified by HPLC and in tumours by scintillation counting using [^{14}C]-dFdC-GemLip.

GemLip was highly active in the BXF 1301 human bladder xenograft at 6 mg/kg, a dose around MTD (maximum tolerated dose) (Figure 6). Complete tumour remission was observed in 4/5 mice three weeks after initiation of the treatment. In contrast, treatment of BXF 1301 with the same dose of the free drug (GemConv, Figure 6) resulted only in a moderate tumour growth inhibition.

This improved *in vivo* potency of GemLip compared to GemConv can be explained by changes in pharmacokinetics and biodistribution. As shown in

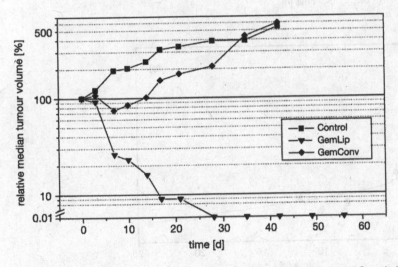

Figure 6 Anti-tumoral activity of conventional (GemConv) versus liposomal Gemcitabine (GemLip) at equimolar doses. Drugs were injected i.v. on days 1, 8, and 15 at a dose of 6 mg/kg. Effects on the s.c. growing human soft tissue sarcoma SXF 1301 in nude mice were determined by serial caliper measurements. The median relative tumour volumes (n = 5 to 6 mice) were calculated. Adapted from ref. 29.

Figure 7, dFdC was eliminated from serum with a terminal half-life of 0.15 h after application of GemConv. In contrast, after application of the dual drug formulation GemLip (35% liposomal entrapped and 65% free dFdC), dFdC was eliminated biphasically with $t_{\frac{1}{2}\alpha} = 0.15$ h (attributed to free dFdC) and $t_{\frac{1}{2}\beta} = 13.3$ h (attributed to the liposomally entrapped dFdC). This change in elimination resulted in a dramatically increased AUC (area under the curve) for GemLip (1680 mg*h/ml for GemLip vs. 47.6 mg*h/ml for GemConv).

Probably due to the long half-life of the liposomal vesicles in the bloodstream, an improved dFdC accumulation in the tumour tissues could be observed (Figure 8). Using the same dose of 6 mg dFdC /kg mice, a four-fold increase in AUC of dFdC in the tumours could be achieved.

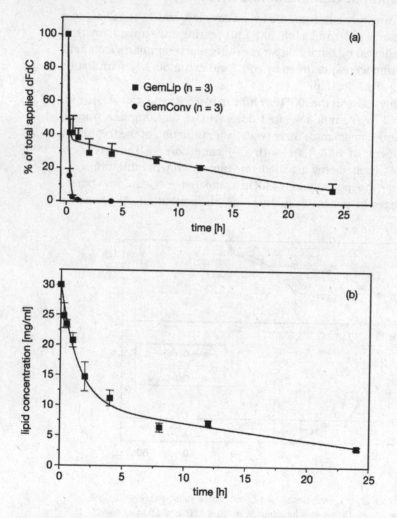

Figure 7 Elimination from plasma of (a) [^{14}C]-dFdC after injection of GemLip or GemConv at a dFdC dose of 6 mg/kg and of (b) ^{3}H-lipid after administration of GemLip (total lipid dose: 2.17 mmol/kg) as determined by scintillation counting. Adapted from ref. 29.

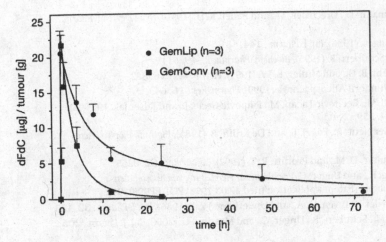

Figure 8 Accumulation of radiolabel in the tumours after administration of [^{14}C]-dFdC given as GemLip or GemConv, respectively (n = 3 to 5). Adapted from ref. 29.

Taken together, our data demonstrate that VPG formulations of dFdC are promising drug delivery systems which may help to overcome common problems of entrapping low molecular weight drugs (as for the most anticancer agents) in conventional small liposomes in terms of trapping efficiency and stable entrapment. In a pilot study the anticancer efficiency of a drug was improved when administered in the form of VPGs—a result which can be explained by:

(a) The prolonged tumour exposure time of dFdC due to its entrapment into liposomes.

(b) The passive tumour targeting due to the EPR-effect as explained above.

References

1. Allen, T. (1994). *Trends Pharmacol. Sci.*, **15**, 215.

2. Liu, D., Mori, A., and Huang, L. (1992). *Biochim. Biophys. Acta*, **1104**, 94.

3. Gerlowski, L. E. and Jain, R. K. (1986). *Microvasc. Res.*, **31**, 288.

4. Dvorak, H. F., Nagy, J. A., Dvorak, J. T., and Dvorak, A. M. (1988). *Am. J. Pathol.*, **133**, 95.

5. Yuan, F., Dellian, M., Fukumara, D., Leunig, M., Berg, D. A., Torchilin, V., *et al.* (1995). *Cancer Res.*, **55**, 3752.

6. Brandl, M., Bachmann, D., Reszka, R., and Drechsler, M. *Liposomale Zubereitung, ihre Herstellung und ihre Verwendung.* DE 44 30 592.3 (filed 18. 08.95). PCT WO 96/05808.

7. Brandl, M., Tardi, C., Drechsler, M., Bachmann, D., Reszka, R., Bauer, K. H., *et al.* (1997). *Adv. Drug Deliv. Rev.*, **24**, 161.

8. Brandl, M., Drechsler, M., Bachmann, D., and Bauer, K. H. (1997). *Chem. Phys. Lipids*, **87**, 65.

9. Small, D. M. (1967). *J. Lipid Res.*, **8**, 551.

10. Klose, G., König, B., Meyer, H. W., Schulze, G., and Degovics, G. (1988). *Chem. Phys. Lipids*, **47**, 225.

11. Brandl, M., Bachmann, D., Drechsler, M., and Bauer, K. H. (1993). In *Liposome technology* 2nd edn (ed. G. Gregoriadis), p. 49. CRC Press Inc., Boca Raton.

12. Brandl, M., Bachmann, D., Drechsler, M., and Bauer, K. H. (1990). *Drug Dev. Ind. Pharm.*, **16**, 2167.

13. Sorgi, F. and Huang, L. (1996). *Int. J. Pharm.*, **144**, 131.

14. Hellwich, U. and Schubert, R. (1995). *Biochem. Pharmacol.*, **49**, 511.

15. Balon, K., Riebesehl, B. U., and Müller, B. W. (1999). *Pharm. Res.*, **16**, 882.

16. Ottiger, C. and Wunderli-Allenspach, H. (1999). *Pharm. Res.*, **16**, 643.

17. Skalko, N., Brandl, M., Becirevic-Lacan, M., Filipovic-Grcic, J., and Jalsenjak, I. (1996). *Eur. J. Pharm. Sci.*, **4**, 359.

18. Nicolay, K., Van der Neut, R., Fok, J. J., and De Kruiff, B. (1985). *Biochim. Biophys. Acta*, **819**, 55.

19. Forssen, E. A., Coulter, D. M., and Proffitt, R. T. (1992). *Cancer Res.*, **52**, 3255.

20. Massing, U., Moog, R., and Unger, C. *Verfahren zur Herstellung von liposomalen Wirkstoffformulierungen.* (Patent application filed 27.03.1998) PCT/EP99/01992.

21. Beijnen, J. H., Van der Houwen, O. A., and Underberg, W. J. (1986). *Int. J. Pharm.*, **32**, 123.

22. Moog, R., Brandl, M., Schubert, R., Unger, C., and Massing, U. (2000). *Int. J. Pharm.*, **206**, 43.

23. Grit, M., Underberg, W., and Crommelin, D. (1991). *J. Pharm. Sci.*, **82**, 362.

24. Grit, M. and Crommelin, D. (1993). *Biochim. Biophys. Acta*, **1167**, 49.

25. Tardi, C., Drechsler, M., Bauer, K. H., and Brandl, M. (2001). *Int. J. Pharm.*, **217**, 161.

26. Brandl, M., Drechsler, M., Bachmann, D., Tardi, C., Schmidtgen, M., and Bauer, K. H. (1998). *Int. J. Pharm.*, **170**, 187.

27. Bender-Fuxius, J. (2000). Diss. rer. nat. (PhD-thesis) Fakultät für Chemie und Pharmazie, Albert-Ludwigs-Universität, Freiburg.

28. Tardi, C., Brandl, M., and Schubert, R. (1998). *J. Contr. Rel.*, **55**, 261.

29. Moog, R. (1998). Diss. rer. nat. (PhD-thesis) Fakultät für Chemie und Pharmazie, Albert-Ludwigs-Universität, Freiburg.

30. Bachmann, D., Brandl, M., and Gregoriadis, G. (1993). *Int. J. Pharm.*, **91**, 69.

31. Brandl, M. and Gregoriadis, G. (1994). *Biochim. Biophys. Acta*, **1196**, 65.

32. Güthlein, F. (2001). Diss. rer. nat. (PhD-thesis) Fakultät für Chemie und Pharmazie, Albert-Ludwigs-Universität, Freiburg.

33. Tardi, C. (1999). Diss. rer. nat. (PhD-thesis) Fakultät für Chemie und Pharmazie, Albert-Ludwigs-Universität, Freiburg.

34. Grohganz, H., Hansen, E., and Brandl, M. (2000). *J. Liposome Res.*, **10**, 223.

Chapter 15
Liposome-based DNA vaccines: procedures for entrapment

Gregory Gregoriadis

The School of Pharmacy, University of London; and Lipoxen Technologies Ltd., 29–39 Brunswick Square, London WC1N 1AX, UK.

Brenda McCormack, Yvonne Perrie[a], Andrew Bacon, Wilson Caparros-Wanderley, and Brahim Zadi

Lipoxen Technologies Ltd., 29–39 Brunswick Square, London WC1N 1AX, UK.

[a]Present address: Aston School of Pharmacy, Aston University, Aston Triangle, Birmingham B4 7ET, UK.

1 Introduction

Numerous workers (1–3) have shown that intramuscular injection of naked plasmid DNA elicits humoural and cell-mediated immune responses against the encoded antigen. It appears (2, 3) that promotion of immunity is the result of DNA uptake by muscle cells which leads to the expression and extracellular release of the antigen to be subsequently taken up by antigen-presenting cells (APC). It is also believed (3) that some of the injected DNA is taken up directly by APC. There are two main disadvantages of immunization with naked DNA. First, DNA is taken up by only a minor fraction of muscle cells which, at any rate, are not professional APC. Secondly, naked DNA is exposed to deoxyribonuclease in the interstitial fluid thus necessitating the use of relatively large quantities of DNA. It is not unusual that injection into regenerating muscle is also required in order to enhance immunity. It has been recently proposed (1, 4) that DNA immunization via liposomes could circumvent the need of muscle involvement and facilitate (5) instead uptake of DNA by APC infiltrating the site of injection or in the lymphatics (where many liposomes will end up), at the same time protecting DNA from nuclease attack (6). Moreover, transfection of APC with liposomal DNA and subsequent immune responses to the expressed antigen could be promoted by the judicial choice of vesicle surface charge, size, and lipid composition, or by the co-entrapment, together with DNA, of plasmids expressing appropriate cytokines (e.g. interleukin 2 or interferon-γ) or immunostimulatory sequences.

To that end, methods have been developed which allow for the quantitative entrapment of a number of plasmid DNAs into large (6) or small (7) neutral, anionic, and cationic liposomes that are capable of transfecting cells *in vitro* with varying efficiency (6). Using this technology, we have shown (1, 4, 8, 9) that immunization of Balb/c and outbred (T.O.) mice by a variety of routes, including the oral route (10), with (cationic) liposomal DNA leads to much greater humoral and cell-mediated (splenic IFN-γ) immune responses to the encoded antigen than those obtained with naked DNA or DNA complexed to preformed similar liposomes. Here we describe methodology for the incorporation of plasmid DNA into liposomes of varying lipid composition, vesicle size, and surface charge. Entrapment of DNA within the liposomes (as opposed to complexing) was verified by gel electrophoresis in the presence of sodium dodecyl sulfate (8).

2 Materials

Egg phosphatidylcholine (PC), distearoylphosphatidylcholine (DSPC), egg phosphatidylethanolamine (PE), phosphatidic acid (PA), phosphatidylglycerol (PG), and phosphatidylserine (PS) (more than 99% pure) were from Lipoid GmBH, Ludwigshaten, Germany. Dioleoylphosphatidylcholine (DOPE), stearylamine (SA) were from Sigma Chemical Co., Poole, Dorset, UK. The sources of 1,2-bis (hexadecylcycloxy)-3-trimethylamino propane (BisHOP), N[1-(2,3-dioleyloxy) propyl]-N,N,N-triethylammonium (DOTMA), 1,2-dioleyloxy-3-(trimethylamonium propane) (DOTAP), 1,2-dioleyl-3-dimethyl-ammonium propane (DODAB), and 3β(N,N,-dimethylaminoethane)-carbamyl cholesterol (DC-Chol) have been described elsewhere (4, 6, 8, 9). Sepharose (CL) 4B and poly(ethylene glycol) 6000 were obtained from Pharmacia.

Plasmid DNAs used were pRc/CMV HBS encoding the S (small) protein of the hepatitis B virus surface antigen (HBsAg, subtype ayw) (4), pGL2 encoding luciferase (6), pRSVGH encoding human growth hormone, PCMV 4.65 encoding *Mycobacterium* leprosy protein (a gift from Dr R. Tascon), CMV 4.EGFP encoding enhanced fluorescent green protein, VR1020 encoding Schistosome protein, pCI-OVA encoding ovalbumin, and p1.17/SichHA encoding the haemagglutinin antigen of influenza virus (Sichuan strain). All other reagents were of analytical grade.

3 Entrapment of plasmid DNA into liposomes by the dehydration–rehydration procedure

The outlined dehydration/rehydration procedure is characterized by its mildness and is thus compatible with most labile materials.

3.1 Solutions

(a) PC (16 μmoles) and DOPE (or PE) (8 μmoles) are dissolved in about 2–5 ml chloroform. For charged liposomes 4 μmoles of PA, PG, or PS (anionic) or

4 μmoles of SA, BisHOP, DOTMA, DOTAP, DODAB, or DC-Chol (cationic) are also added. Greater amounts of charged lipids can be added depending on the amount of vesicle surface charge required.

(b) Up to 500 μg of plasmid DNA (for the amount of PC shown above) is dissolved in 2 ml distilled water, or 10 mM sodium phosphate buffer pH 7.2 (phosphate buffer; PB) if needed. The nature of buffer in respect to composition, pH, and molarity can be varied as long as this does not interfere with liposome formation or DNA entrapment yield. Amounts of added DNA can be increased proportionally to the total amount of lipid used. For cationic liposomes, the amount of added DNA can also be increased by employing more cationic lipid.

3.2 Procedure steps

Entrapment of plasmid DNA into liposomes entails the preparation of a lipid film from which multilamellar vesicles (MLV) and, eventually, small unilamellar vesicles (SUV) are produced. SUV are then mixed with the plasmid DNA destined for entrapment and dehydrated. The dry cake is subsequently broken up and rehydrated to generate multilamellar 'dehydration–rehydration' vesicles (DRV) containing the plasmid DNA. On centrifugation, liposome-entrapped DNA is separated from non-entrapped DNA. When required, DNA-containing DRV are reduced in size by microfluidization in the presence or absence of non-entrapped DNA or by employing a novel alternative method (7) which utilizes sucrose (see below).

Protocol 1

Preparation of MLV and SUV

Equipment and reagents

- 50 ml round-bottomed spherical Quick-fit flask
- Rotary evaporator
- Glass beads
- Sonicator
- See Section 3.1

A. Preparation of the lipid film

1 The chloroform solution of lipids is placed in a 50 ml round-bottomed spherical Quick-fit flask.

2 Following evaporation of the solvent in a rotary evaporator at about 37 °C, a thin lipid film is formed on the walls of the flask.

3 The film is flushed for about 60 sec with oxygen-free nitrogen (N_2) to ensure complete solvent removal and to replace air.

Protocol 1 continued

B. Preparation of MLV

1   2 ml of distilled water (H_2O) and a few glass beads are added into the flask, the stopper is replaced, and the flask shaken vigorously by hand or mechanically until the lipid film has been transformed into a milky suspension.

2   This process is carried out above the liquid-crystalline transition temperature (Tc) of the phospholipid (>Tc) by pre-warming the water before its placement into a pre-warmed flask.

3   The suspension is allowed to stand at >Tc for about 1–2 h whereupon multilamellar liposomes are formed.

C. Preparation of SUV

1   The milky suspension (without the glass beads) is sonicated at >Tc (with frequent intervals of rest) using a titanium probe slightly immersed into the suspension which is under N_2 (achieved by the continuous delivery of a gentle stream of N_2 through thin plastic tubing). This step is meant to produce a slightly opaque to clear suspension of SUV of up to 80 nm in diameter.

2   The time required to produce SUV varies, depending on the amount of lipid used and the diameter of the probe. For the amounts of lipid mentioned above, a clear or slightly opaque suspension is usually obtained within up to four sonication cycles, each lasting 30 sec with 30 sec rest intervals in between, using a probe of 0.75 inch diameter.

3   The process of sonication is considered successful when adjustment of the settings in the sonicator is such that the suspension is agitated vigorously.

4   The sonicated suspension of SUV is centrifuged for 2 min at $1700 \times g$ to remove titanium fragments and the supernatant is allowed to rest at >Tc for about 1–2 h.

Protocol 2

Entrapment of plasmid DNA into liposomes

Equipment and reagents

- See Protocol 1
- Freeze-dryer
- Centrifuge

A. Dehydration of SUV in the presence of added plasmid DNA

1   SUV mixed with solution 3.1b, are rapidly frozen in liquid nitrogen while the flask is rotated, and freeze-dried overnight under vacuum (<0.1 torr) in a freeze-dryer.

2   If necessary, the suspension can be transferred into an alternative Pyrex container prior to freezing and drying.

Protocol 2 continued

B. Rehydration of the freeze-dried material

1 To the freeze-dried material 0.1 ml H_2O (per 16 μmoles of PC) pre-warmed at >Tc is added and the mixture is swirled vigorously at >Tc. The volume of H_2O added must be kept at a minimum, i.e. enough H_2O to ensure complete hydration of the powder under vigorous swirling.

2 The sample is kept at >Tc for about 30 min.

3 The process is repeated with 0.1 ml H_2O and, 30 min later at >Tc, with 0.8 ml PB (pre-warmed at >Tc).

4 The sample is then allowed to stand for about 30 min at >Tc.

C. Removal of non-entrapped DNA

1 The liposomal suspension, now containing multilamellar DRV with entrapped and non-entrapped plasmid DNA, is centrifuged at 40 000 g for 60 min (4 °C).

2 The pellet obtained (DNA-containing DRV) is suspended in H_2O (or PB) and centrifuged again under the same conditions. The process is repeated at least once to remove the remainder non-entrapped material.

3 The final pellet is suspended to an appropriate volume (e.g. 2 ml) of H_2O or PB. When the liposomal suspension is destined for *in vivo* use (e.g. intramuscular or subcutaneous injection), NaCl is added to a final concentration of 0.9%.

4 The z-average mean diameter of the suspended vesicles measured by photon correlation spectroscopy (PCS) is about 600–700 nm (8).

Protocol 3

Estimation of DNA entrapment

Equipment and reagents

- See Protocol 1
- Radiolabelled DNA
- Triton X-100, isopropanol

Method

1 DNA entrapment in DRV liposomes is monitored by measuring the DNA in the suspended pellet and combined supernatants. The most convenient way to monitor DNA entrapment is by using radiolabelled (^{32}P or ^{35}S) DNA.

2 If a radiolabel is not available or cannot be used, appropriate quantitative techniques should be employed. To determine DNA by such techniques a sample of the liposome suspension is mixed with Triton X-100 (up to 5% final concentration) or, preferably, with isopropanol (1:1 volume ratio) so as to liberate the DNA.

Protocol 3 continued

3   However, if Triton X-100 or the solubilized liposomal lipids interfere with the assay of the DNA, liposomal lipids or the DNA must be extracted using appropriate techniques (e.g. ref. 6). Entrapment values range between 29–99%, depending on the DNA used and the presence or absence of a cationic charge. Values are highest when DNA is entrapped into cationic DRV (Table 1).

Table 1 Incorporation of plasmid DNA into liposomes by the dehydration–rehydration method

Liposomes	Incorporated plasmid DNA[a] (% of used)							
	pGL2	pRc/CMV/ HBS	pRSVGH	pCMV4.65	pCMV4. EGFP	VR1020/	pCI-OVA	p1.17/ SichHA
PC, DOPE[b]	44.2[d]	55.4	45.6	28.6				
PC, DOPE[c]	12.1		11.3					
PC, DOPE, PS[b]	57.3[d]							
PC, DOPE, PS[c]	12.6							
PC, DOPE, PG[b]			53.5					
PC, DOPE, PG[c]			10.2					
PC, DOPE, SA[b]	74.8[d]							
PC, DOPE, SA[c]	48.3							
PC, DOPE, BisHOP[b]	69.3[d]							
PC, DOPE, DOTMA[b]	86.8							
PC, DOPE, DC-Chol[b]		87.1	76.9					
PC, DOPE, DC-Chol[c]			77.2					
PC, DOPE, DOTAP[b]		80.1	79.8	52.7	71.9	89.6	91.4	98.6 (93.0)[e]
PC, DOPE, DOTAP[c]		88.6	80.6	67.7		81.6		
PC, DOPE, DODAP[b]			57.4					
PC, DOPE, DODAP[c]			64.8					

[a] Plasmid DNAs used encoded luciferase (pGL2), hepatitis B surface antigen (S region) (pRc/CMV HBS), human growth hormone (pRSVGH), *Mycobacterium* leprosy protein (pCMV 4.65), 'fluorescent green protein' (pCMV 4.EGFP), Schistosome protein (VR1020), ovalbumin (PCI-OVA) and haemagglutinin antigen (p1.17/SichHA).

[b, c] ^{35}S-labelled plasmid DNA (10–500 μg) was incorporated ([b]) into or mixed ([c]) with neutral (PC, DOPE), anionic (PC, DOPE, PS, or PG), or cationic (PC, DOPE, SA, BisHOP, DOTMA, DC-Chol, DOTAP, or DODAP) dehydration–rehydration vesicles (DRV). Incorporation values for the different amounts of DNA used for each of the liposomal formulations did not differ significantly and were therefore pooled (values shown are means of values obtained from three to five experiments). PC (16 μmoles) was used in molar ratios of 1:0.5 (neutral) and 1:0.5:0.25 (anionic and cationic liposomes).

[d] Entrapment values for microfluidized DRV were 12–83% depending on the vesicle charge and amount of DNA used (6).

[e] Entrapment value in parentheses was obtained by the dehydration–rehydration method carried out in the presence of sucrose. z-Average vesicle size was 200 nm.

The following procedures are needed when DNA-containing DRV liposomes are to be converted to smaller vesicles (down to about 100 nm z-average mean diameter), still retaining a considerable proportion of the DNA, most of it in the case of cationic DRV.

Protocol 4

Size reduction of DNA-containing DRV liposomes

Equipment and reagents

- See Protocol 1
- Microfluidizer 110S (Microfluidics, Newton, MA, USA)
- Sepharose CL-4B column
- Dialysis equipment
- Sucrose
- Poly(ethylene glycol)

A. Microfluidization of DRV-entrapped DNA

1 The liposomal suspension obtained in Protocol 2B (prior to the separation of entrapped from the non-entrapped drug in Protocol 2C) ('unwashed liposomes') is diluted to 10 ml with H_2O and passed for a number of full cycles through a Microfluidizer 110S. The pressure gauge is set at 60 psi throughout the procedure to give a flow rate of 35 ml/min.

2 The number of cycles used depends on the vesicle size required (6) or on the sensitivity of the plasmid DNA. In the case of pGL2, microfluidization for more than three cycles resulted in progressive smearing of the DNA and failure to transfect cells *in vitro* (6). It is likely that other plasmid DNAs will behave similarly on extensive microfluidization.

3 Microfluidization of the sample can also be carried out after the removal of non-entrapped DNA as in Protocol 2C ('washed liposomes'), although DNA retention in this case may be reduced. The presence of unentrapped DNA during microfluidization (a process that destabilizes liposomes which then re-form as smaller vesicles) is expected (6) to diminish DNA leakage, perhaps by reducing the osmotic rupture of vesicles (11). Again, with cationic DRV, DNA is unlikely to leak significantly as it is associated with the cationic charges of the bilayers.

B. Preparation of DNA-containing small liposomes by the 'sucrose' method

Quantitative entrapment of DNA into small (about 200 nm diameter) liposomes in the absence of microfluidization can be carried out by a novel one-step method (7) as follows.

1 SUV (e.g. cationic) prepared as in Protocol 1C are mixed with sucrose to give a weight/weight ratio of 1.0 (e.g. 21 mg total lipid for 21 mg sucrose) and the appropriate amount of plasmid DNA (e.g. 10–500 µg).

2 The mixture is then frozen and dehydrated by freeze-drying. Rehydration of the cake obtained is carried out as in Protocol 2B.

3 For the separation of the entrapped from non-entrapped DNA the suspension is centrifuged as in Protocol 2C.

Protocol 4 continued

C. Separation of entrapped from non-entrapped DNA

1   When the number of cycles required has been completed, the microfluidized sample (about 10 ml) can, if needed, be reduced in volume by placing the sample in dialysis tubing which is then covered in a flat container with poly(ethylene glycol) 6000 flakes. Removal of excess H_2O from the tubing is relatively rapid and it is therefore essential that the sample is inspected regularly.

2   When the required volume has been reached, the sample is treated for the separation of entrapped from free DNA. This is carried out either by molecular sieve chromatography using a Sepharose CL-4B column, or, for cationic liposomes, by centrifugation as in Protocol 2C.

D. Measurement of DNA retention by microfluidized DRV and vesicle characteristics

1   The content of DNA within liposomes is estimated as in Protocol 3 and is expressed as % of DNA in the original preparation obtained in Protocol 2C.

2   When the sample is microfluidized following Protocol 2B, i.e. before the estimation of entrapment, it is necessary that a small portion of the sample to be microfluidized is kept aside for the estimation of entrapment according to Protocol 3.

3   Vesicle size measurements (after Protocol 2B, Protocol 4B, and 4C) are carried out by photon correlation spectroscopy as described elsewhere (6, 8, 12).

4   Liposomes with entrapped DNA can also be subjected to microelectrophoresis in a Zetasizer to determine their zeta potential. This is often required in order to determine the net surface charge of DNA-containing cationic liposomes.

References

1. Gregoriadis, G. (1998). *Pharm. Res.*, **15**, 661.
2. Davis, H. L., Whalen, R. G., and Demeneix, B. A. (1993). *Hum. Gene Ther.*, **4**, 151.
3. Lewis, P. J. and Babiuk, L. A. (1999). *Adv. Virus Res.*, **54**, 129.
4. Gregoriadis, G., Saffie, R., and de Souza, J. B. (1997). *FEBS Lett.*, **402**, 107.
5. Gregoriadis, G. (1995). *Trends Biotechnol.*, **13**, 527.
6. Gregoriadis, G., Saffie, R., and Hart, S. L. (1996). *J. Drug Target.*, **3**, 469.
7. Zadi, B. and Gregoriadis, G. (2000). *J. Liposome Res.*, **10**, 73.
8. Perrie, Y. and Gregoriadis, G. (2000). *Biochim. Biophys. Acta*, **1475**, 125.
9. Perrie, Y., Frederik, P. M., and Gregoriadis, G. (2001). *Vaccine*, **19**, 3301.
10. Perrie, Y., Obrenovic, M., McCarthy, D., and Gregoriadis, G. (2002). *J. Liposome Res.*, **12**, 185.
11. Kirby, C. and Gregoriadis, G. (1984). *Biotechnology*, **2**, 979.
12. Skalko, N., Bouwstra, J., Spies, F., and Gregoriadis, G. (1996). *Biochim. Biophys. Acta*, **1301**, 249.

Appendix

Abbott Laboratories, Animal Health Division, North Chicago, IL 60064, USA
Tel: 1 888 299 7416
URL: http://www.animalhealth.abbott.com
Abbott Laboratories Ltd,
Abbott House, Norden Road,
Maidenhead SL6 4XE, UK
Tel: 44 1628 773355

ADAC Laboratories, 540 Adler Drive, Milpitas, CA 95035, USA
Tel: 1 408 321 9100
Fax: 1 408 321 9686
URL: http://www.adaclabs.com
ADAC Laboratories UK, Unit 3,
Rycote Lane, Milton Common,
Oxford OX9 2NP, UK
Tel: 44 1844 278011
Fax: 44 1844 278211

Alltech Associates, 2051 Waukegan Road, Deerfield, IL 60015–1899, USA

Amersham Pharmacia Biotech UK Ltd, Amersham Place, Little Chalfont, Buckinghamshire HP7 9NA, UK
(see also Nycomed Amersham Imaging UK; Pharmacia)
Tel: 800 515313
Fax: 800 616927
URL: http//www.apbiotech.com/

Anderman and Co. Ltd, 145 London Road, Kingston-upon-Thames, Surrey KT2 6NH, UK
Tel: 44 181 5410035
Fax: 44 181 5410623

APV Systems, 500 Research Drive, Wilmington Technology Park, Wilmington, MA 01887, USA
URL: http://www.apv.invensys.com
APV Deutschland GmbH,
Zechenstr. 49, D-59425 Unna,
Germany
Tel: 49 230 3 108000
Fax: 49 230 3 108210

Avanti Polar Lipids, Inc., 700 Industrial Park Drive, Alabaster, AL 35007, USA
Tel: 1 800 227 0651 or 1 205 663 2494
Fax: 1 205 663 0756
URL: http://www.avantilipids.com

Avestin Inc., 2450 Don Reid Drive, Ottawa, Ontario K1H 1E1, Canada
Tel: 1 613 736 0019
Fax: 1 613 736 8086

Axis-Shield PoC AS, PO Box 6863 Rodelokka, N-0504 Oslo, Norway
Tel: 47 2 2042000
Fax: 47 2 2042001

Aztech Trading, 12 Kernan Drive, Swingbridge Trading Estate, Loughborough, Leicestershire LE11 5JF, UK
Tel: 44 1509 214722
Fax: 44 1509 610650

Bayer Corporation, Pharmaceutical Division, 400 Morgan Lane, West Haven, CT 06516–4175, USA
URL: http://www.bayerpharma-na.com

381

Beckman Coulter (UK) Ltd, Oakley Court, Kingsmead Business Park, London Road, High Wycombe, Buckinghamshire HP11 1JU, UK
Tel: 44 1494 441181
Fax: 44 1494 447558
URL: http://www.beckman.com/
Beckman Coulter Inc., 4300 N. Harbor Boulevard, PO Box 3100, Fullerton, CA 92834–3100, USA
Tel: 001 714 871 4848
Fax: 001 714 773 8283
URL: http://www.beckman.com/

Becton Dickinson and Co., 21 Between Towns Road, Cowley, Oxford OX4 3LY, UK
Tel: 44 1865 748844
Fax: 44 1865 781627
URL: http://www.bd.com/
Becton Dickinson and Co., 1 Becton Drive, Franklin Lakes, NJ 07417–1883, USA
Tel: 001 201 8476800
URL: http://www.bd.com/
Becton Dickinson, Life Science Research, 2350 Qume Drive, San Jose, CA 95131–1807, USA
Tel: 800 448 2347
Fax: 1 408 954 2007

Bio 101 Inc., c/o Anachem Ltd, Anachem House, 20 Charles Street, Luton, Bedfordshire LU2 0EB, UK
Tel: 01582 456666
Fax: 01582 391768
URL: http://www.anachem.co.uk/
Bio 101 Inc., PO Box 2284, La Jolla, CA 92038–2284, USA
Tel: 1 760 598 7299
Fax: 1 760 598 0116
URL: http://www.bio101.com/

BIODEX Medical Systems, Brookhaven Technology Center, 20 Ramsay Road Box 702, Shirley,

NY 11967–0702, USA
Tel: 1 631 924 9000
Fax: 1 631 924 9241
URL: http://www.biodex.com

Bio-Rad Laboratories Ltd, Bio-Rad House, Maylands Avenue, Hemel Hempstead, Hertfordshire HP2 7TD, UK
Tel: 0181 3282000
Fax: 0181 3282550
URL: http://www.bio-rad.com/
Bio-Rad Laboratories Ltd, Division Headquarters, 1000 Alfred Noble Drive, Hercules, CA 94547, USA
Tel: 1 510 724 7000
Fax: 1 510 741 5817
URL: http://www.bio-rad.com/

Boehringer-Mannheim (see Roche)

Branson Ultrasonics Corp., 41 Eagle Road, Danbury, CT 06813, USA
Tel: 1 203 796 0339
Fax: 1 203 796 0320

Brinkmann Instruments Inc., One Cantiague Road, PO Box 1019, Westbury, NY 11590–0207, USA
Tel: 1 800 645 3050 or 1 516 334 7500
Fax: 1 516 334 7506

Calbiochem-Novabiochem GmbH, PO Box 1167, D-65796 Bad Soden, Germany
Tel: 800 6931000
Fax: 800 62361 00

Canberra Industries, 800 Research Parkway, Meriden, CT 06450, USA
Tel: 1 203 238 2351

Fax: 1 203 235 1347
URL: http://www.canberra.com

Capintec, Inc., 6 Arrow Road,
Ramsey, NJ 07466, USA
Tel: 1 201 825 9500
Fax: 1 201 825 4829
URL: http://www.capintec.com

Christison Scientific Equipment Ltd,
Albany Road, Gateshead NE8 3AT, UK
Tel: 44 191 478 8120
Fax: 44 191 490 0549
URL: http://www.Christison.com

CP Instrument Co. Ltd, PO Box 22,
Bishop Stortford, Hertfordshire
CM23 3DX, UK
Tel: 44 1279 757711
Fax: 44 1279 755785
URL: http//:www.cpinstrument.co.uk/

Dupont (UK) Ltd, Industrial Products
Division, Wedgwood Way,
Stevenage, Hertfordshire SG1 4QN, UK
Tel: 44 1438 734000
Fax: 44 1438 734382
URL: http://www.dupont.com/
Dupont Co. (Biotechnology Systems
Division), PO Box 80024,
Wilmington, DE 19880–002, USA
Tel: 1 302 774 1000
Fax: 1 302 774 7321
URL: http://www.dupont.com/

Eastman Chemical Co., 100 North
Eastman Road, PO Box 511, Kingsport,
TN 37662–5075, USA
Tel: 1 423 229 2000
URL: http//:www.eastman.com/

Eli Lilly Canada, Inc., 3650 Danforth
Avenue, Toronto, ON M1N 2E8,
Canada
Tel: 1 416 694 3221
Fax: 1 416 694 0487
URL: http://www.lilly.ca

Eppendorf Vertrieb Deutschland GmbH,
Friedensstrasse 116, D-51145 Koeln,
Germany
Tel: 49 180 325 5911
Fax: 49 220 3927655

Fisher Scientific UK Ltd, Bishop
Meadow Road, Loughborough,
Leicestershire LE11 5RG, UK
Tel: 44 1509 231166
Fax: 44 1509 231893
URL: http://www.fisher.co.uk/
Fisher Scientific, Fisher Research,
2761 Walnut Avenue, Tustin,
CA 92780, USA
Tel: 1 714 669 4600
Fax: 1 714 669 1613
URL: http://www.fishersci.com/

Fluka, PO Box 2060, Milwaukee,
WI 53201, USA
Tel: 1 414 273 5013
Fax: 1 414 273 4979
URL: http://www.sigma-aldrich.com/
Fluka Chemical Co. Ltd, PO Box 260,
CH-9471 Buchs, Switzerland
Tel: 41 81 7452828
Fax: 41 81 7565449
URL: http://www.sigma-aldrich.com/

Gibco-BRL (see Life Technologies)

Greiner bio-one b.v., PO Box 280,
2400 AG Alpen a/d Rijn,
The Netherlands
Tel: 31 17 2420900
Fax: 31 17 2443801

Heto-Holten A/S, Gydevang 17-19,
DK-3450 Allerod,
Denmark
Tel: 45 4 8166200
Fax: 45 4 8166297

Hull Company, 3535 Davisville Road,
Hatboro, PA 19040–4296, USA
Tel: 1 215 672 7800

Fax: 1 215 672 7807
URL: http://www.hullcompany.com

Hybaid Ltd, Action Court, Ashford
Road, Ashford, Middlesex TW15 1XB,
UK
Tel: 44 1784 425000
Fax: 44 1784 248085
URL: http://www.hybaid.com/
Hybaid US, 8 East Forge Parkway,
Franklin, MA 02038, USA
Tel: 001 508 5416918
Fax: 001 508 5413041
URL: http://www.hybaid.com/

HyClone Laboratories, 1725 South
HyClone Road, Logan, UT 84321,
USA
Tel: 1 435 753 4584
Fax: 1 435 753 4589
URL: http//:www.hyclone.com/

Inex Pharmaceuticals Corporation,
100–8900 Glenlyon Parkway,
Burnaby, BC V5J 5J8, Canada
Tel: 1 604 419 3200
Fax: 1 604 419 3201
URL: http://www.inexpharm.com

Invitrogen Corp., 1600 Faraday
Avenue, Carlsbad, CA 92008, USA
Tel: 1 760 603 7200
Fax: 1 760 603 7201
URL: http://www.invitrogen.com/
Invitrogen BV, PO Box 2312,
9704 CH Groningen,
The Netherlands
Tel: 800 53455345
Fax: 800 78907890
URL: http://www.invitrogen.com/

Kinetics Group, Inc., 2805 Mission
College Blvd., Santa Clara, CA 95054,
USA
Tel: 1 408 727 7740
Fax: 1 408 727 9774
URL: http://www.kineticsgroup.com

Labcongo Corporation, 8811 Prospect
Avenue, Kansas City, Missouri
64132–2696, USA
Tel: 1 816 333 8811
Fax: 1 816 363 0130
URL: http://www.labconco.com

Leica Microsystems, International
Headquarter, Ernst-Leitz-Strasse 17-37,
D-35578 Wetzlar, Germany
Tel: 49 6441 290000
Fax: 49 6441 2925990

Life Technologies Ltd, PO Box 35, 3
Free Fountain Drive, Inchinnan
Business Park, Paisley PA4 9RF,
UK
Tel: 800 269210
Fax: 800 243485
URL: http://www.lifetech.com/
Life Technologies Inc.,
9800 Medical Center Drive,
Rockville, MD 20850,
USA
Tel: 1 301 610 8000
URL: http://www.lifetech.com/

Lipoid GmbH, Manufacturing Plant and
Sales Office, Frigenstr. 4, D-67065
Ludwigshafen, Germany
Tel: 49 62 153819 0
Fax: 49 62 1553559
Lipoid AG, Sales Office, Alte
Steinhauserstr. 19 , CH-6330 Cham,
Switzerland
Tel: 41 41 7417408
Fax: 41 41 7417336
URL: http://www.lipoid.com

Malvern UK, Malvern Instrument Ltd,
Enigma Business Park, Grovewood
Road, Malvern, Worcester WR14 1XZ,
UK
Tel: 44 1684 892456
Fax: 44 1684 892789
URL: http://www.malvern.co.uk

Marconi Medical Systems, 595 Miner Road, Cleveland, OH 44143, USA
Tel: 440 483 3000
URL: http://www.marconimed.com
Marconi, Ground Floor,
Saffron Ground, Ditchmore Lane,
Stevenage, Hertfordshire SG1 3LD, UK
Tel: 44 1438 311777
Fax: 44 1438 311888

**Martin Christ
Gefriertrocknungsanlagen GmbH**, PO Box 1713, D-37507 Osterode am harz, Germany
Tel: 49 552 2 5007 00
Fax: 49 552 2 5007 12
URL: http://www.martinchrist.de

Merck Fine Chemicals, Frankfurter Str. 250, 64293 Darmstadt, Germany
Tel: 49 615 1 72 0000
Fax: 49 615 1 72 2000

Merck Sharp & Dohme Research Laboratories, Neuroscience Research Centre, Terlings Park, Harlow, Essex CM20 2QR, UK
URL: http://www.msd-nrc.co.uk/
MSD Sharp and Dohme GmbH,
Lindenplatz 1, D-85540, Haar, Germany
URL: http://www.msd-deutschland.com/

Mettler-Toledo Ltd, 64 Boston Road, Beaumont Leys, Leicester LE4 1AW, UK
Tel: 44 1662 35 7070/44 1162 350888
Fax: 44 1162 365500
URL: http://www.mt.com/na/

MicroCal Inc., 22 Industrial Drive East, Northampton, MA 01060–2327, USA
Tel: (800) 633 3115 or (413) 586 7720
Fax: (413) 9586 0149
URL:
http://www.microcalorimetry.com

MicroCal LLC (HSDSC), Fortuna House South 5th Street,
Central Milton Keynes MK9 2EU, UK
Tel: 44 1908 309490
Fax: 44 1908 309499
URL: http://www.bindingconstants.com/index.html

Millipore (UK) Ltd, The Boulevard, Blackmoor Lane, Watford, Hertfordshire WD1 8YW, UK
Tel: 44 1923 816375
Fax: 44 1923 818297
URL: http://www.millipore.com/local/UKhtm/
Millipore Corp., 80 Ashby Road, Bedford, MA 01730, USA
Tel: 1 800 6455476
Fax: 1 800 6455439
URL: http://www.millipore.com/

Molecular Probes, 4849 Pitchford Avenue, Eugene, OR 97402–9165, USA
Tel: 1 541 465 8300
Fax: 1 541 344 6504
PoortGebouw, Rijnsburgerweg 10, 2333 AA Leiden, The Netherlands
Tel: 31 71 5233378
Fax: 31 71 5233419

Nattermann Phospholipid GmbH, Nattermannallee 1, D-50829 Koeln, Germany
Tel: 49 221 5092714
Fax: 49 221 5092816

New England Biolabs, 32 Tozer Road, Beverley, MA 01915–5510, USA
Tel: 1 978 927 5054

Nicomp, 75 Aero Camino, Suite B, Santa Barbara, CA 93117, USA
Tel: 1 805 968 1497
Fax: 1 805 968 0361
URL: http://www.pssnicomp.com

Nikon Inc., 1300 Walt Whitman Road, Melville, NY 11747-3064, USA
Tel: 1 516 547 4200
Fax: 1 516 547 0299
URL: http://www.nikonusa.com/
Nikon Corp., Fuji Building, 2-3, 3-chome, Marunouchi, Chiyoda-ku, Tokyo 100, Japan
Tel: 81 3 32145311
Fax: 81 3 32015856
URL: http://www.nikon.co.jp/main/index_e.htm/

Northern Lipids Inc., BC Research Complex, 3650 Westbrook Mall, Vancouver, BC V6S 2L2, Canada
Tel: 1 604 222 2548
Fax: 1 604 222 2563
URL: http://www.northernlipids.com

Nycomed Amersham Imaging, Amersham Labs, White Lion Road, Amersham, Buckinghamshire HP7 9LL, UK
Tel: 0800 558822 (or 01494 544000)
Fax: 0800 669933 (or 01494 542266)
URL: http//:www.amersham.co.uk/
Nycomed Amersham, 101 Carnegie Center, Princeton, NJ 08540, USA
Tel: 1 609 514 6000
URL: http://www.amersham.co.uk/

Perkin Elmer Ltd, Post Office Lane, Beaconsfield, Buckinghamshire HP9 1QA, UK
Tel: 44 1494 676161
URL: http//:www.perkin-elmer.com/

Perkin Elmer-Life Science Inc., 549 Albany Street, Boston, MA 02118, USA
Tel: 1 617 482 9595
URL: http://www.lifesciences.perkinelmer.com

Perkin Elmer (DSC MTDSC), 710 Bridgeport Avenue, Shelton, Connecticut 06484-4794, USA
Tel: 1 203 925 4600
Toll Free (USA Only): 800 762 4000
Fax: 1 203 925 4654
URL: http://instruments.perkinelmer.com/index.asp
Perkin Elmer, Chalfont Road, Seer Green, Beaconsfield, Bucks HP9 2FX
Tel: 44 1494 874515
Fax: 44 1494 679331
URL: http://instruments.perkinelmer.com/index.asp

Pharmacia Corporation Worldwide Headquarters, 100 Rte. 206 North, Peapack, NJ 07977, USA
Tel: 908 901 8000
Fax: 908 901 8379

Pharmacia, Davy Avenue, Knowlhill, Milton Keynes, Buckinghamshire MK5 8PH, UK (also see Amersham Pharmacia Biotech)
Tel: 44 1908 661101
Fax: 44 1908 690091
URL: http//www.eu.pnu.com/

Phoenix Scientific, Inc., 3915 South 48th Terrace, Saint Joseph, MO 64503, USA
Tel: 1 816 364 3777

Promega UK Ltd, Delta House, Chilworth Research Centre, Southampton SO16 7NS, UK
Tel: 0800 378994
Fax: 0800 181037
URL: http://www.promega.com/
Promega Corp., 2800 Woods Hollow Road, Madison, WI 53711-5399, USA
Tel: 1 608 274 4330
Fax: 1 608 277 2516
URL: http://www.promega.com/

Qiagen UK Ltd, Boundary Court,
Gatwick Road, Crawley,
West Sussex RH10 2AX, UK
Tel: 44 1293 422911
Fax: 44 1293 422922
URL: http://www.qiagen.com/
Qiagen Inc., 28159 Avenue Stanford,
Valencia, CA 91355, USA
Tel: 001 800 4268157
Fax: 001 800 7182056
URL: http://www.qiagen.com/

Roche Diagnostics Ltd, Bell Lane,
Lewes, East Sussex BN7 1LG, UK
Tel: 44 808 1009998 (or 01273 480044)
Fax: 44 808 1001920 (01273 480266)
URL: http://www.roche.com/
Roche Diagnostics Corp.,
9115 Hague Road, PO Box 50457,
Indianapolis, IN 46256, USA
Tel: 001 317 8452358
Fax: 001 317 5762126
URL: http://www.roche.com/
Roche Diagnostics GmbH,
Sandhoferstrasse 116, 68305
Mannheim, Germany
Tel: 49 621 7594747
Fax: 49 621 7594002
URL: http://www.roche.com/

Schleicher & Schuell, Inc., 10 Optical
Avenue, Keene, NH 03431, USA
Tel: 1 603 352 3810
Fax: 1 603 357 3627
URL: http://www.s-und-s.de
Schleicher & Schuell UK Ltd,
Unit 11, Brunswick Park Industrial
Estate, London N11 1JL, UK
Tel: 44 208 361 3111
Fax: 44 208 361 6352

Sedere, Parc Volta-BP27,
94141 Alfortville Cedex, France
Tel: 33 14 5180518
Fax: 33 14 5180525

Setaram (HSDSC),
Brookhaven Instruments Ltd, Chapel
House, Stock Wood, Redditch,
Worcestershire B96 6ST, UK
Tel: 44 1386 792727
Fax: 44 1386 792720
URL: http://www.setaram.com/

Serail Freeze Drying Systems, 680
Hollow Road, Unit 4 R.D.
1, Phoenixville, PA 19460, USA
Tel: 1 610 983 0260
Fax: 1 610 983 0268
URL: http://www.serail.com

Shandon Scientific Ltd, 93–96
Chadwick Road, Astmoor,
Runcorn, Cheshire WA7 1PR, UK
Tel: 44 1928 566611
URL: http//www.shandon.com/

Siemens Nuclear Medicine Group,
2501 North Barrington Road,
Hoffman Estates, IL 60195–5203, USA
Tel: 1 847 304 7700
Fax: 1 847 304 7707
URL: http://www.siemensmedical.com
Siemens plc, Siemens House,
Oldbury, Bracknell RG12 8FZ, UK
Tel: 44 1344 396000
Fax: 44 1344 396133

Sigma–Aldrich Co. Ltd, The Old
Brickyard, New Road,
Gillingham, Dorset SP8 4XT, UK
Tel: 0800 717181 (or 01747 822211)
Fax: 0800 378538 (or 01747 823779)
URL: http://www.sigma-aldrich.com/
Sigma Chemical Co., PO Box 14508, St
Louis, MO 63178, USA
Tel: 1 314 771 5765
Fax: 1 314 771 5757
URL: http://www.sigma-aldrich.com/

Spectrum Laboratories, Inc., 18617
Broadwick Street, Rancho Dominguez,

CA 90220–6435, USA
Tel: 1 310 885 4600
Fax: 1 310 885 4666

Stratagene Inc., 11011 North Torrey
Pines Road, La Jolla, CA 92037,
USA
Tel: 001 858 5355400
URL: http://www.stratagene.com/
Stratagene Europe,
Gebouw California, Hogehilweg 15,
1101 CB Amsterdam Zuidoost,
The Netherlands
Tel: 800 91009100
URL: http://www.stratagene.com/

Structure Probe Inc., PO Box 656,
West Chester, PA 19381–0656,
USA
Tel: 1 610 436 5400
Fax: 1 610 436 5755

Syncor International Corporation,
6464 Canoga Avenue, Woodlands
Hills, CA 91367, USA
Tel: 1 818 737 4000
Fax: 1 818 737 4826
URL: http://www.syncor.com

TA Instruments (DSC, MTDSC),
Corporate Headquarters, 109 Lukens
Drive, New Castle, DE 19720, USA
Tel: 1 302 427 4000
Fax: 1 302 427 4001
URL: http://www.tainst.com/
TA Instruments Ltd, Europe House,
Bilton Centre, Cleeve Road,
Leatherhead, Surrey KT22 7UQ, UK
Tel: 44 1372 360363

Fax: 44 1372 360135
URL: http://www.tainst.com

Thermometrics New Jersey, 808 US
Highway 1, Edison, NJ 08817–4695,
USA
Tel: 1 732 287 2870
Fax: 1 732 2878847
Thermometrics UK, Crown Industrial
Estate, Priorswood Road, Taunton,
Somerset TA2 8QY, UK
Tel: 44 1823 335200

United States Biochemical (USB),
PO Box 22400, Cleveland, OH 44122,
USA
Tel: 1 216 464 9277

Virtis, 815 Route 208, Gardiner,
NY 12525–9989,
USA
Tel: 800 765 6198 or 1 845 255 5000
Fax: 1 845 255 5338

Waters Corporation, 34 Marple Street,
Milford, MA 01767, USA
Tel: 1 508 478 2000
Fax: 1 508 872 1990
URL: http://www.waters.com

Whatman International Ltd, Whatman
House, St. Leonards Road, 20/20
Maidstone, Kent, UK
Tel: 44 1622 676670
Fax: 44 1622 677011
Whatman Inc., 9 Bridewell Place,
Clifton, NJ 07014, USA
Tel: 1 973 773 5800
Fax: 1 973 472 6949
URL: http://www.whatman.com

Index

389

Printed in the United States
By Bookmasters